Handbook
of Health Care
Management

Handbook
of Health Care
Management ❧

W. Jack Duncan • Peter M. Ginter • Linda E. Swayne

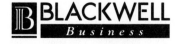

BLACKWELL
Business

Copyright © Blackwell Publishers, 1998

Blackwell Publishers Inc.
350 Main Street
Malden, MA
02148

Blackwell Publishers Ltd.
108 Cowley Road
Oxford OX4 1JF
UK

Library of Congress Cataloging-in-Publication Data

Handbook of health care management / [edited by] W. Jack Duncan, Linda
  E. Swayne, Peter M. Ginter.
      p.   cm.
    Includes bibliographical references and index.
    ISBN 1-55786-833-6
    1. Health services adminstration--United States.   I. Duncan, W.
  Jack (Walter Jack)   II. Swayne, Linda E.   III. Ginter, Peter M.
  RA971.H274   1997
  362.1'068—dc21   97-13926
                                                          CIP

British Library of Congress Cataloging-in-Publication Data

Manufactured in the USA.

Contents

❧ **PART II   TOOLS OF HEALTH CARE MANAGEMENT   153**

Chapter 5.   Financial Accounting and Management in Health Service Organizations   155

Preface

An interest in health care could be justified solely on the basis of the fact that it is one of largest and most dynamic industries in our domestic and global economies. Important though this may be, what brings most of us to an interest in health care is personal—a personal encounter with a complex system that is sometimes caring and comforting and sometimes unfriendly and bureaucratic. Few people would seriously argue that that the US health care system is not a good one. Technologically, few can match it. It is not uncommon, for example, to have multiple facilities capable of procedures such as heart surgery in American cities with less than half a million people.

In spite of its technological sophistication, however, all is not well with US health care. Public health officials point out that in many areas of the United States, health indicators such as infant mortality compare more readily with the Third World than highly industrialized nations. The obverse of the wealth of heart surgery facilities in metropolitan areas is the appalling lack of primary health care facilities and providers in rural areas and the inner cities. The purpose of this *Handbook* is not to praise technological superiority, although it is certainly worthy of praise; nor is it to criticize maldistributions of health resources at the macro level, although these too are deserving of criticism. The focus, instead, is on the *management of the system.*

Regardless of where one encounters the health care system—the emergency room, the hospital, the family planning clinic, or the physician's office—there is an increasing expectation that the system should respond in a way not unlike any other business. People should be respected as customers, services should be dispensed in a caring and efficient manner, and the price of the services should bear, if not an obvious, at least a comprehensible relationship to the value of the services rendered and received. In other words, we have come to expect and demand a health care system that is well managed. And that is as it should be, because health care has become more competitive. Competition is inevitably the *engine* that drives a focus on customers and attention to cost and value calculations.

This *Handbook*, as the title clearly states, is about management and the manager's real and potential contribution to a more effective and efficient health care system. Physicians, nurses, technicians, and support personnel provide the critical nucleus for the health care system; but managers are responsible for much of the system's real and imagined success and failure. Strategically, managers must keep an eye to the future, read the signs, and do the best they can to ensure that health care organizations are effective by *doing the right things*. Operationally, they must keep their eye on the present, see to details, and ensure that activities are accomplished as efficiently as possible—so the right things *must be done right*. This is no small task. It may not rival heart surgery in complexity and challenge, but it is very hard work.

Ironically, while managers are struggling with decision making, a network of consultants, scholars, and researchers interested in the health care industry are analyzing, studying, and documenting experiences that could be of tremendous value to the larger audience of health care managers. The problem is one of linkage—the lack of readily available, practically presented, and adequately summarized material. Facilitating this linkage is the primary objective of the *Handbook of Health Care Management*.

It was recognized early in the planning stage that the relevance of this *Handbook* would be determined by two factors: (1) the contributing authors and (2) the topics included for discussion and examination. The following pages are written by experts in a number of areas of health care management and leadership. Some have pioneered various subfields of health care management. All have made important and significant contributions to our understanding of their areas through their research and writing. This *Handbook* provides a unique opportunity for this group of experts to share their ideas, state them in a concise manner, and offer useful suggestions to present and prospective health care managers.

Just as the authors were carefully chosen, the topics for inclusion were carefully evaluated. As one might imagine, in an industry as complex and diverse as health care, hundreds of issues are worthy of discussion. However, pages are limited and decisions had to be made as to what to include and what to omit. Rather than making that decision alone, we went to the market and asked a number of practicing managers, researchers, and consultants what they believed were the essential topics that should be included in a book of this nature. The 14 topics included in this *Handbook* represent the consensus of this diverse and informed group.

The *Handbook of Health Care Management* is organized in three major parts. Part I deals with the management of relationships. Chapters are included on managing stakeholder relations, customer relations, relations with other organizations (alliances), and relations with the external environment (strategic management). Part II focuses on the tools managers possess in developing and maintaining efficient and effective organizations. Chapters are included on health care finance, health economics, health information systems, health care marketing, and total quality management. Part III examines key organizational processes with chapters on team building, visionary leadership, change and innovation, designing effective health care organizations and motivation.

As editors, we are especially grateful to the contributing authors who agreed to write chapters for this *Handbook*. All are highly productive researchers and teachers of health administration and face many demands on their limited time. Their willingness to alter their own priorities to contribute a chapter is personally very gratifying. We are also grateful to the deans, department chairs, and other academic administrators in the institutions these contributors represent for providing the environment and support that makes such contributions possible. We wish we could recognize each one by name, but limited space makes such personal recognitions impractical.

We appreciate very much the willingness of the approximately 50 health care managers, consultants, and researchers who responded to our survey and assisted us in deciding which topics to include. Our job was made much easier because of the support we received from Blackwell Publishers. Rolf Janke's vision of the usefulness of this *Handbook* and his involvement in conceptualizing and guiding the project not only kept us on schedule but added excitement and fun to the project. Ms. Dana Silliman was with us every step of the way. The electronic highway between her office and ours was busy day and night; and her assistance was always timely, useful, and much appreciated.

We wish to offer a special note of thanks for the advice and support of our colleagues at the University of Alabama at Birmingham and the University of North Carolina at Charlotte. At UAB, former Dean M. Gene Newport (School of Business/ Graduate School of Management), Dean Eli I. Capilouto (School of Public Health), Stuart A. Capper, chair of the Department of Health Care Organization and Policy, and Michael A. Morrisey, Director of the Lister Hill Center for Health Policy provided resources and encouragement. At UNCC, Dean Edward E. Mazzey (Belk College of Business) was equally skillful in creating an environment and generous in providing the support that are both necessary to transform a project of this nature from an idea into a reality.

Last, but certainly not least, we wish to thank our families, who inevitably bear a major part of the cost of yet another project. The costs are most often forgone opportunities and are, therefore, neither recognized nor appreciated as much as they deserve to be. Although we have failed to acknowledge such sacrifices on their part, we take this opportunity to say how grateful we are for their support and encouragement.

W. Jack Duncan and Peter M. Ginter, Birmingham, Alabama
Linda E. Swayne, Charlotte, North Carolina

About
the Authors

Arrington, Barbara. "Quality Management and Improvement." Ph.D. Saint Louis University. Associate Professor of health administration. Arrington received her undergraduate training in nursing and has over 15 years of governance experience in health care organizations, including 11 years in hospital and health system governance. She is a regular consultant to health care organizations and maintains active teaching, consulting, and research interests in strategic planning, leadership, and continuous quality improvement. Dr. Arrington is a fellow of the American College of Healthcare Executives.

Ashmos, Donde P. "Building Effective Health Care Teams." Ph.D. University of Texas at Austin. Associate professor of management and marketing at the University of Texas at San Antonio. Served as a visiting associate professor in the Graduate School of Business at the University of Texas at Austin. Research interests include strategic decision making, participation, and organizational systems and health care strategy. Her scholarly research has been published in the *Academy of Management Journal, Organizational Behavior and Human Decision Processes, Decision Sciences, Health Services Research, Journal of Applied Behavioral Sciences, Human Resource Management*, and other journals.

Austin, Charles J. "Health Information Systems." Ph.D. University of Cincinnati. Professor of health administration at the Medical University of South Carolina. Formerly President of East Texas State University, vice president for academic affairs at Georgia Southern College, Dean of Graduate Studies at Trinity University, and chair of the Department of Health Services Administration at the University of Alabama at Birmingham. Author of leading texts on health information systems and numerous scholarly articles and papers on management and health care issues. For a decade he was the chair of the editorial board of the *Journal of Health Administration Education.*

Blair, John D. "Effective Stakeholder Management." Ph.D. University of Michigan. Professor of management and Professor of health organization and management in the College of Business Administration and the School of Medicine at Texas Tech University. Senior research fellow with the Institute for Management and Leadership Research. Author of numerous scholarly articles and former Associate Editor of the *Journal of Management* and the founding coeditor of the *Yearly Review of Management.* Coauthor with Myron Fottler of *Challenges in Health Care Management: Strategic Perspectives for Managing Key Stakeholders.*

Bramble, J. D. "Strategic Hospital Alliances." Ph.D. candidate in health services organization and research at the Medical College of Virginia. Currently a Research Associate in the Williamson Institute for Health Studies. His research focuses on organization structures of local hospital systems and networks.

Broyles, Robert W. "Financial Accounting and Management in Health Service Organizations." Ph.D. University of Michigan. Professor of health care administration and policy in the College of Public Health at the University of Oklahoma Health Sciences Center. He is the author or coauthor of ten books and 80 articles in journals such as the *Journal of Health Politics, Policy and Law, Medical Care, Medical Care Review, Inquiry,* and *Health Care Management Review.* His primary research interests are in health care economics and finance. Dr. Broyles is a consultant to numerous hospitals and state agencies.

Duncan, W. Jack. "Strategic Management." Ph.D. Louisiana State University. Professor and university scholar in the Graduate School of Management and Professor of health care organization and policy and Senior Scholar in the Lister Hill Center for Health Policy in the School of Public Health at the University of Alabama at Birmingham. Fellow of the Academy of Management and Fellow of the International Academy of Management. Author of 13 books, including *Strategic Management of Health Care Organizations*, and more than 150 articles and papers on management and health care issues. Past president of the Southern Management Association and the Southwest Division of the Academy of Management.

Falcone, David. "Financial Accounting and Management in Health Service Organizations." Ph.D. in political science from Duke University. Professor and chair of the Department of Health Administration and Policy, College of Public Health, University of Oklahoma Health Sciences Center. Falcone is also codirector of the Oklahoma Center on Aging and a Senior Fellow in the Center for the Study of Aging and Human Development at Duke University. He has published books and monographs as well as articles in journals such as *Health Services Research, The Journal of Health Politics, Policy and Law, Journal of Politics, Journal of Rural Health, Aging and Social Policy,* and others.

Fottler, Myron D. "Effective Stakeholder Management." Ph.D. Columbia University. Professor of management in the Graduate School of Management, Professor of health services administration in the School of Health Related Professions, and Senior Scholar in the Lister Hill Center for Health Policy in the School of Public Health at the University of Alabama at Birmingham. He is also Director of the Ph.D. program in administration-health services at UAB. Author of numerous scholarly articles on the prospective payment system, strategic management of human resources, and human resource management. Coauthor with John D. Blair of *Challenges in Health Care Management: Strategic Perspectives for Managing Key Stakeholders.*

Ginter, Peter M. "Strategic Management." Ph.D. University of North Texas. Professor of management in the Graduate School of Management, Professor of health care organization and policy and Senior Scholar in the Lister Hill Center for Health Policy in the School of Public Health at the University of Alabama at Birmingham. Author of eight books, including *Strategic Management of Health Care Organizations,* and numerous articles, papers, and cases on management and health care issues. Past president of the Southwest Federation of Administrative Disciplines.

Kurz, Richard S. "Quality Management and Improvement." Ph.D. University of North Carolina at Chapel Hill. Dean of the School of Public Health and Professor of health administration at Saint Louis University. Past chairman of the board of the Association of University Programs in Health Administration and current editor of *Hospital and Health Services Administration,* an international journal published by the Foundation of the American College of Healthcare Executives. Widely published author in health services management, especially on topics of leadership and quality improvement.

Longest, Beaufort B., Jr. "Organizational Change and Innovation." Ph.D. Georgia State University. Professor of health services administration in the Graduate School of Public Health and Professor of business administration in the Joseph M. Katz Graduate School of Business, and Director of the Health Policy Institute at the University of Pittsburgh. A coauthor of one of the most widely used books in health services administration and author of several texts and numerous scholarly articles and papers on management and health care issues. Fellow of the American College of Health Care Executives.

Luke, Roice. "Strategic Hosptial Alliances." Ph.D. University of Michigan. Professor of health administration at the Medical College of Virginia and a member of the Williamson Institute for Health Studies. A recognized expert on local hospital systems and an active speaker and author in his field. His current research projects include a corporately sponsored national study of the rapidly restructuring health care and local systems and a federally funded study of the performance of strategic hospital alliances.

McDaniel, Reuben R., Jr. "Strategic Leadership: A View from Quantum and Chaos Theories." Ed.D. Indiana University. Holds the Charles and Elizabeth Prothro Regent's chair of health care management and is Professor of management science and information systems in the Graduate School of Business at the University of Texas at Austin. A widely published and respected researcher on strategic decision-making processes, organizational design, and information systems, he has published articles in numerous journals, including the *Academy of Management Journal, Health Care Management Review, Health Services Research, Health Progress, The Journal of Applied Behavioral Sciences,* and *Organizational Behavior and Human Decision Processes.*

O'Connor, Stephen J. "Motivating Effective Performance." Ph.D. University of Alabama at Birmingham. Associate Professor of Health Care Management in the School of Business Administration at the University of Wisconsin at Milwaukee. His articles have been published in *Journal of Health Care Marketing, Hospital and Health Services Administration, Medical Care Review, Health Services Management Research, Journal of Hospital Marketing,* and the Proceedings of the Academy of Management.

Olden, Peter C. "Strategic Hospital Alliances." Ph.D. Medical College of Virginia. Assistant Professor at the University of Scranton in the Department of health administration and human resources. Dr. Olden speaks and writes about the health care delivery system and health service organizations.

Rohrer, James E. "Designing Effective Health Care Organizations for the Future." Ph.D. University of Michigan. Head of the graduate program in health administration and Director of the Center for Health Services Research at the University of Iowa. His research interests are health services planning and monitoring patient outcomes. His research has appeared in *Medical Care, Health Services Research, Social Science and Medicine,* and other scholarly journals. Dr. Rohrer serves on the editorial board of the *American Journal of Public Health.*

Swayne, Linda E. "Strategic Management." Ph.D. University of North Texas. Professor of marketing in the Belk College of Business Administration and Codirector of the Physicians' Management Institute at the University of North Carolina at Charlotte. Dr. Swayne has served as Executive Director of the Carolinas Task Force on Health Care and is the author of six books, including *Strategic Management of Health Care Organizations*, and numerous articles, papers, and cases on marketing and health care issues. She is also Past President of the Southwest Federation of Administrative Disciplines and the Southern Marketing Association.

Taylor, Steven A. "Managing Customer Relations." Ph.D. Florida State University. Assistant professor of marketing at Illinois State University. Dr. Taylor's research interests lie in services marketing and relationship marketing. His articles have been published in *Journal of Marketing, Journal of Retailing, International Journal of Services Industry Management, Hospital and Health Services Administration,* and *Journal of Health Care Marketing.*

Valdmanis, Vivian. "Health Economics." Ph.D. Vanderbilt University. Assistant Professor in the College of Public Health at the University of Oklahoma Health Sciences Center. She previously held positions at Mathematical Policy Research, Inc. and Tulane University. Dr. Valdmanis teaches courses on health care economics, microeconomics, and operations research. Her research interests focus on assessing hospital productivity and efficiency. She has published articles in numerous health care, economics, and operations research journals and has presented the results of her research at national and international meetings.

Wager, Karen A. "Health Information Systems." MHA Medical University of South Carolina. Assistant professor and Director of the Master of Health Sciences program in health information systems at the Medical University of South Carolina. A registered records administrator and an active member of the American Health Information Management Association, she is currently a candidate for the DBA in information systems.

Wrenn, Bruce. "Health Care Marketing." Ph.D. Northwestern University. Associate professor of marketing at Indiana University at South Bend. Dr. Wrenn participated in research with Philip Kotler and Stephen Shortell looking at the marketing practices of hospitals and health care systems. In addition to writing publications in health care marketing, he is the coauthor of books on marketing research and marketing planning. He is interested in marketing for religious organizations and is coauthor of *Marketing for Congregations*.

Introduction

This *Handbook of Health Care Management* attempts to achieve an ambitious goal: to provide a series of essays that will be of value both to students of health care management and students of related disciplines who wish to know more about selected topics in health care. The term *students* is used intentionally to include anyone and everyone interested in learning more about one of our most complex and exciting global industries. Every society must, in one way or another, attend to the health care needs of its citizens. Seeing to health care needs is an expensive proposition. In terms of personal consumption expenditures, Americans spend more for health care than for any other items except housing and food. Ensuring efficiency and effectiveness in health care is indeed a monumental management task.

Each society approaches the problem in its own way, with varying degrees of success. In most societies health care is one of the most rapidly changing sectors, if not the most rapidly changing one. That fluidity suggests the need for ongoing, lifelong learning on the part of those who provide health services and those who manage the organizations within which these services are provided. Therefore, this *Handbook* is directed both to those who presently lead health care organizations and those who aspire to lead them in the future.

Each of the chapters contained in this *Handbook* is a delicate mixture of theory and practice and has been written by experts who are grounded in the theory. Some have been health care managers, and all have systematically observed and studied health care organizations and their leaders. All of the contributors have been asked to translate the theory relative to their specific topic into terms that will be instructive both to traditionally defined students preparing to enter positions of health care leadership and nontraditionally defined students who are attempting to stay abreast of developments in the field. The task is a formidable one. Perhaps it is more than should be asked of any writer. However, each contributor has courageously accepted the challenge and performed magnificently. Some emphasize theory more than practice; others focus on practice more than theory. To a great extent the approach is a function of the topic being addressed and the unique background and experience of each contributor. We believe that collectively, the chapters contained in this *Handbook* paint an interesting, accurate, and relatively comprehensive picture of health care management theory and practice that will be useful to students in all stages of learning.

This *Handbook of Health Care Management* could have been organized in many ways. Each option offered some advantages and some disadvantages, and even though there were choices, organization was not an unimportant consideration. To achieve an effective organization providing continuity, ease of reading, and consistency, we decided to structure this book in three major parts, each representing an area with significant impact on the job of health care management. The figure on page 3 provides an illustration of the logic of this structure.

Part I deals with the management of relationships as illustrated in the upper left-hand portion of the triangle in the figure. It includes chapters on managing stakeholder relations, customer relations, relations with other organizations (alliances), and relations with the external environment (strategic management). Part II looks at some important tools health care managers use to do their jobs. It contains chapters on health care finance, health economics, health information systems, health care marketing, and total quality management. Part III examines selected organizational processes in health care and includes chapters on effective health care teams, visionary leadership, organizational change and innovation, designing effective health care organizations and ways to motivate effective performance.

& Managing Relationships

A great deal of the health care manager's job involves managing relationships with other organizations and anticipating and responding to external changes. Because such organizations and forces are inherently less controllable than forces inside the

Figure 1   Dimensions of Health Care Management

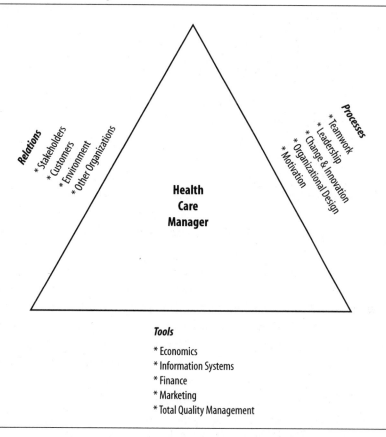

Relations
* Stakeholders
* Customers
* Environment
* Other Organizations

Processes
* Teamwork
* Leadership
* Change & Innovation
* Organizational Design
* Motivation

**Health
Care
Manager**

Tools

* Economics
* Information Systems
* Finance
* Marketing
* Total Quality Management

organization, the manager loses certain options when attempting to manage these relationships. Legitimate authority is no longer the coordinator of last resort because managers have no authority over suppliers, customers, government regulators, competitors, or even members of the same network who join together to compete more effectively with other organizations. They likewise lack the controls necessary to direct environmental forces like technology, social and demographic trends, and political philosophies. Managing external relations offers unique challenges. Part I includes four chapters that address different groups and forces in the environment of health care organizations.

Effective Stakeholder Management

Chapter 1 is written by John D. Blair of Texas Tech University and Myron D. Fottler of the University of Alabama at Birmingham, who have defined much of the field of stakeholder management in health care (as the bibliography of their chapter illustrates). This chapter summarizes and integrates their prior work and provides fresh insights into stakeholder relationships in the future based on their study of 580 health care experts' perceptions of the relative importance of hospital stakeholders in 1994 compared with their forecasts for 1999. This survey confirms the importance that respondents attached to the integrated health care networks and systems. A specific example of community-oriented primary care networks is provided in Chapter 13, which deals with effective organizational structures for the future.

For the purposes of Chapter 1, Blair and Fottler argue that health care networks and systems will require leaders who can effectively manage increasingly complex and changing stakeholder relations. For example, the panel of experts who participated in this study indicated their belief that in 1994 the most important key hospital stakeholders were patients, physicians as individual caregivers, government agencies, and medical practices—in that order. These same experts believed that in 1999 the most important key hospital stakeholders will be integrated systems and networks, managed care organizations, government agencies, employers, and patients.

Like that of any forecast, the accuracy of these expert's predictions will require time to validate. However, the points made in the chapter are appropriate regardless of the exact order of the importance of key hospital stakeholders—stakeholders are important, and it is likely that the relative importance of key hospital stakeholders will change over the next five years as a reflection of the overall changes in health care. For these reasons, it is necessary to develop a process of effectively managing stakeholder relations. Blair and Fottler provide us with a useful approach to *strategic stakeholder management.* It is interesting to note that the panel of experts in the study believed that all of the most powerful hospital stakeholders in 1999 will be external.

Managing Customer Relations

Every economic organization has customers, and the existence of competition makes customers important stakeholders. Although historically attempts have been made to determine precisely who are the customers in health care and arguments have been presented as to why patients are not customers in one sense or another, most agree that this argument is largely irrelevant. The fact remains that all reforms taking place in health care suggest increasing competition, and increasing competition suggests understanding and serving patients better as health care customers.

In Chapter 2 Steven A. Taylor of Illinois State University offers a comprehensive discussion of *relationship marketing* as it applies to health care organizations. This chapter is an extension of the work Taylor and his colleagues have done on the relationship between service quality and customer satisfaction in business and health care organizations.

Taylor argues that historically, marketing has focused on individual transactions and encounters with customers without considering the cumulative or long-term impact of marketing actions. Relationship marketing, by contrast, is concerned with attracting, developing, and retaining customer relationships and thereby results in "true customers" who believe they have received genuine value and are likely to be loyal to the organization and resistant to defection to competitors. True customers are beneficial to organizations because they are more profitable than new customers and cost less to retain. Customers benefit from the long-term relationship because it provides a more personalized, satisfying, and predictable association.

Relationship marketing is based on commitment and trust. Commitment occurs when the partners to the exchange believe that an ongoing association is worth either the price or the effort required to maintain the association. Trust occurs when the parties have confidence that the other partners will perform with reliability and integrity. However, although commitment and trust are necessary conditions for relationship marketing, service quality and customer satisfaction are also needed if the relationship is to endure. The challenge, as Taylor notes, is how to ensure patient satisfaction and a positive quality image. This is the foundation of relationship marketing.

Strategic Hospital Alliances

Strategic alliances are emerging in all industries, as Roice Luke, Peter C. Olden, and J. D. Bramble point out in the introduction to chapter 3. Health care in general, and hospitals in particular, are no exceptions. The chapter notes that in 1995 over 60 percent of all urban, acute care, general hospitals were involved in one or more systems or networks. Strategic hospital alliances (SHAs) are defined as two or more hospitals in a market that unite in order to generate critical competitive advantages and pursue their collective survival in a managed care marketplace.

These contributors are all affiliated with the Williamson Institute at the Medical College of Virginia at Virginia Commonwealth University, and they have been collecting data and studying hospital alliances for almost a decade. Using a classification scheme based on organizational independence and the degree of tightness of coupling, they develop an interesting typology of hospital alliances.

Chapter 3 provides an in-depth discussion of the dimensions and details of the SHA. In addition, it addresses two of the most fundamental and practical questions facing decision makers relative to strategic alliances: (1) With which hospitals should a hospital affiliate and (2) how tight should the coupling be between and among the aligning partners? When a hospital decides to enter an SHA, it places its long-term survival in the hands of other hospitals. Sometimes the partners are the hospital's closest competitors. It is argued that the most important single factor in deciding whether or not to enter an alliance is the extent to which the partnership reduces strategic uncertainties in the environment. Therefore, alliances should be carefully evaluated in light of a clear understanding of such existing uncertainties and the extent to which alignment and partnering with other hospitals can reduce them.

Strategic Management

The final chapter in Part I deals with strategic management or managing external relations in the most general sense. A great deal of strategic management is, after all, ensuring that the organization "fits" the demands of the external environment. Effective strategic management, therefore, requires managing a number of relationships with competitors, government regulators, customers, and other organizations.

The purpose of Chapter 4, written by Peter M. Ginter, Linda E. Swayne, and W. Jack Duncan, is to provide an overview of the strategic management process, not an in-depth treatment of the theory and practice of strategic management. It is also intended to offer the reader a process for actually accomplishing strategic management. The chapter begins with the argument that the behavior or strategy of a health care organization is the result of interaction among three important factors.

The external environment provides the strategic decision maker with an indication of what he or she *should be doing.* The rules of success are written outside the organization, and carefully assessing external environmental forces is an important element in situation analysis. An organization's internal environment, resources, competencies, and capabilities determine to a great extent what the organization *can do* in response to the demands of the external environment. Although this is generally true, it should be noted that a great deal of recent strategic management theory is devoted to illustrating how some of the most successful organizations in all industries are those that can effectively *stretch and leverage* their resources in a manner that allows them to exceed resource limitations. The third and final element in situation analysis is determining what an organization, its leadership, and its employees *want to do*, as reflected in their vision, values, and mission statements.

When strategic decision makers understand these three factors, they are in a better position to formulate successful strategies. Chapter 4 provides a useful classification of strategic options along with examples of each. However, it is important to note that strategic decision making does not stop with strategy formulation. Even though we may choose to differentiate carefully between strategic and tactical action, it is important to note that implementation and strategic control are extremely important stages in the overall strategic management process.

✒ TOOLS OF HEALTH CARE MANAGEMENT

The second part of the *Handbook,* comprising five chapters, deals with selected "tools" health care managers have at their disposal when they attempt to build and maintain effective and efficient organizations. Many of the topics in these chapters will be less familiar to some health care managers because tools are developed by specialists in a particular area and used by managers who are not specialists in finance, economics, information systems, marketing, or total quality management. However, even though the topics may be less familiar, they are useful aids to managers in leading their organizations.

Health Care Finance

Chapter 5, by Robert W. Broyles and David Falcone (University of Oklahoma Health Sciences Center), provides an enlightening discussion of the ever-evolving field of health care finance. Broyles and Falcone explore some of the recommended changes in the format of health care organization financial statements. Since financial statements are critically important factors in determining the attractiveness of alliances, the wisdom of mergers, and the success of a variety of strategic decisions, it is important for all health care managers to understand the latest interpretations and presentations of these documents.

After discussing and providing examples of the traditional ways of evaluating financial performance along such dimensions as profitability, liquidity, debt structure, and intensity of resource utilization, the chapter presents a review of the management of the major operating assets. It offers a number of useful ideas and techniques for health care managers who are attempting to improve management of working capital assets like cash, accounts receivable, and inventories. As a result of cost containment pressures and resource limitations, these basic financial management techniques remain important tools.

The chapter concludes with discussions of two additional topics—the evaluation of capital expenditures and the effective financial control of operations. Health care organizations are indeed labor-intensive operations. Most, however, require high-technology equipment and specialized facilities. Evaluating capital needs and selecting critical projects in the face of limited capital resources represent significant challenges for health care managers. At the same time, the pricing of services and development of strategic portfolios of services require an understanding of the costs involved in service delivery. Activity-based costing is introduced as an effective way of accounting for these costs.

Health Economics

In Chapter 6, Vivian Valdmanis (University of Oklahoma Health Sciences Center) provides an overview of health economics. Many, if not most, of the trends in health care management can be traced to the underlying economics of the industry. At the national level, the United States now spends about 14 percent of its gross national product on health care, and the economic incentives within the system are likely to lead to even higher health care costs. This primer on health economics, therefore, begins with an analysis of why there has been such rapid growth in the demand for health care services.

The chapter proceeds with an examination of some major factors in health economics. Health insurance, it notes, has played a unique role in the American health care market. The philosophy upon which health insurance is based is a key determinant of expenditures for health care and the behavioral incentives for patients and providers. In addition to discussing health insurance, the chapter goes on to paint an economic picture of the health care system and examines changes in hospitals and in the role of physicians in terms of both incentives and financial realities.

Valdmanis argues that the present health care system threatens the standard of living of Americans by draining resources from more efficient uses, increasing the federal deficit , reducing national savings, and locking people into their present jobs out of fear of losing the security of health insurance. Health economics thus involves serious social consequences that cannot and should not be ignored. The economics of health care at first glance seem abstract and beyond the comprehension of most people who have access to, are denied access to, or must manage this complex system. Upon reflection, however, it is clear that there is little genuine promise of effectively managed health care organizations until the underlying incentives of patients and providers are understood and management policies are developed to facilitate economically rational behavior that also increases the overall welfare of society.

Health Information Systems

Charles J. Austin and Karen A. Wagner (Medical University of South Carolina) discuss health information systems in Chapter 7. This chapter presents an overview of the different types of information systems, describes current uses of the various systems, and offers some informed speculation about the future course of health information systems.

Most computer applications in health care relate to one of the following: (1) clinical information systems such as those aiding the work in laboratories and pharmacies, as well as clinical decision support systems designed to aid clinicians in making decisions; (2) administrative and financial systems, which were the first used in health delivery organizations; and (3) strategic decision support systems, which are executive information systems that aid health care executives in making competitive and other kinds of strategic decisions. The growth of integrated delivery systems such as those mentioned in Chapters 1, 3, and 4, for example, presents major strategic information system challenges. Interestingly, one of the most often discussed topics in health information systems today is the computer-based patient record (CPR).

Health information systems of the future must deal with increasingly complex health care systems. Integrated delivery systems will demand community information networks to support them. The expanded use of electronic data interchange applications will make it technically feasible to exchange clinical and financial data across regions and national networks. Voice recognition, imaging, and telemedicine should have a major positive impact on the improvement of access and the standardization of care. The reality of CPRs will have a significant impact on the cost of health services; perhaps more than anything else, CPRs should aid greatly in conducting large sample outcomes research.

Health Care Marketing

Of all the major "business" disciplines, marketing has been among the last to be applied to health care organizations. Bruce Wrenn (Indiana University at South Bend) begins Chapter 8 with the observation that it was not until the 1970s that marketing had a significant presence in any health care organization. Among some health care providers, marketing remains a controversial topic, although increasing competition has caused most to recognize its importance.

Much of the delay and skepticism concerning the use of marketing can be traced to the nature of health care organizations. The *marketing concept* is based on the need to identify and satisfy customer wants and needs, accomplish organizational goals while satisfying those needs, and adopt a customer focus in all areas of the organization. The degree to which an organization has implemented the marketing concept is referred to as the organization's marketing *orientation*. Development of a genuine marketing orientation has been difficult in health care, which has always operated on the assumption that professionals were in the best position to determine customer needs and how they should be satisfied.

When adopted as a philosophy, marketing is an effective tool for identifying, under-standing, and exploiting competitive advantages and should be thought of in this con-text rather than simply as a means of stimulating demand. When regarded in this way, marketing is an integral part of all areas of the health care organization because it is a way of thinking, a philosophy of management based on customer service. Wrenn ren-ders the reader an additional service by concluding the chapter with a bibliography in which he provides an essential reading list on health care marketing, a useful resource for those who want to know more about health care services marketing.

Quality Management and Improvement

Much of management in business or health care is a matter of attitude. This is nowhere better illustrated than in the area of total quality management. Since quality is a "race without an end" and a goal that is never fully achieved, it is appropriate to include a discussion of quality management in the *Handbook.*

Chapter 9, by Barbara Arrington and Richard J. Kurz (Saint Louis University), examines the subject of quality management and improvement. The contemporary interest in this subject makes the writing of such a chapter a demanding and contro-versial task—demanding because so much is happening in the area, and controversial because so many people have their own views and biases about what quality is and how it can and should be achieved.

Health care managers and medical providers have always been concerned about quality. In health care the "quality related stakes" are even higher than in most other industries. Survival and quality-of-life issues are directly related to the quality of ser-vices provided. Only in recent years, however, has the issue of quality been applied to the health care organization as a whole.

This chapter clearly links quality and strategy through resource leveraging. Resource leveraging occurs when the most focused and efficient actions are taken to bring about lasting improvements in organizational structures, processes, and outcomes. Health care organizations, it is argued, can leverage quality by concentrating on strategy, focusing on evaluating performance in a way that stretches the organization to high lev-els of accomplishment, and enhancing the organization's ability to learn. Organizational learning is particularly important to quality improvement because organizations actu-ally become more competent by learning from their own and others' experiences. In this way quality improvement can be affected by removing barriers to learning and using knowledge gained in one area to improve organizational performance.

In addition to linking strategy and organizational learning to quality manage-ment and improvement, this chapter introduces the essential concept of total quality management and discusses the impact of quality improvement programs on health care organizations. In the end, commitment to quality is a matter of faith. There is no compelling set of data to prove beyond a doubt that an investment in quality provides incremental financial returns. However, when quality becomes an automatic criterion for action, it can lead to important strategic and competitive advantages.

❧ ORGANIZATIONAL PROCESSES IN HEALTH CARE MANAGEMENT

In addition to overseeing external relations, health care managers are responsible for ensuring that internal operations contribute to the achievement of their organization's goals. Managing internal operations is a multifaceted task of providing leadership, motivating performance, building teamwork, and creating an environment that encourages change and innovation. When these processes are functioning properly, organizations are efficient and "do things right." When they are combined with an understanding of the external environment, organizations are effective and also "do the right things." The five chapters in Part III all relate to organizational processes.

Building Effective Health Care Teams

Chapter 10, by Donde P. Ashmos (University of Texas at San Antonio), is an exciting alternative view for those who are tired of reading the "same old things" about team building. Ashmos reacts against the machine model and focuses on teams as complex adaptive systems. In doing so, she challenges a number of conventional assumptions and suggests a number of interesting revisions to our way of thinking about teams in health care organizations.

Much of this chapter is built around the importance of revising our assumptions about teams and understanding their essential functions so that they may become more productive aids in accomplishing organizational goals. It is noted, for example, that the effectiveness of teams can be improved by recognizing some of their most important functions, such as increasing participation and involving more people in decision making. This broader participation and resulting diversity of perspectives in turn improves our understanding of complex problems. Teams that interact in an ongoing manner may evolve into groups and satisfy members' social needs. Teams sometimes help members reach a collective mind, develop certain patterns of behavior, and eventually make fewer organizational errors than individuals acting alone or in less developed teams. Finally, teams, when properly organized and used, can outperform individuals making decisions alone.

Ashmos concludes that in many cases the problems teams experience are caused by outdated command and control assumptions. When leaders view teams as complex adaptive systems, however, their potential is greatly increased. Teamwork is a high-performance possibility. It is also a high-maintenance proposition. Building effective health care teams is hard work and requires skill and perseverance.

Strategic Leadership

No *Handbook of Health Care Management* would be complete without a discussion of leadership. In Chapter 11 Reuben R. McDaniel, Jr., (University of Texas at Austin) provides a discussion of leadership that is anything but traditional. Borrowing from concepts of quantum and chaos theories, McDaniel provides an analysis of strategic leadership. Like Chapter 10, this analysis begins by questioning our most cherished assumptions about leadership and organizations. It notes, for example, that much of leadership theory in the past has been built on equilibrium models in which the leader's role was assumed to be helping organizations adapt to change through setting goals, building commitment to goals, and reducing uncertainty. According to this view, the focus of leadership was on planning and control. In fact, this view was more about management than leadership.

This chapter presentes the alternative view that strategic leaders perform best when they keep their organizations on the edge of chaos, because it is only at this point that the creative forces needed to deal with the complex strategic issues facing health care managers can be recognized and developed. This approach makes the strategic leadership of health care organizations more a matter of sensemaking, learning, and designing than of planning and control. So much for traditional discussions of the sources and styles of leadership.

The chapter defines the strategic leadership problem in health care organizations and presents the traditional and alternative views of leadership along with their implications. McDaniel concludes that managers should recognize that they cannot be in control, predict the future, or even plan for success. Successful strategic leaders in health care organizations, he argues, should instead give up trying to control and focus on designing new organizational forms that tolerate fluctuations as individuals and groups adjust to change. These new organizational forms need to facilitate organizational learning, enhance the quality of connections among individuals and groups, emphasize cooperation rather than competition, and be driven by clearly understood values and visions. Ultimately this view, as the chapter notes, forces strategic leaders in health care organizations to answer difficult questions and encourages them to reach beyond a single organization and look to the health of communities and entire populations. "Who should be better off as health systems improve?" "Whom should strategic leaders in health care represent?"

Organizational Change and Innovation

A common theme throughout every chapter in this *Handbook* is the present rate and projected increased rate of changes in health care environments. In Chapter 12, Beaufort B. Longest, Jr., (University of Pittsburgh) develops a decision-making orientation to the organizational change and innovation process. This approach should help health care leaders understand change and innovation as the process of identifying and carefully defining change issues, analyzing them, developing alternative approaches, and ultimately selecting a course of action.

Organizational change is defined as a discernible modification in an organization's purpose, culture, strategies, tasks, technologies, people, or structures. Many of these changes are borrowed from other organizations or from a specific place in a larger and more complex organization. Some changes, however, are the result of new ideas, inventions, and innovations. Both are capable of taking health care organizations to new heights of organizational performance; and both are capable of creating uncertainty and resistance.

Much of this chapter is devoted to the practical question of implementing organizational changes. This emphasis is important, because ultimately the success of any strategic change or organizational innovation depends on how well it is implemented. While some leaders are good at generating changes, few are really good at implementing them. Generating changes and encouraging chaos are fun and exciting tasks. Implementing change is just hard work. However, even for those who are good at implementation, the task is not complete when the proposed changes become reality. Changes, and people's responses to them, have to be evaluated and effective leaders learn from successes and failures. The comprehensive model of organizational change and innovation presented in this chapter should be a useful guide for health care managers.

Designing Effective Health Care Organizations for the Future

In the initial planning stage of the *Handbook of Health Care Management*, the topic of designing effective health care organizations for the future had a traditional internal orientation. The idea was to look at different structures and see how traditional and modern organizational concepts applied or did not apply to health care organizations. As the planning developed and the importance of stakeholder relations and alliances became more evident, it was clear that some of the most, if not *the* most, important determinants, of effective organizational design in health care in the future will involve networks and systems rather than hierarchy and chain of command. Certainly, the survey reported in Chapter 1 would support this argument.

In Chapter 13, James E. Rohrer of the University of Iowa discusses an additional important stakeholder in health care: the community. The effective health care organization of the future, he argues, will embrace a mission of community service.

In community-oriented primary care (COPC) organizations, community assessment is a key factor, and the mix of health services provided reflects community health needs. The success of these organizations is measured in terms of their positive effects on the patient and the community. The chapter concludes with a set of principles for developing successful community-oriented health systems and some practical guidelines for action. To be successful, COPC systems should, among other things, provide a shared vision of how the local system should function, expand participation beyond health care providers, carefully evaluate the scope of health services in light of community needs, and take advantage of internal problems and external threats in constructive ways so as to build cooperation within the system.

Turning a fragmented local health delivery system into a COPC system, difficult at best, represents a fundamental challenge for community and health care leaders. Moreover, it is a promising approach to building effective health care organizations in the future.

Motivation

Chapter 14, by Stephen J. O'Connor (University of Wisconsin at Milwaukee), discusses the ever-present management challenge of motivating effective performance in health care organizations. Like all industries, health care is undergoing restructuring, downsizing, and related changes that make motivation a more demanding and difficult task for health care managers. After providing an interesting historical overview of motivation in management theory, O'Connor surveys a number of motivation theories that even well-informed and experienced managers should find useful. He then applies these theories, especially Herzberg's two-factor theory, to the quintessential problem of motivating professional employees.

O'Connor relates the characteristics of a profession to issues of intrinsic rewards and examines the power of a sense of accomplishment, recognition, and other nonmonetary rewards. He notes that we should "never ridicule a recognition" and proceeds to illustrate how factors that might appear childish and silly to outsiders can be enormous motivators to members of a particular organization. Most professionals have high achievement needs as a result of their training. Regardless of how these needs develop, achievement represents a major opportunity for motivating high-level professional performance if leaders recognize and understand motivational approaches that take advantage of the opportunity.

There is not at present, nor is there likely to be in the future, a single "grand theory" of motivation that applies to all health care employees. Every individual and every profession and occupational group are distinct. The best strategy is to think about motivation from a variety of perspectives. This chapter helps illustrate and itemize some of the important perspectives.

We believe that this *Handbook of Health Care Management* is a useful survey of a complex and exciting field, which will be even more dynamic and demanding in the future. The experts whose chapters make up this book provide valuable and timely discussions and tools that can help to ensure an ongoing supply of leaders in this critically important field.

Managing Relationships in Health Care

I

Effective Stakeholder Management:

Challenges, Opportunities and Strategies

1

John D. Blair, Texas Tech University
*Myron D. Fottler, University of Alabama at Birmingham**

T he health care environment is undergoing fundamental and somewhat revolutionary changes. A sweeping restructuring of the health care industry is currently taking place, even without proposed governmental changes. Significant
reforms *are* occurring. The effects of these reforms—whether government-mandated
or driven by private sector initiatives such as managed care or powerful buyer groups
demanding more health care for less money—are unknown. However, they *will* have
an impact the future of the industry as they drive the development of increasingly
complex, integrated organization networks and systems (Arthur Andersen, 1993;
Blair, Rock, Rotarius, Fottler, Bosse, and Driskill, 1996; Burns and Thorpe, 1993; Coddington, Moore, and Fischer, 1993; Coddington, Moore, and Fischer, 1994; Coile, 1994;
Conrad and Hoare, 1994; Gillies, Shortell, Anderson, Mitchell, and Morgan, 1993;
Kongstvedt and Plocher, 1995; Rotarius, Paolino, McMurrough, Fottler, and Blair,

*The authors express their special thanks to their long-term colleagues John A. Buesseler, MD,
MSBA, and Timothy M. Rotarius, MBA, PhD, whose insightful comments and suggestions were
most appreciated.

1995; Shortell, Gillies, Anderson, Mitchell, and Morgan, 1993; Watson, Kimberly, and Burns, 1995).

One characteristic of these new networks is that leaders of health care organizations must manage relationships with a growing number of active, powerful, and sometimes competing stakeholders—any individuals, groups, or organizations that have a stake in the decisions and actions of an organization and attempt to influence those decisions and actions. These stakeholders exert an influence on every health care management issue and must be recognized and evaluated for their potential to support or threaten the organization and its competitive goals.

These new networks and systems magnify the need for managers to engage in effective strategic stakeholder management (Blair and Fottler, 1990; Appendix A). Figure 1.1 shows the key stakeholders for hospitals as perceived by 580 health care experts who were surveyed in 1994 (Blair, Fottler, Paolino, and Rotarius, 1995; see Appendix B for a detailed description of the Facing the Uncertain Future expert study). These experts included medical practice executives, physician executives, hospital executives, insurance and managed care executives, and health care industry suppliers. We asked each respondent who were the *current* (1994) key stakeholders for hospitals *and* who will be the *future* key stakeholders in 1999. Key stakeholders are defined as those whom at least 25 percent of the respondents defined as one of their five most important stakeholders.

As noted in the figure title, there is both stability and change in the key stakeholders over the five-year period. The bold arrow shows the range of stakeholder importance reported by the experts. The top portion of each side of the figure shows the "most important" key stakeholders, identified as such by at least 50 percent of the respondents. The middle third shows key stakeholders identified by from 25 to 50 percent of respondents. The bottom third shows the marginal stakeholders identified by less than 25 percent of respondents as key stakeholders.

In 1994 the most important key stakeholders of hospitals as identified by our expert panel were patients (73 percent), physicians as individual caregivers (65 percent), governments (64 percent), and medical practices (50 percent). Other key stakeholders of hospitals were managed care organizations, employers, other independent hospitals, and other hospitals in the same system.

These same experts predicted that by 1999 the most important hospital key stakeholders will be integrated delivery systems/networks (IDS/Ns) (81 percent), managed care organizations (80 percent), government (65 percent), employers (57 percent), and patients (53 percent). Other projected key stakeholders include system hospitals, physicians as individual caregivers, and medical practices.

An examination of Figure 1.1 indicates several significant changes in the relative importance of key stakeholders predicted for the future. The smaller arrows

Figure 1.1 Stability and Change in Hospital Stakeholder Importance (As Seen by a Combined Sample of Health Care Industry Experts)

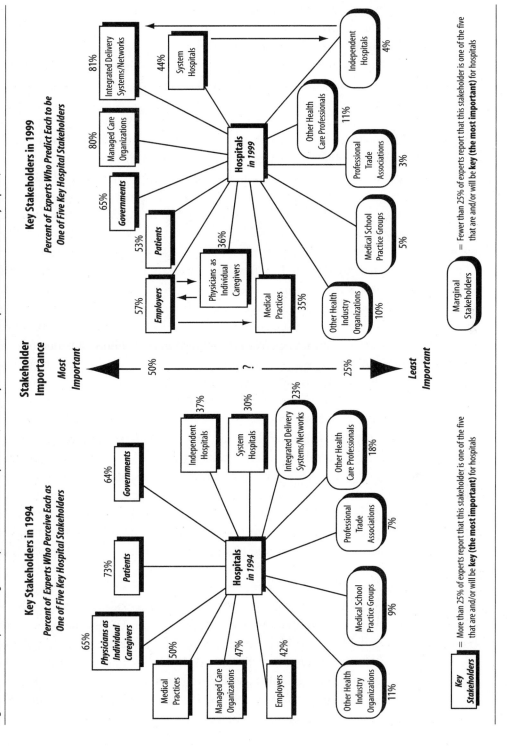

draw attention to how certain key stakeholders are expected to change in importance. First, IDS/Ns (marginal stakeholders in 1994) are predicted to be *the* most important key stakeholder of hospitals in 1999. In other words, our expert panel predicted that IDS/Ns will develop quickly over the five-year period so that the average hospital will be part of such a system in 1999 and subject to its rules, regulations, incentives, and constraints.

Second, managed care organizations (MCOs) are expected to increase in importance from being key stakeholders in 1994 to being the second most important key stakeholders in 1999 by virtue of their role in providing a capitated insurance product for the IDS/Ns. Managed care organizations are insurance-based organizations designed to "manage" care provided to patients. From the hospital's perspective, the terms and conditions of the capitated insurance product offered by the MCO affect patient access to its services, the quantity and quality of those services provided, and the hospital's income.

Third, employers are expected to increase in importance from being key hospital stakeholders in 1994 to being among the five most important stakeholders in 1999. This change is due to the more aggressive stance taken by many employers over the past five years in regard to health care cost containment. Many employers have joined health care coalitions of employers. While the goals and activities of different coalitions vary, most have tried to pressure hospitals to contain their costs, have negotiated contracts with hospitals (and others) to provide specified services to their employees on a capitated basis, and have demanded data from hospitals concerning the costs and outcomes of specific services.

Fourth, patients and governments remain among the most important key stakeholders for both years. Governments are obviously important because of their regulatory powers and their ability to set reimbursement rules and rates for both Medicare and Medicaid patients. Although their overall importance is expected to drop sharply, as the ultimate consumers of health services, patients can choose to use or not use a given provider. In addition, their satisfaction or dissatisfaction with particular providers can influence the acceptability of these providers to a given IDS/N.

Fifth, physicians as individual caregivers and medical practices are expected to be less important in 1999 than they were in 1994. Both are expected to be key stakeholders of hospitals in 1999, but not among the most important. Unless these two stakeholders are part of the IDS/N with which the hospital is associated, they are viewed as competitors unable to provide desired resources. If they are part of the same IDS/N, they offer the potential of patient referrals to the hospital. Likewise, other system hospitals may be complementary to the focal hospital (and thus offer the potential for referrals) or substitutable and, therefore, competitive.

Other stakeholders were viewed by our expert panel as marginal hospital stakeholders in the future. However, it should be noted that any of these could be a key stakeholder for a *particular* hospital. For example, medical school practice groups could be a key stakeholder for an academic medical center, even though they are not key stakeholders for hospitals in general.

The number and types of complex relationships routinely faced by today's health care executives are inadequately presented by this simplified model of key relationships. However, the model does illustrate just how complex health care relationships have become; and it suggests that today's strategic stakeholder management tools need to be sophisticated and powerful if executives are to lead their health care organizations effectively.

Few organizations have fully developed an integrated, articulated strategic approach for managing their key stakeholders At best for most organizations, executives' stakeholder management perspectives are incomplete, and their approaches to stakeholder assessment and management are underdeveloped and haphazard. At worst, they display a total lack of explicit awareness of, and involvement in, a systematic and effective stakeholder management approach. Health care leaders require a detailed, overall approach, along with specific tools and techniques, in order to facilitate managing stakeholders strategically.

The strategic approach to stakeholder management provides a means of properly identifying all the players, their roles, and their level of stake in the network (Freeman, 1984; Mason and Mitroff, 1981; Blair and Fottler, 1990; Appendix A). This chapter outlines the strategic stakeholder management process, provides some detail and examples for each step, and uses data from a recent survey of hospital executives to indicate contemporary reality.

These are some of the steps in this approach to strategic stakeholder management:

- Identify all relevant external, interface, and internal stakeholders.
- Diagnose each stakeholder in terms of potential for threat and potential for cooperation.
- Ensure that the diagnosis for each stakeholder is relevant for the specific issue facing the organization.
- Classify each stakeholder as supportive, mixed-blessing, nonsupportive, or marginal.
- Formulate generic stakeholder management strategies, involve the supportive stakeholder, collaborate with the mixed-blessing stakeholder, defend against the nonsupportive stakeholder, and monitor the marginal stakeholder.
- Implement these generic strategies by developing specific implementation tactics and programs for each strategy-stakeholder combination.

- Determine which employees, as internal stakeholders, should be involved in the implementation process.
- Evaluate managerial implications of effectively managing stakeholders from a strategic point of view.

🍃 IDENTIFYING ORGANIZATIONAL STAKEHOLDERS

Stakeholders are categorized into one of three distinct stakeholder groups: external, interface, and internal. The hospital must respond to a large number and a wide variety of external stakeholders—including suppliers, competitors, related health organizations, government agencies, private accrediting associations, professional associations, labor unions, patients, third-party payers, the media, the financial community, special interest groups, and the local community. Whereas the internal and interface stakeholders are at least partly supportive of the hospital, many of the external stakeholders may be seen as neutral, nonsupportive, or even openly hostile.

External stakeholders fall into three categories in their relationship to the health-care organization. Some provide inputs into the organization, some compete with it, and some have a particular special interest in how the organization functions. Note that all of the most powerful key stakeholders for hospitals in 1999 are expected to be external to the organization (see Figure 1.1).

Interface stakeholders are those who function both internally and externally to the organization, that is, those who are on the interface between the organization and its environment. The major categories of interface stakeholders include the medical staff; the hospital board of trustees; the corporate office of the parent company; and stockholders, taxpayers, or other contributors. These tend to be among the most powerful stakeholders in health care organizations but are easily misunderstood because they are thought of as "us" or "them" when they are both—and neither.

As in the case of internal stakeholders, the organization must offer each interface stakeholder sufficient inducements to continue to make appropriate contributions. However, the inducements can be even more complex than in the case of internal stakeholders because of the lack of such things as a structured human resource system or adequate management authority. Examples include such inducements as professional autonomy (medical staff), institutional prestige or political contacts (hospital board), good financial returns (corporate office), access (taxpayers), and special services or benefits (contributors).

Finally, internal stakeholders operate almost entirely within the generally accepted "bounds" of the organization and typically include management, professional, and nonprofessional staff. Management attempts to manage these internal stakeholders by providing sufficient inducements to obtain ongoing contributions from them. The stakeholders determine whether the inducement is sufficient for the contribution they are required to make, partly by considering the alternative inducement—contribution offers received from competitive organizations.

Unless both the organization and the stakeholder believe such an agreement will be mutually beneficial and of fair value (relative to alternatives), agreement will not be reached and/or sustained. Under conditions of scarce resources, the exchange partners can be expected to attempt to obtain as high an inducement as possible while making as low a contribution as possible.

Once all the stakeholders have been classified into their respective categories, it becomes obvious that health care organizations do not face just one or a few stakeholders. Rather, health care executives must learn to manage a portfolio of stakeholders. It is vital that the leaders of health care organizations see the strategic implications of these stakeholder portfolios. No longer can specific functional managers be concerned only with those stakeholders that obviously fall within their functional responsibilities. Instead, these managers must be cognizant of all the other relationships that are influenced by their one-on-one episodes with specific stakeholders. And the challenge facing health care organization executives is the creation of consistency and effectiveness in all of these individual stakeholder episodes.

DIAGNOSING KEY STAKEHOLDERS IN TERMS OF ʔ☙ POTENTIAL FOR THREAT AND POTENTIAL FOR COOPERATION

To manage stakeholders, health care managers must be involved in a continual process of internal and external scanning when making strategic decisions. They must go beyond the traditional issues in strategic management, such as the likely actions of competitors or the attractiveness of different markets. They must also look for those external, interface, and internal stakeholders most likely to influence the organization's decisions. As mentioned earlier, managers must make two critical assessments about these stakeholders: (1) their potential to threaten the organization and (2) their potential to cooperate with it.

Diagnosing the Stakeholder's Potential for Threat

Hostility or threat appears as a key variable in several formulations of organization-environment-strategy relationships (Miller and Friesen, 1978). Physicians, for example, are often explicitly identified as a group that does or could apply extensive pressure on hospitals, thereby impacting the hospital's effective strategic management

(Blair and Boal, 1991; Shortell, Morrison, and Friedman, 1990). Looking at the current or anticipated threat inherent in the relationship with a particular stakeholder or group of stakeholders is similar to developing a "worst case" scenario and protects managers from unpleasant surprises.

Stakeholder power and its relevance for any particular issue confronting the organization's managers determines the stakeholder's potential for threat. Power is primarily a function of the dependence of the organization on the stakeholder (Pfeffer and Salancik, 1978). Generally, the more dependent the organization, the more powerful the stakeholder. For example, the power of staff physicians is a function of the hospital's dependence on those physicians for patients, alternative sources of patients, the use of hospital beds, and the provision of hospital services.

Figure 1.2 shows the expected relative power of various stakeholders vis-à-vis the typical hospital in 1999. The results are very similar to those found in Figure 1.1 above. IDS/Ns, MCOs, governments, system hospitals, employers, and medical practices are expected to have the most power in relation to the typical hospital. All of these were identified as key future stakeholders in 1999 based upon their control of valued resources (i.e., money or patients), or their ability to impose costs (i.e., regulatory costs and rules restricting reimbursement) on the hospital.

The only anomaly in Figure 1.2 is the ultimate consumer of health services—the patient. The patient is expected to be one of the most important key stakeholders in 1999, but Figure 1.2 indicates that only 27 percent of the experts expect patients to have great power vis-à-vis hospitals in 1999. This view reflects the fact that patients will be represented by others in their dealings with hospitals (i.e., employers, IDS/Ns, MCOs, and governments). These patients' representatives are viewed as more powerful than individual patients because they control reimbursement to the hospital.

We are arguing that the organization's managers need systematically to anticipate and evaluate the actual or potential threats to its relationships with stakeholders and, in some cases, to evaluate threats faced by their supportive stakeholders. These threats may be focused on the stakeholder's attempt to obtain inducements from the organization that may or may not be provided. These desired inducements include financial resources, participation in decision making, and enactment of certain organizational policies versus other possible policies. Alternatively, these threats may focus on undermining the fundamental viability of the organization.

Diagnosing the Stakeholder's Potential for Cooperation

Because stakeholder analyses emphasize the types and magnitude of threats that stakeholders pose to the organization, the second dimension of level of cooperation in

Figure 1.2 Experts Predict Expected Power of Hospital Stakeholders in 1999

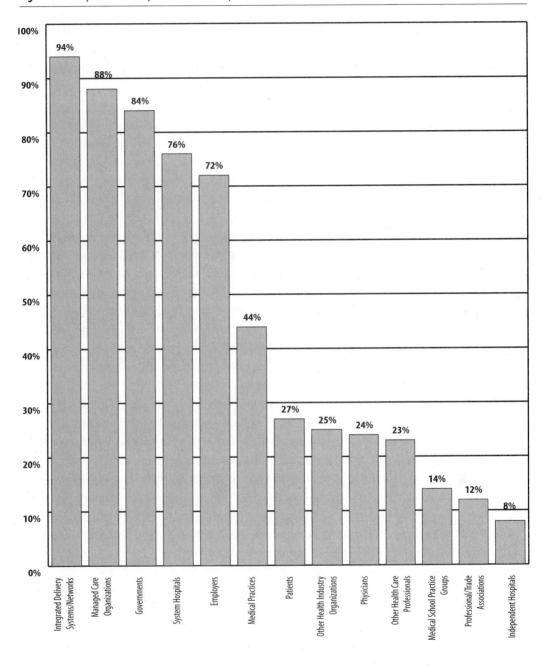

Percentage of experts predicting great stakeholder power relative to hospitals in 1999.

the organization's relationship with its stakeholders is easily ignored. We feel that this dimension should be emphasized equally as managers attempt stakeholder diagnosis, to direct attention more clearly to potential stakeholder management strategies that go beyond the merely defensive or offensive in confronting stakeholder pressures. Diagnosing this dimension suggests the potential for using more cooperative strategies, which focus on cooperation in stakeholder relationships in terms of the actual or potential contributions needed and valued by the organization.

Understanding each stakeholder's values and the priority placed on each value by the stakeholder ensures that the hospital can correctly assess the stakeholder. Figure 1.3 shows the priority values of the six most powerful stakeholders in 1999. All of these stakeholders view cost containment as the most important priority value for hospitals in 1999. Access is the least important value and quality of care is in the middle for most of these powerful stakeholders.

An example of competitors joining together against a common enemy is occurring as hospitals merge to reduce the bargaining power of preferred provider organizations (PPOs). PPOs are a type of managed care organization. They create networks of providers (hospitals, physicians, medical equipment suppliers, etc.) who are "preferred" in terms of how much the PPO will reimburse the cost of receiving care from that provider. Patients who receive care from providers outside the network will pay more of the bill themselves. PPOs have been able to demand price concessions from hospitals in markets where several hospitals compete for market share. However, with unprofitable hospitals falling by the wayside, the remaining hospitals can merge. The PPO then has only one dominant organization left with which to negotiate, and its position becomes very weak, since it cannot threaten to send its patient members elsewhere.

However, stakeholder management does not end for hospital administrators planning to implement this strategy. While the Antitrust Division of the Justice Department is carefully monitoring these types of mergers, both the public and regulators are becoming increasingly aware that these types of mergers may be necessary to meet the three criteria of cost, quality, and access. Health care executives need to anticipate the likely reaction of regulators—who represent the "public's" stake—regarding prospective mergers (Fottler and Malvey, 1995).

Health care organizations today should find cooperative potential particularly relevant because it may allow them to join forces by creating networks and other health care systems with other stakeholders and thus better manage their respective environments. One may look at the cooperation or cooperative potential of a relationship in parallel with looking at actual or potential threat. In this case, however, one is looking at a "best case" scenario and may therefore discover new possibilities otherwise ignored because of fundamental assumptions and perspectives.

Figure 1.3   Experts Predict Priority Values of the Most Powerful Hospital Stakeholders by 1999

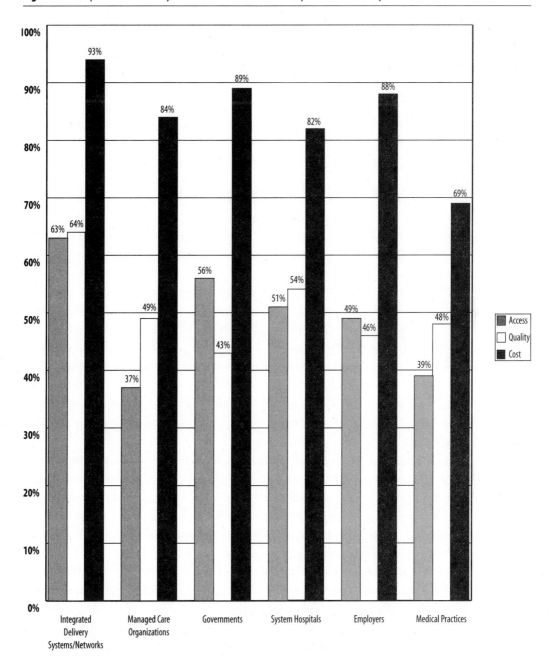

Percentage of experts responding that each value will be a higher priority for the stakeholder by 1999.

The stakeholder's dependence on the organization and its relevance for any particular issue facing the organization determines the stakeholder's cooperative potential. Generally, the more dependent the stakeholder on the organization, the higher the potential for cooperation. Often, however, the organization and the stakeholder may be very interdependent, as in the case of a small town with a limited number of physicians and one hospital. Although the hospital may encounter potential threats from some physicians who send patients to another hospital in a larger city, it is also likely to receive cooperation from most other physicians who want to keep their patients in the community.

Factors Affecting the Potentials for Threat and Cooperation

Besides power and dependence, other factors also affect the level of a stakeholder's potential for threat or cooperation. Figure 1.4 provides a list of the stakeholder characteristics health care executives should examine when diagnosing the potential for threat or cooperation.

Exactly how a factor will affect the potential for threat or cooperation depends on (1) the specific context and history of the organization's relations with that stakeholder and (2) the historical and contextual relations with other key stakeholders influencing the organization. For example, a hospital manager may be able to assess the cooperative or threat potential of the medical staff only in the context of how competing institutions are managing their medical staffs *and* in the context of how the organization has treated its medical staff in the past. By carefully considering the factors in Figure 1.4, executives can fine-tune their analyses and management of stakeholders.

As an example of the potentials for threat and/or cooperation, consider federal, state, and local governments. They can influence organizations in at least two different ways: through political actions and as regulators. Governments use political activities to alter the strategic decisions organizations make (e.g., antitrust issues vis-à-vis physician-hospital alliances). On the other hand, regulations cause organizations to change operational activities (e.g., Medicare forms and rules).

A more in-depth analysis in our book (Blair and Fottler, 1990) discusses the specifics of stakeholder diagnosis and also provides tool kits that illustrate how to effectively diagnose the potentials for threat and cooperation.

The next section of this chapter introduces several different levels of health care organization integration, ranging from the traditional system of independent health care providers through the typical physician-hospital organizational (PHO) form all the way to fully integrated health care delivery systems.

Figure 1.4   Factors Affecting the Potential for Threat and Cooperation of Hospital Stakeholder

	Increases or Decreases Stakeholder's Potential for Threat?	Increases or Decreases Stakeholder's Potential for Cooperation?
Stakeholder controls key resources (needed by hospital)	*Increases*	*Increases*
Stakeholder does not control key resources	*Decreases*	*Either*
Stakeholder more powerful than hospital	*Increases*	*Either*
Stakeholder as powerful as hospital	*Either*	*Either*
Stakeholder less powerful than hospital	*Increases*	*Increases*
Stakeholder likely to take action (supportive of the hospital)	*Decreases*	*Increases*
Stakeholder likely to take nonsupportive action	*Increases*	*Decreases*
Stakeholder unlikely to take any action	*Decreases*	*Decreases*
Stakeholder likely to form coalition with other stakeholders	*Increases*	*Either*
Stakeholder likely to form coalition with hospital	*Decreases*	*Increases*
Stakeholder unlikely to form any coalition	*Decreases*	*Decreases*

Source: Typology adapted and extended from J. Blair & M. Fottler, *Challenges in Health Care Management: Strategic Perspectives for Managing Key Stakeholders* (Jossey-Bass: 1990): 126.

🐍 CLASSIFYING DIFFERENT TYPES OF STAKEHOLDERS

The two dimensions—potential for threat and potential for cooperation—map stakeholders into a diagnostic framework. As discussed previously, these two dimensions of classification serve as summary measures of stakeholder supportiveness or lack thereof and incorporate information from multiple factors. Using these two dimensions, we can characterize four types of health care stakeholders, as shown in Figure 1.5.

There is a dynamic process occurring at all times. Stakeholders initially categorized in one cell might be moved to another cell as a result of what the organization does or fails to do, what stakeholders do or fail to do, what new information the organization

Figure 1.5   Diagnostic Typology of Hospital Stakeholders

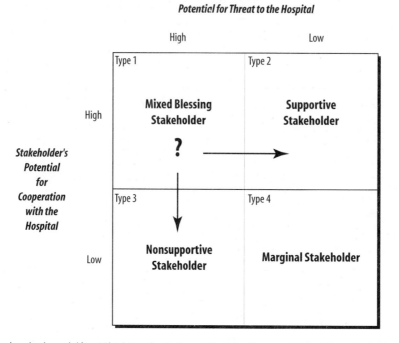

Source: Typology adapted and extended from J. Blair & M. Fottler, *Challenges in Health Care Management: Strategic Perspectives for Managing Key Stakeholders* (Jossey-Bass: 1990): 126.

has that would change the classification, and what issue is currently facing the organization and its stakeholders.

Before discussing the four types of stakeholders, we should make clear that one stakeholder can be both a direct and indirect stakeholder. By direct, we mean that the stakeholder deals directly with the organization. An indirect stakeholder is still a stakeholder but exerts influence through an intermediary. For example, governments and patients can be both direct and indirect stakeholders of a hospital. We will discuss the implications of these "double distinction" stakeholders later in this chapter.

Type 1: The Mixed-Blessing Stakeholder

The mixed-blessing stakeholder plays a particularly key role. With mixed-blessing stakeholders, the health care executive faces a situation in which the stakeholder registers high on both types of potential: threat and cooperation. Normally, stakeholders of the mixed-blessing type would include not only the medical staff but other physicians not on the staff, insurance companies, insured patients, and hospitals with complementary but not competing services. Physicians are probably the clearest example of this type of stakeholder. Although physicians can and do much that benefits hospitals, they can also threaten hospitals because of their general control over admissions, the use and provision of different services, and the quality of care.

Some special interest groups are also a mixed blessing. For example, substance abuse programs at hospitals are influenced by such groups as Alcoholics Anonymous. These groups have a significant stake in the hospital's program and its therapeutic approach. Such groups can either enhance referrals to the program or can undermine the program, thereby greatly influencing its clinical and financial viability.

Figure 1.5 also shows a question mark under the mixed-blessing stakeholder type with two arrows. One is directed toward the type 2: supportive stakeholder. The other is pointed at the type 3: nonsupportive stakeholder. These arrows imply that a mixed-blessing stakeholder could become either more or less supportive. Later on, this chapter looks at appropriate stakeholder management strategies for each type of stakeholder and emphasizes how to manage this mixed-blessing stakeholder most effectively.

Type 2: The Supportive Stakeholder

The ideal stakeholder supports the organization's goals and actions. Managers wish all their stakeholders were of this type. Such a stakeholder presents a low potential threat but a high potential for cooperation. Usually, a well-managed hospital's board of trustees, managers, staff employees, parent company, local community, and nursing homes will be of this type. In many large medical centers with multiple health care facilities, a common support facility such as a power plant, laundry, or parking consortium typifies the concept of the supportive stakeholder.

Type 3: The Nonsupportive Stakeholder

Stakeholders of this type are the most distressing for an organization and its managers. They have a high potential for threat but a low potential for cooperation. Typical nonsupportive stakeholders for hospitals include competing hospitals, freestanding alternatives such as urgi- or surgicenters, employee unions, the federal government, other governmental regulatory agencies, indigent patients, the news media, and employer coalitions.

Interestingly, the managed care organizations, even though they may be nonsupportive stakeholders for a hospital, are one of the two necessary organizations a hospital requires to form a fully integrated health care delivery system (the other one being some kind of physician group). This presents the major strategic issues facing today's health care executives: how to manage nonsupportive stakeholders effectively today so that in the future those same stakeholders will be less threatening and more cooperative. We will return to this issue later in this chapter.

Type 4: The Marginal Stakeholder

Marginal stakeholders are high on neither threat nor cooperative potential. Although they potentially have a stake in the organization and its decisions, they are generally not relevant for most issues. For a well-run hospital, typical stakeholders of this kind may include volunteer groups in the community, stockholders or taxpayers, and professional employee associations. However, certain issues such as cost containment or access to care could activate one or more of these stakeholders, causing their potential for either threat or cooperation to increase.

Issue-Specific Stakeholder Diagnosis

Not everyone will agree with the set of stakeholders we have used as examples for each type. There is a very good reason to be uncomfortable with such global classifications of particular stakeholders. The most important issues facing organizations and their managers at any given time change constantly. Of all the possible stakeholders for a given health care organization, the ones that will be relevant to their managers depend on the corporate/competitive strategies being pursued as well as on the particular issue. If the issue is cost containment, the stakeholders concerned will be different than if the issue is access to health care. The diagnosis of the relevant stakeholders in terms of the four stakeholder types will probably be different on these two issues as well.

Moreover, whatever the classification of a particular stakeholder on a specific issue, managers should explicitly classify stakeholders to surface inadvertent managerial biases. For example, if a manager identifies all stakeholders for any particular issue as nonsupportive, that manager should also critically examine his or her assessment of the relationship between the organization and its stakeholders. And if a particular stakeholder is always thought of as the same in terms of threat and cooperation, the manager may be both missing opportunities for capitalizing on the potential for cooperation and also running the risk of being blindsided by underestimating the potential for threat on a specific issue. For a thorough, step-by-step guide to identifying and assessing stakeholders, see our book (Blair and Fottler, 1990), which develops and presents tool kits that facilitate this important step in the strategic stakeholder management process.

Figure 1.6 shows how the experts diagnose IDS/Ns and MCOs in terms of their degree of supportiveness to hospitals in both 1994 and 1999. For both years the largest proportion of experts viewed IDS/Ns as mixed-blessing stakeholders for hospitals. Moreover, the proportion increased from 44 percent in 1994 to 64 percent in 1999, and the increase was associated with a decline in the proportion who viewed IDS/Ns as either supportive or marginal. Most experts, therefore, view the IDS/N as having a high potential for both cooperation and threat. Similar results are shown for the MCO.

Figure 1.6 Integrated Delivery Systems/Networks as Types of Hospital Stakeholders—Now and in the Future (Health Care Experts' Perceptions and Predictions)

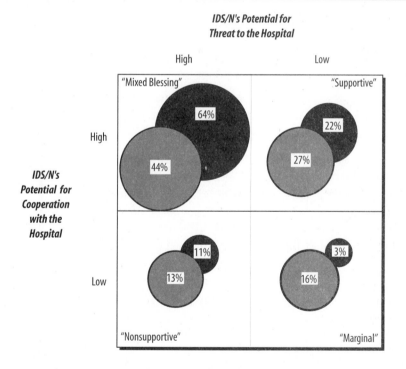

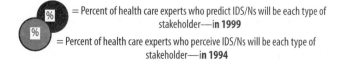

Formulating and Implementing
〜 **Generic Strategies for Stakeholder Management**

Stakeholder diagnosis of the type attempted in Figure 1.5 suggests some generic strategies for managing stakeholders with different levels of potential for threat and cooperation respectively. Figure 1.7 presents a fourfold typology of such strategies, each of which can be either proactive or reactive. Since executives continually manage a wide variety of stakeholders (in terms of their potential for cooperation and threat), all executives need to use a combination of strategies at any one time.

Strategy 1: Collaborate with the Mixed-Blessing Stakeholder

The mixed-blessing stakeholder, high on the dimensions of both potential threat and potential cooperation, may best be managed through collaboration. The goal of this

Figure 1.7   Generic Stakeholder Management Strategies for Hospitals

Stakeholder's
Potential for Threat to the Hospital

	High	Low
	Strategy 1 **Collaborate** *with the* *Mixed Blessing* *Stakeholder*	**Strategy 2** **Involve** *the* *Supportive* *Stakeholder*
	Strategy 3 **Defend** *against the* *Nonsupportive* *Stakeholder*	**Strategy 4** **Monitor** *the* *Marginal* *Stakeholder*

Stakeholder's Potential for Cooperation with the Hospital — High (top row), Low (bottom row)

Source: Typology adapted and extended from J. Blair & M. Fottler, *Challenges in Health Care Management: Strategic Perspectives for Managing Key Stakeholders* (Jossey-Bass: 1990): 133.

strategy is to turn mixed-blessing stakeholders into supportive stakeholders. If executives seek to maximize their stakeholders' potential for cooperation, these potentially threatening stakeholders will find that their supportive endeavors make it more difficult for them to oppose the organization.

For example, a proposed strategic alliance between a hospital and a medical group represents a collaborative strategy. If this alliance were to take the form of building a freestanding surgi-center or imaging center, such collaboration would effectively stop the physicians (mixed-blessing stakeholders) from building a center themselves and thus competing with hospital-based surgery or diagnostic procedures. The hospital can contribute its name and capital resources, while the physicians will presumably send their patients to the hospital when inpatient services are needed. Both the hospital and the physicians potentially will benefit.

Regional hospitals represent another mixed-blessing stakeholder to an urban hospital. If the urban hospital can use creative contracting covenants to ensure some form of referral pattern from the regional hospitals, the urban hospital has used the collaborative strategy effectively. However, these contractual covenants *could* be viewed as a defensive posture on the organization's part. The use of this kind of collaborative strategy indicates the caution with which this strategy must be used.

The caution is warranted because of the inherent instability of mixed-blessing stakeholders vis-à-vis the organization. Therefore, an effective collaboration strategy with them may well determine the long-term stakeholder-organization relationship. In other words, if this type of stakeholder is not properly managed through a collaborative strategy, the instability of these types of stakeholders could lead a mixed-blessing stakeholder to become a nonsupportive stakeholder.

Collaboration may be implemented through a variety of joint ventures, up to and including mergers (Fottler, Money, Schermerhorn, and Wong, 1982). Various approaches to physician "bonding" by hospitals and the development of referral networks between urban and rural hospitals are other examples.

Strategy 2: Involve the Supportive Stakeholder

By involving supportive stakeholders in relevant issues, health care executives can maximally capitalize on these stakeholders' cooperative potential. Because these stakeholders pose a low threat potential, both their need to be managed and their cooperative potential are likely to be ignored.

Involvement differs from *collaboration* in two ways: (1) Involvement further activates or enhances the supportive capability of an already supportive stakeholder, and (2) collaboration includes an element of caution due to the high potential for threat inherent in mixed-blessing stakeholders. The involvement strategy does not emphasize reducing threat, since its potential is low, but instead attempts to capitalize on the already existing potential for cooperation by converting even more of the *potential* into *actual*. Collaboration, on the other hand, involves much more of a give-and-take on the part of the organization and the stakeholder respectively. Collaboration may require the organization to give up or expend certain key resources or change important policies to gain stakeholder support either by lowering threat or increasing cooperation. As mentioned earlier, collaboration strategies contain an element of caution that involvement strategies do not.

Managers can operationalize the involvement strategy by using participative management techniques, by decentralizing authority to clinical managers, or by engaging in other tactics to increase the decision-making participation of these stakeholders. For example, hospital managers may invite clinical managers to participate in the analysis and planning for eliminating redundant programs. The clinical managers will more likely become committed to achieving such an organizational objective than if they had not been involved in establishing it. A key requirement for the success of this type of strategy is the ability of the managers to enlarge their vision of ways to involve supportive stakeholders further in higher levels of cooperation.

Now many group practices and hospitals are explicitly involving their supportive employees and in-house volunteer stakeholders by training them to manage mixed-blessing stakeholders such as funded patients, patients' families, and physicians. They are doing this through "guest" or "customer" relations programs designed to manage more effectively one or more of their potentially threatening stakeholders (e.g., funded patients) by increasing the cooperative potential of a key internal stakeholder (e.g., employees).

Another use of involvement is explicitly strategic and focuses on systematically linking human resource management systems and practices to overall strategic management. Called strategic human resource management (SHRM), it has only recently been introduced into the field of health care management (Fottler, Hernandez, and Joiner, 1994). SHRM is very consistent with our strategic stakeholder management approach, since it increases involvement of generally supportive internal stakeholders (employees) in furthering the strategic goals of the organization through effective and strategically linked human resource management (Fottler, Phillips, Blair, and Duran, 1990).

Regarding employee management strategies, hospital executives need to be aware of physicians' perceptions when entering into alliances with them. Physicians are generally mixed-blessing stakeholders from a hospital perspective. However, hospital executives often use involvement strategies to manage them. This can strain the hospital-physician relationship. For example, assume a hospital buys a physician practice, thereby making all the physicians employees of the hospital. If hospital executives try to exert typical hierarchical authority and typical involvement strategies in regard to the newly acquired physicians, they will most likely rebel. Even though the physicians are hospital employees, they may still view themselves as partners in the venture, who would thus expect to be involved in strategic decision making at the highest levels. This example is a classic case of the hospital misdiagnosing the physicians as non-threatening supportive stakeholders, when in fact the physicians are powerful mixed-blessing stakeholders.

Strategy 3: Defend Against the Nonsupportive Stakeholder

Stakeholders who pose a high threat but a low potential for cooperation are best managed with a defensive strategy. The federal government and indigent patients are good examples of this nonsupportive stakeholder group for most health care organizations. In Kotter's (1979) framework on external dependence, the defense strategy tries to reduce the dependence that forms the basis for the stakeholders' interest in the organization. In our terms, a defensive strategy involves preventing the stakeholder from imposing costs—or other disincentives—on the organizations.

However, health care executives should *not* attempt to eliminate totally their dependence on nonsupportive stakeholders. Such efforts are either doomed to failure or may result in a negative image for the organization. For example, trying to sever all ties with the federal government is counterproductive if a hospital hopes to market to older patients. And a public hospital that tries to deny access to all indigent patients will almost surely be viewed negatively by the public and the local government.

Let us consider an example of this defensive strategy in action, using the federal government's regulatory agencies as the stakeholder. For example, given the regulations hospitals face, their most appropriate tactic is to explore ways of complying with the demands imposed by the federal government at the least possible cost. Diagnosis-Related Groups (DRGs) that produce a surplus for hospitals define their areas of distinctive competence. Hence, hospital executives might adopt a case-mix approach to the delivery of health care, modifying the services they offer based on cost and process accounting. Investment in more effective management information systems, specialized medical records "grouper" software, and recruiting and paying for more highly skilled medical records personnel are all part of this defensive strategy vis-à-vis a nonsupportive, demanding third-party payer and/or regulator.

The best defensive strategy for managing nonsupportive stakeholders is to shift the organization's dependencies (where possible) from nonsupportive to mixed-blessing or supportive stakeholders. For example, if government reimbursement is restricted, the organization can attract more private patients.

Strategy 4: Monitor the Marginal Stakeholder

Monitoring helps manage those marginal stakeholders whose potential for both threat or cooperation is low. For example, numerous special interest groups are opposed to certain procedures such as abortion or artificial implants or are concerned about certain patient groups such as the aged. Typically, these groups have only a marginal stake in the activities of the organization, affecting operations indirectly through advocating a moral or ethical standpoint. Taxpayers and stockholders also represent marginal stakeholders. They are unlikely to be either of much help or much hindrance unless the organization takes actions that activate them. In essence these stakeholders are unstable when viewed by the organization. They can move into any one of the other three categories of stakeholder if the issue is of enough importance to them.

Patient families are often considered marginal stakeholders. But failing to monitor these key marginal stakeholders ignores the possibility of their becoming supportive stakeholders that can make a decisive difference to the course of patient care. On the other hand, dissatisfied patient families that go unnoticed can wreak havoc in an organization. Assigning specific responsibility for monitoring this stakeholder to a member of the patient care team can avert disaster for the organization's management.

The underlying philosophy for managing these marginal stakeholders is proactively maintaining the status quo, while keeping finances and management time to a minimum. Executives address issues on an ad hoc basis. The general thrust of this approach is, "Let sleeping dogs lie." Keeping them asleep, however, may require an organization to engage in ongoing public relations activities and be sensitive to issues that could turn them into an actual threat.

Marginal stakeholders should—in general—be *minimally satisfied*. What it takes to keep a particular marginal stakeholder minimally satisfied may increase over time, thus demanding more managerial time and other organizational resources. Managers must monitor such expenditures of inducements or disinducements to determine whether they have become excessive or are perhaps inadequate at this time because the marginal stakeholder has become a key stakeholder, either in general or on a particular issue.

Figure 1.8 shows the experts' perceptions of the generic strategies hospitals were using to manage IDS/Ns and MCOs in 1994 and the strategies they will use in 1999. The experts perceived hospitals as primarily collaborating with (46 percent) or defending against IDS/Ns (25 percent) in 1994. However, they predicted that by 1999 hospitals will either involve (56 percent) or collaborate with (31 percent) IDS/Ns. This is a major change for the five-year period, even though the same experts predicted that IDS/Ns will continue to be mixed-blessing stakeholders in 1999, that is, they

Figure 1.8 Stakeholder Strategies for Integrated Delivery Systems/Networks—Now and in the Future (Health Care Experts' Perceptions and Predictions)

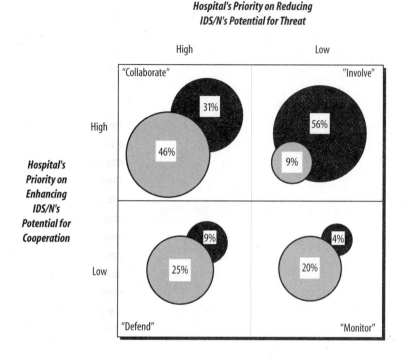

expected hospitals to act *as though* the IDS/Ns are *supportive* stakeholders for which the most appropriate generic strategy is *involvement*. In effect, the experts were predicting that hospitals will follow a "self-fulfilling prophecy" approach whereby they will treat the mixed-blessing IDS/N as though it is already supportive in order to develop such supportiveness in the future.

Somewhat similar results were found for MCOs. In 1994 approximately equal proportions of the experts viewed hospitals as either collaborating with (40 percent) or defending against (41 percent) MCOs. By 1999, they predicted, hospitals will either be collaborating with (59 percent) or involving (31 percent) MCOs. In other words, their strategies assume that MCOs ought to be managed as though they will be more supportive of hospitals in the future than they have been in the past.

The risk in pursuing a strategy that assumes a key stakeholder is more supportive than is actually the case is that the hospital will fail to defend itself against any threat that a mixed-blessing IDS/N or MCO may pose. For example, the MCO may attempt to renegotiate the existing contract with a hospital in order to lower the prices paid and the reimbursement for particular services. If the hospital has failed to anticipate this threat and to develop appropriate data to justify its current prices and reimbursement, it may be forced to reduce/eliminate services and/or cut staff because it viewed the MCO as a supportive stakeholder when it was in reality a mixed-blessing stakeholder whose goals were only partially supportive of the hospital's goals.

An Overarching Stakeholder Management Strategy

In addition to using the four strategies specifically tailored for stakeholders who are classified into one of the four diagnostic categories, health care executives may also employ an overarching strategy. This overarching strategy moves the stakeholder from a less favorable to a more favorable category. The stakeholder can then be managed using the generic strategy most appropriate for that "new" diagnostic category.

For example, rather than simply defend against the news media as a nonsupportive stakeholder, a hospital could implement an aggressive program of external relations with openness to the media. If successful, the program would transfer the news media to the less threatening category of marginal stakeholder, allowing it to be managed through a monitoring strategy. If the hospital is willing to invest more time, energy, skill, and money in the effort, the media might even be coopted enough to become a supportive stakeholder.

For example, if a hospital is contemplating a strategic alliance with a mixed-blessing stakeholder (such as a medical group), we see an opportunity for the hospital. For if the hospital effectively manages the medical group with a collaborative strategy such as building a surgi-center for the group of physicians, it may also successfully turn a mixed-blessing stakeholder into a less threatening supportive stakeholder.

However, it is important to recognize that even if mixed-blessing stakeholders are collaboratively managed, they do not necessarily become supportive stakeholders. Not every player in this new era of health care delivery will voluntarily become involved and integrated. Therefore, stakeholders do not always react as the strategy suggests. Additionally, if long-term strategic goals are pursued without ensuring tactical success, stakeholder management will not work effectively. For example, organizations can create structural integration (i.e., strategic integration) fairly easily. However, if social/cultural integration (i.e., tactical integration) is not achieved, the new structure may not work.

Of course, stakeholders generally will not just sit still and be managed. Stakeholders who are powerful and, hence, threatening are as likely to try to manage organizations as vice versa. Many organizations and their stakeholders continually engage in management and countermanagement strategies. To manage these stakeholders effectively, executives should continually identify stakeholders and match their diagnosis with appropriate strategies. In other words, we suggest periodically repeating the prior steps to ensure that key assumptions still apply.

ॐ IDENTIFYING MANAGERIAL RESPONSIBILITY FOR DIFFERENT STAKEHOLDERS

While the previous sections have shown the variety of stakeholders that have an interest in today's health care organization (and, specifically, in today's hospitals and hospital systems), it would be a mistake to assume that the chief executive officer (CEO) or any other single individual manages all of these diverse stakeholders. Instead, the evolution of some of these organizations has seen the development of management specialists whose major purpose is to manage particular stakeholders. For example, in some organizations a medical staff director, or vice president for medical affairs, has the major responsibility for managing the medical staff. Nonetheless, others, including the CEO, are also available to help handle nonroutine problems.

In the following stakeholder management examples, we discuss four executives who also typically devote much of their time to managing several key stakeholders. These roles were chosen as selected examples of managers who have responsibility for several stakeholders.

The director of Physician Practice Management Services (PPMS) is responsible for developing a physician/provider network capable of delivering health care to the insured patient base in an efficient, cost-effective manner. This person is also integrally involved in medical staff development and recruiting. The director of Regional Services (RS) has been discussed previously (recall all of our earlier examples involving RS). Here it is important to note that RS can work collaboratively with PPMS by creating joint RS/PPMS teams to provide service to regional physicians affiliated with rural hospitals in a given hospital's regional network.

The chief financial officer (CFO) and the vice president of marketing (VPM) will work closely with the hospital's new network partner, the health plan as MCO. Since the hospital formed this health care delivery network, it has assumed a much greater portion of the financial risk than before. For example, with capitation, the hospital agrees to treat all the patients in a given population for a preset amount of money. If the patient's medical bills exceed this preset amount, the health care providers absorb the excess cost. Due to this increased financial risk, the CFO is quite involved with the new network risk-contracting functions. The VPM has direct responsibility for promoting the hospital's interests (both individually and in the network). The "all in one" concept of health care delivery is still new to the purchasers of health care. A key responsibility of the VPM is to counteract any steps taken by competing health care networks.

A required characteristic of these specific hospital executives is that each one of them must let go of the old hospital mentality of "filling beds" and "if we own it, we can control it." Instead, they must embrace the new "health care network mentality" of providing the easiest access to the highest quality, most cost-effective health care for a given population. As previously mentioned, physicians are generally reluctant to be managed or controlled by hospital executives, who therefore need to develop an approach that allows physicians to remain an important part of the strategic direction of the new health care delivery network, while also ensuring that the new system runs well.

Stakeholder maps showing the potential opportunities and responsibilities of each stakeholder manager can help managers understand the strategic stakeholder process. They can then use this technique to go from a general stakeholder map developed during stakeholder assessment to incorporating stakeholder management into an executive's job description. Such maps are a tool for clarifying and communicating unique and overlapping managerial roles and responsibilities. Obviously, development of these maps requires some agreement among the various managers concerning *who* (singular or plural) will manage which *stakeholders* on *which issues*. This process typically involves internal negotiations and the development of organizational policies and procedures. The advantage of the stakeholder map is to *clarify* relationships and responsibilities.

Figure 1.9 shows expert perceptions of the relative effectiveness of various specific structural relationships and management skills hospitals could use to achieve a very sustainable competitive advantage in 1999. These tactics relate to both the structure of network relationships *and* the management expertise needed to manage these network relationships successfully. The most effective structural relationship will be for hospitals to form partnerships or joint organizations with medical groups, other hospitals, and health plans (i.e., MCOs). Fifty-seven percent of the experts surveyed felt that the development of such a *comprehensive* structural system will be the most important structural approach for hospitals to achieve a very sustainable competitive advantage.

The most important management skill hospitals need to achieve a sustainable competitive advantage is the ability of their executives to work collaboratively with

Figure 1.9 Experts Predict Actions and Expertise Required to Implement Hospital Stakeholder Strategies

	Percentage
Knowing how to work collaboratively with medical groups, hospitals and health plans (fully integrated)	61%
Forming partnerships or joint organizations with medical groups, hospitals and health plans (fully integrated)	57%
Knowing how to work collaboratively with health plans	48%
Knowing how to work collaboratively with medical groups	47%
Managing diverse network interests through skills in creating a common vision and purpose	45%
Forming partnerships or joint organizations with health plans	41%
Building referral sources through formal provider network affiliations	37%
Forming partnerships or joint organizations with medical groups	37%
Managing diverse network interests through skills in negotiation and conflict management	36%
Knowing how to work collaboratively with hospitals	36%
Managing diverse network interests through skills in planning and organizing	34%
Building referral sources through direct contracting with employers	30%
Forming partnerships or joint organizations with hospitals	29%
Building referral sources through long standing but informal networks	5%

Percentage of experts predicting that relationship or expertise provides a very competitive advantage.

all three components of an IDS/N (i.e., medical groups, hospitals, and MCOs). In addition, the ability to create a common vision and purpose across a range of different functions involved in an IDS/N is also viewed as an important skill. In sum, hospitals wishing to achieve a very sustainable competitive advantage need to develop structural relationships (via contracts) with all of the major components of an IDS/N. Then they need to develop a common vision and purpose to guide all of the individual activities and relationships in the organization.

❧ DISCUSSION

To survive the turbulent and revolutionary changes facing the health care industry, health care executives must better manage their external, interface, and external stakeholders. Organizations have to rethink their strategies and operations as they face increasing, and potentially conflicting, demands for effectiveness and efficiency from these stakeholders. Executives must minimally satisfy the needs of marginal stakeholders while maximally satisfying the needs of key stakeholders.

To satisfy key stakeholders, managers must make two critical assessments about these stakeholders: their potential to threaten the organization and their potential to cooperate with it. When determining the stakeholder's orientation, managers should account for such factors as control of resources, relative power, likelihood and supportiveness of potential stakeholder action, and coalition formation. These factors should be interpreted in light of the specific context and history of the organization's relations with it, and the influence of other key stakeholders on the organization as well as on that stakeholder.

Stakeholder management integrates in a systematic way what managers have often dealt with separately: strategic management, marketing, human resources management, public relations, and social issues. To manage stakeholders, health care executives need to be involved in a continuing process of internal and external scanning when making strategic decisions. They must go beyond the traditional issues of strategic management such as the attractiveness of different markets and the likely actions of competitors. They must be helped to develop their skills in identifying, assessing, and managing their key stakeholders.

The process of integrated strategic and stakeholder management can be implemented through the following steps:

1. Formulate a business strategy consistent with the organization's mission, goals, strengths, weaknesses, opportunities, and threats.
2. Identify all external, interface, and internal stakeholders relevant for the implementation of the business strategy.
3. Assess each stakeholder in terms of core values, power sources, and power relative to the organization.
4. Categorize all stakeholders as either key or marginal in general and in relation to the issue being considered in particular, based upon their respective potentials for threat and cooperation.
5. On the basis of the above diagnosis, classify all key stakeholders as supportive, mixed-blessing, or nonsupportive.
6. Formulate generic stakeholder management strategies to involve the supportive stakeholder, collaborate with the mixed-blessing stakeholder, defend against the nonsupportive stakeholder, and monitor the marginal stakeholder.
7. Implement each of these generic strategies by developing specific implementation tactics and programs for each.
8. Assign responsibility to internal stakeholders who will be responsible for implementing particular generic strategies and tactics.
9. Evaluate the success of both the business strategy and the management of key stakeholders on a continual basis.

10. Modify each strategy based upon these evaluations and changes in the environment.

11. Repeat this process on a continual basis.

Until recently, there has been a gap between the respective literatures of strategic and operational management. The gap has resulted in a failure to consider the role of stakeholder management and how to do it comprehensively and systematically. Strategic plans do not typically drive the day-to-day activities of most managers and other organizational participants. The most important reason is a failure to consider implementation issues that require the management of key stakeholders. For better or worse, stakeholder management is what managers *actually do*. The aim of this chapter, and the research upon which it is based, has been to provide clear guidelines for managing key stakeholders and to close the gap between strategy formulation and strategy implementation.

🙢 REFERENCES

Arthur Andersen & Co. *Best Practices Report on Physician/Hospital Integration—An Overview,* 1993.

Blair, J. D. and K. B. Boal. "Strategy Formation Processes in Health Care Organizations: A Context-Specific Examination of Context-Free Strategy Issues." *Journal of Management* 17: 2 (1991): 305–344.

Burns, L. R. and D. P. Thorpe. "Trends and Models in Physician-Hospital Organization." *Health Care Management Review* 18: 4 (1993): 7–20.

Coddington, D. C., D. D. Moore, and E. A. Fischer. "Integrated Health Care Systems: The Key Characteristics." *Medical Group Management Journal* (November/December 1993): 76–80.

Coddington, D. C., D. D. Moore, and E. A. Fischer. *Making Integrated Health Care Work.* MGMA, Englewood, CO, 1996.

Coile, R. S., Jr. *The New Governance: Strategies for an Era of Health Reform.* Ann Arbor, MI: Health Administration Press, 1994.

Conrad, D. A. and G. A. Hoare (eds.). *Strategic Alignment: Managing Integrated Health Systems.* Ann Arbor, MI: Health Administration Press, 1994.

Fottler, M. D., S. R. Hernandez, and C. L. Joiner (eds.). *Strategic Management of Human Resources in Health Services Organizations.* 2nd ed. Albany, NY: Delmar Publishers, 1994.

Fottler, M. D. and D. Malvey. "Multiprovider Systems." In L. Wolper (ed.), *Health Care Administration: Principles, Practices, Structure and Delivery.* 2nd ed. Gaithersburg, MD: Aspen Publishers, 1995: 489–515.

Fottler, M. D., W. Money, J. R. Schermerhorn, and J. Wong. "Multi-Institutional Arrangements in Health Care." *Academy of Management Review* 6: 3 (1982): 397–409.

Freeman, R. E. *Strategic Management: A Stakeholder Approach.* Marshfield, MA: Pitman Publishing, 1984.

Gillies, R., S. Shortell, D. Anderson, J. Mitchell, and K. Morgan. "Conceptualizing and Measuring Integration: Findings from the Health Systems Integration Study." *Hospital and Health Services Administration* 38: 4 (1993): 467–489.

Kongstvedt, P. R. and D. W. Plocher. "Integrated Health Care Delivery Systems." In Kongstvedt, P. R. (ed.), *Essentials of Managed Care.* Gaithersburg, MD: Aspen Publishers, 1995.

Kotter, J. P. "Managing External Dependence." *Academy of Management Review* 4:1 (1979): 87–92.

Mason, R. O. and I. I. Mitroff. *Challenging Strategic Planning Assumptions.* New York: Wiley, 1981.

Miller, D. and P. H. Friesen. "Archetypes of Strategy Formulation." *Management Science* 24 (1978): 921-933.

Pfeffer, J. and G. Salancik. *The External Control of Organizations: A Resource Dependence Perspective.* New York: Harper & Row, 1978.

Shortell, S. M., R. Gillies, D. Anderson, J. Mitchell, and K. Morgan. "Creating Organized Delivery Systems: The Barriers and Facilitators." *Hospital and Health Services Administration* 38: 4 (1993): 447–466.

Shortell, S. M., E. M. Morrison, and B. Friedman. *Strategic Choices for American's Hospitals: Managing Change in Turbulent Times.* San Francisco: Jossey-Bass Publishers, 1990.

Watson, S. I., J. Kimberly, and L. R. Burns. "Vertical Integration in Health Care: Promise and Performance." Paper presented at the 1995 Academy of Management, Vancouver, BC (August 1995).

Strategic Stakeholder Management Research and Practice Applications by Us and Our Colleagues

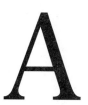

The following book, book chapters, and journal articles reflect our ongoing commitment to the development and application of strategic stakeholder management concepts, strategies and techniques. Together with our talented colleagues, we have looked at stakeholder issues in many types of health care organizations and outside health care. Some of the articles focus on parts of the stakeholder management process, for example, negotiation or assessment. Others look at different types of organizations or at different roles, for example, the role of the physician executive.

Overview of Strategic Stakeholder Management Theory and Practice

Blair, J. D. and M. D. Fottler. *Challenges in Health Care Management: Strategic Perspectives for Managing Key Stakeholders*. San Francisco: Jossey-Bass, 1990.

Hospitals

Blair, J. D., T. M. Rotarius, K. B. Shepherd, C. J. Whitehead, and E. G. Whyte. "Strategic Stakeholder Management for Health Care Executives." In L. Wolper (ed.), *Health*

Care Administration: Principles, Practices, Structure and Delivery. 2nd ed. Gaithersburg, MD: Aspen Publishers, 1995: 302-326.

Blair, J. D., G. T. Savage, and C. J. Whitehead. "A Strategic Approach for Negotiating with Hospital Stakeholders." *Health Care Management Review* 14: 1 (1989): 13–23.

Blair, J. D. and C. J. Whitehead. "Too Many on the Seesaw: Stakeholder Diagnosis and Management for Hospitals." *Hospital and Health Services Management* 33: 2 (Summer 1988): 153–156.

Fottler, M. D., J. D. Blair, C. J. Whitehead, M. D. Laus, and G. T. Savage. "Assessing Key Stakeholders: Who Matters to Hospitals and Why?" *Hospital and Health Services Administration* 34: 4 (Winter 1989): 525–546.

Fottler M. D., R. L. Phillips, J. D. Blair, and C. A. Duran. "Achieving Competitive Advantage Through Strategic Human Resource Management. *Hospital and Health Service Administration* 35 (1990): 341–363.

Managed Care Organizations

Whitehead, C. J., J. D. Blair, R. R. Smith, T. W. Nix, and G. T. Savage. "Stakeholder Supportiveness and Strategic Vulnerability: Implications for the HMO Industry's Competitive Strategy." *Health Care Management Review* 14: 3 (1989): 65–76.

Medical Groups

Blair, J. D., M. D. Fottler, A. R. Paolino, and T. M. Rotarius. *Medical Group Practices Face the Uncertain Future: Challenges, Opportunities and Strategies.* Englewood, CO: Center for Research in Ambulatory Health Care Administration, 1995.

Blair, J. D., M. D. Fottler, and C. J. Whitehead. "Diagnosing the Stakeholder Bottom Line for Medical Group Practices: Key Stakeholders' Potential to Threaten and/or Cooperate." *Medical Group Management Journal* 43: 2 (March/April, 1996): 40–50, 74.

Blair, J. D., T. T. Rock, T. M. Rotarius, M. D. Fottler, G. C. Bosse, and J. M. Driskill. "The Problematic Fit of Diagnosis and Strategy for Medical Group Stakeholders—Including Integrated Delivery Systems and Networks." *Health Care Management Review* 21: 1 (Winter 1996): 7–28.

Dymond, S. B., T. W. Nix, T. M. Rotarius, and G. T. Savage. "Why Do Key Integrated Delivery Stakeholders Really Matter? Assessing Control, Coalitions, Resources, and Power." *Medical Group Management Journal* 42: 6 (November/December, 1995): 26–38.

Fottler, M. D., J. D. Blair, T. M. Rotarius, and M. R. Youngblood. "Strategic Choices for Medical Group Practices: Managing Key Strategic Relationships in the Integrated Future." *Medical Group Management Journal* 43: 2 (May/April, June): 32–50.

Paolino, A. R., J. M. Greaves, J. D. Blair, M. D. Fottler, and T. M. Rotarius. "Medical Practice and Physician Executives Face the Uncertain Future: Strategic Stakeholder Management III." *Medical Group Management Journal* (September, October 1995).

Rotarius, T. M., A. R. Paolino, B. M. McMurrough, M. D. Fottler, and J. D. Blair. "Integrated Delivery Systems/Networks in the Uncertain Future: Strategic Stakeholder Management II." *Medical Group Management Journal* (July/August 1995): 22–31.

Physician Leaders

Blair, J. D., J. A. Buesseler, S. Y. Stanton, and C. J. Whitehead. "Stakeholder Issues for the Physician Executive." *Physician Executive* 15: 3 (May-June 1989): 9–14.

Whitehead, C. J., S. Y. Stanton, J. A. Buesseler, and J. D. Blair. "Stakeholder Strategies for the Physician Executive." *Physician Executive* 15: 4 (July-August 1989): 2–6.

Organizations Outside the Health Care Industry

Blair, J. D., J. Stanley, and C. J. Whitehead. "A Stakeholder Management Perspective on Military Health Care." *Armed Forces and Society* 18: 4 (Summer 1992): 548–575.

Savage, G. T., T. W. Nix, C. J. Whitehead, and J. D. Blair. "Strategies for Assessing and Managing Stakeholders." *Academy of Management Executive* 5: 2 (1991): 61–75.

The Facing the Uncertain Future Study

B

The results depicted in this chapter are from the Facing the Uncertain Future (FUF) study, a project jointly conducted by the Center for Research in Ambulatory Health Care Administration (CRAHCA), the research and development arm of the Medical Group Management Association (MGMA), Englewood, Colorado, and the Institute for Management and Leadership Research (IMLR) at Texas Tech University, Lubbock, Texas. MGMA's professional credentialing arm, the American College of Medical Practice Executives (ACMPE), and faculty of Texas Tech University's Ph.D. and MBA Programs in Health Organization Management (HOM) and faculty from the University of Alabama at Birmingham are also collaborating in the project. Abbott Laboratories, Abbott Park, Illinois, is the funding sponsor.

The FUF study was designed to capture the type of data necessary to (1) understand the uncertain future facing health care organizations, (2) use this new information to identify challenges and opportunities for health care organizations, and (3) propose strategies to aid the survival of health care systems. This study consisted of two distinct rounds of questionnaire development and data collection. The first round was administered in mid-1994. The second round followed approximately one year later. The 1994 survey collected data from five different panels of health care experts: (1) medical practice executives (MPEs), (2) physicians who are active in administration, (3) hospital executives, (4) insurance and managed care executives, and (5) health care industry supplier executives. Collectively, these five panels of respondents represent an expert group of 580 health care executives. Their responses were used in this chapter.

A brief profile of the 580 health care experts from the 1994 questionnaire follows.

Respondent panel analysis:

Medical Practice Executives	47%
Physician Executives	16
Hospital Executives	12
Insurance and Managed Care Executives	7
Health Care Industry Supplier Executives	18
Total Health Care Expert Respondents	100%

Of the expert respondents, 20 percent were female and 80 percent were male. The average respondent

- was 47 years old
- had worked for his/her organization for 9.2 years
- had been in his/her current position for 8.4 years

Sixty-nine percent of the experts were at the top two levels of their organization's hierarchy. Of the physician experts, 40 percent were in primary care.

Managing Customer Relations

2

Steven A. Taylor, Illinois State University

❧ INTRODUCTION

The health care industry in the United States continues to become increasingly competitive. One way in which health service organizations have responded to increasing competitive pressures is to become more market-oriented (Peter and Donnelly, 1995). A market-oriented firm is one that develops marketing objectives and implements strategies based on the wants and needs of its customers. Thus, one way for a market-oriented firm to differentiate itself from the competition would be on the basis of how well the firm satisfies its customers in efforts to meet its organizational objectives (Kotler, 1994).

However, emerging marketing thought suggests that focusing on customers through a market orientation without considering how marketing actions impact customers' overall perceptions of the firm over time can be shortsighted. In other words, marketers have historically focused on individual transactions with customers without considering the cumulative impact of their marketing actions. The relationship marketing paradigm has recently emerged as a mechanism for focusing marketers' attention on the overall relationship a customer has with an organization over time. General descriptions of the relationship marketing paradigm include the following: (1) "Relationship marketing concerns attracting, developing, and retaining customer relationships" (Berry and Parasuraman, 1991, p. 133); or (2) "The fundamental tenet of relationship marketing is the creation of 'true customers': customers who are glad they selected a company, who perceive they are receiving genuine value from the relationship, who feel valued by the company and are unlikely to defect to a competitor" (Berry, 1995, p. 172). The primary objective of this chapter is to demonstrate how a market orientation and relationship marketing techniques, when implemented through customer relations programs, can contribute to outcomes leading to competitive advantage.

Specifically, the way in which many health service organizations attempt to implement a market orientation is through their customer relations programs. The subject of customer relations appears to evoke a broad range of interpretations from managers of health service organizations. For example, some managers may interpret customer relations as merely providing information to patients and guests, while others may cite the handling of patient complaints as the key role of managing customer relations. Still others appear to consider quality control or patient satisfaction as the primary purview of customer relations programs. What is clear is that most customer relations programs in operation today appear to share a similar orientation toward focusing solely on solving patients' episodic problems as they arise. This chapter demonstrates that while each of the identified functions above can be an important part of the process of managing customer relations in health service organizations, the appropriate handling of an organization's relationships with its customers will increasingly require a multitude of strategically planned managerial actions directed toward developing and maintaining relationships with customers *over time.*

There are a couple of reasons for marketers' increasing efforts to keep customers through relationship marketing techniques as opposed to trying to attract new customers. First, repeat purchasers are often more profitable than new customers (Berry and Parasuraman, 1991; Hawkins, Best, and Coney, 1995; Heskett, Sasser, and Hart, 1990). Reichheld and Sasser (1990) suggest that dedicated repeat customers spend more money at and stay with an organization longer than other customers, tend to spread more favorable word-of-mouth recommendations, and are often even willing to pay a premium to organizations with whom they have a satisfactory standing relationship. Heskett, Sasser, and Hart (1990) support this argument by noting that (1) it costs less to serve repeat customers, particularly in health care, where there are usually large costs associated with establishing service relationships in terms of time, effort, and information transfer; (2) repeat customers know a service and therefore have established expectations; and (3) the cost of retaining a loyal customer is generally one-fifth that of attracting new customers.

Second, Berry and Parasuraman (1991) assert that customers also benefit from relationship marketing because (1) relationship marketing can serve to make intangible services more tangible and therefore easier to evaluate; and (2) many customers appear to desire closer, more personalized relationships with service providers. These customer benefits would appear particularly relevant for health services, which tend to be highly involving and personally relevant. In fact, Wagner, Fleming, Mangold, and LaForge (1994) specifically call for the application of relationship marketing principles to the practice of delivering health services.

The purpose of this chapter is to provide a framework that will assist health service practitioners in developing their own customer relations programs based on a market orientation and relationship marketing techniques. The following discussion is divided into four sections. The first section defines *customer relations* based on the weight of the evidence in the literature and in practice. The second section explores the existing literature to identify (1) the key constructs involved in an organization's relationship with its customers and (2) how the identified components of an organization's relationship with its customers interact to form desirable judgments, attitudes, and behaviors. In short, the management of an organization's relationships with its customers cannot begin until there is a clear understanding of the process by which these customers develop the traits health services marketers wish to foster through a customer relations program. In the third section, the chapter presents a proposed framework for customer relations programs, identifying specific managerial actions that can translate relationship marketing principles into competitive advantage. It concludes by considering the likely future directions and developments in the area of managing customer relations.

❧ CUSTOMER RELATIONS WITHIN THE CONTEXT OF HEALTH SERVICES

As stated previously, the term *customer relations* appears to refer to different functions in different health service organizations. Some health service organizations appear to consider the customer relations function as essentially including either the dispensing of general information or the handling of patient complaints. These firms tend to limit their management of customer relations to such services as on-site customer service representatives (e.g., an information desk in the lobby of a hospital), or customer information and/or complaint desks or phone numbers. Some firms appear to view the customer relations function as including patient advocates (Henthorne, Henthorne, and Alcor, 1994) who serve as representatives of patients in the process of navigating the organization's bureaucratic structure. Still other health service organizations appear to emphasize patient satisfaction research protocols. In fact, some marketers have recently gone so far as to argue for limiting customer relations to the use of database marketing techniques for the purpose of retaining existing customers (Vavra 1992).

Given the myriad of approaches to customer relations in the practice of health services, a useful place to begin this discussion is to identify what should be considered within the term's domain. At least two factors are important in considering the appropriate domain for customer relations programs. The first is identifying the "customers" of health service organizations, and the second involves settling on what constitutes a relationship (i.e., "relations").

The process of identifying an organization's customers can begin by noting that each of the above customer relations examples shares an emphasis on the relationship between individual patients and the health service organization. Clearly, patients should be considered a key customer base of health service organizations. However, health service organizations often serve a number of additional customers, including physicians, employees, payers, suppliers, and other stakeholders (Furse, Burcham, Rose, and Oliver, 1994). This argument is particularly important given the growing emphasis on cost control and managed care in the United States. Therefore, it is argued here that effective customer relations should capture the concerns of all the stakeholders or customers of a particular health service organization. That is, any managerial actions taken as part of a customer relations program should be broadly applicable to any potential customer of a health services firm. The framework proposed herein purports to meet this standard.

A second consideration in developing the domain of customer relations in health services involves the nature of the relationship between a customer and the health service organization. In other words, what is the "relations" part of customer relations? We can begin to address this issue by examining patient relationships. In very broad terms, patients generally present to providers of health services for treatment of either acute illnesses or long-term, chronic conditions. However, Williams and Torrens (1984) suggest that chronic illnesses represent the predominant health problems of American people, underscoring the importance of managing relationships with patients in such a way as to ensure patient satisfaction over time. Health services marketers should also recognize that today's acute care patient is tomorrow's acute care and/or chronically ill patient. Thus, the idea that health service providers should consider the impact of their actions over time *from the perspective of patients* appears an appropriate base for customer relations programs.

This base, however, is not enough in today's competitive health services environments. An orientation toward the development of positive, long-term relationships with patients can *and should* also be extended to the organization's relationships with its other customer bases. Health service organizations are increasingly finding competitive advantages in developing and maintaining positive, long-term relationships with suppliers, other health service organizations, government agencies, and even local communities at large through alliances, contracting, and other forms of cooperation. Thus, the relationship marketing paradigm appears as useful a philosophy for the practice of health care marketing as it is in other industries and areas of marketing practice.

In summary, the preceding section has presented two key points to help managers of health services identify the appropriate domain of the customer relations function.

1. Effective customer relations should capture the concerns of all the stakeholders or customers of a particular health service organization.
2. Positive, long-term relationships with all of an organization's stakeholders or customers should be sought through relationship marketing practices.

The next section more formally defines *relationship marketing* and then reviews the existing literature to identify the constructs managers of health services should consider in developing customer relations programs, as well as the ways in which these constructs interact within the context of an organization's relationship with its customers.

❧ RELATIONSHIP MARKETING AND HOW IT WORKS IN HEALTH SERVICES

As stated previously, the emerging marketing literature advocates relationship marketing as a primary organizational emphasis of many of today's successful service firms. Morgan and Hunt (1994, p. 22) review the existing literature and propose the following formal definition of relationship marketing, which is adopted for purposes of the current discussion:

> Relationship marketing refers to all marketing activities directed toward establishing, developing, and maintaining successful relational exchanges.

Morgan and Hunt suggest that relational exchanges are different from discrete transactions in that they involve previous agreements and are longer in duration, thus reflecting an ongoing process.

A reasonable premise appears to be that health services marketers must understand *which* constructs operate in customer relationships, as well as *how* they operate, in order to identify appropriate objectives for a customer relations program in support of relationship marketing practices. A number of constructs identified in the literature appear important to an organization's relationships with its various stakeholder groups, and four of them seem particularly significant for the purposes of the current discussion.

The first two constructs believed to be central to an organization's relationships with its various stakeholder groups are *relationship commitment* and *trust* (Morgan and Hunt, 1994, p. 23):

Relationship commitment—"...an exchange partner believing that an ongoing relationship with another is so important as to warrant maximum efforts at maintaining it; that is, the committed party believes the relationship is worth working on to ensure that it endures indefinitely."

Trust—"...conceptualize trust as existing when one party has confidence in an exchange partner's reliability and integrity."

Morgan and Hunt (1994) present a proposed model of relationship marketing that identifies how relationship commitment and trust operate in relations between an organization and its customers. Trust contributes to marketing relationships by decreasing uncertainty, increasing functional conflict and cooperation, and increasing relationship commitment. Relationship commitment, which again is based on trust, contributes positively to cooperation and acquiescence and reduces a customer's propensity to leave.* Interested readers are directed to Morgan and Hunt (1994) for a more comprehensive discussion of their proposed model of relationship marketing.

However, a health service organization's relationship with its customers requires more than trust and commitment. It is also critical for the continuation of successful long-term relationships between organizations and their customers to ensure the provision of *service quality* and *customer satisfaction* (Taylor, 1993, 1994; Taylor and Cronin, 1994; Wagner, Fleming, Mangold, and LaForge, 1994). Specifically, service quality and customer satisfaction have been found to be critical to the success of today's health service organizations through the positive relationship between these constructs and word-of-mouth behaviors (Berry and Parasuraman, 1991; Hawkins, Best, and Coney,

---

*Morgan and Hunt (1994, pp. 25–26) offer definitions for each of the following constructs: (a) *acquiescence*–"...the degree to which a partner accepts or adheres to another's specific requests or policies"; (b) *propensity to leave*–"...the perceived likelihood that a partner will terminate the relationship in the (reasonably) near future"; (c) *cooperation*–"...refers to situations in which parties work together to achieve mutual goals"; (d) *functional conflict*–"...when disputes are resolved amicably..."; and (e) *uncertainty*–"...refers to the extent to which a partner (1) has enough information to make key decisions, (2) can predict the consequences of those actions, and (3) has confidence in those decisions."

1995), loyalty (Fisk, Brown, Cannizzaro, and Naftal, 1990), and future purchase intentions (McAlexander, Kaldenberg, and Koenig, 1994; Taylor, 1994; Taylor and Cronin, 1994; Woodside, Frey, and Daly, 1989).

Taylor (1994) recently demonstrated that even though quality of care and patient satisfaction have emerged as core to many marketing strategies in health services, these two constructs have been largely confounded in the health services literature. Fortunately, the emerging services marketing literature is beginning to distinguish quality from satisfaction, which forms the basis for the following definitions for the purposes of the current discussion:

Service quality—a long-term attitude reflecting a consumer's perception of service-firm excellence in performance (Oliver, 1993a; Taylor, 1994).

Customer satisfaction—a summary cognitive and affective reaction to a service incident (or sometimes a long-term service relationship) resulting from a comparison between the service encounter and what was expected (Rust and Oliver, 1994).

A great deal of discussion has recently emerged in the services marketing literature concerning how service quality attitudes and customer satisfaction judgments interact to produce desirable customer outcomes such as future purchase intentions. For example, Cronin and Taylor (1992) test an empirical model across four unique service industries with results suggesting that customer satisfaction is a superordinate construct to service quality (i.e., service quality → customer satisfaction). This position has been supported conceptually for general services by Oliver (1993a) and is empirically specific to health services in the seminal work of Woodside, Frey, and Daly (1989). More recently, Taylor and Cronin (1994) evaluate a similar model specific to health services and identify a nonrecursive relationship between the service quality and customer satisfaction constructs in the formation of patients' stated future purchase intentions (i.e., service quality ⇄ satisfaction).

Taylor (1994) most recently suggests that the weight of the existing evidence concerning the relationship between patient satisfaction and service quality in health services supports the position that patient satisfaction influences service quality attitudes over time. That is, the patient's perception of how satisfied he or she is following every interaction with the health service organization either increases or decreases the individual's overall quality attitude toward the organization. Once a service quality attitude drops below the patient's particular threshold of tolerance, he or she will likely engage in undesirable behaviors such as negative word-of-mouth reporting and/or seeking alternative sources of care for future health service needs.

In summary, four constructs appear to be particularly important for the development and maintenance of an organization's relationship with its customers or stakeholder groups: trust, commitment, service quality, and customer satisfaction. An effective customer relations program should consider all four of these constructs and their interactions within the context of an organization's relationships with all of its customers. Once health services marketers understand how these constructs interact with one another, they can begin to develop recommendations for managing customer relationships toward competitive advantage.

Figure 2.1 presents a model of how quality attitudes, customer satisfaction judgments, trust, and commitment all interact over the course of a customer's relationship with a health service organization based on what is currently known from the services marketing literature. The model is divided into three sections based on how these constructs interact over time.

The first section of the model in Figure 2.1 is entitled Preservice Encounter and refers to that period of time *preceding* a customer's first encounter with a health service organization (time t–1). That is, people have quality attitudes about health service organizations *even before they first interact with the health service facility*, which we will call Quality Image$_{t-1}$. These quality attitudes are based not on personal experience but rather, generally, on word-of-mouth communications and/or the organization's marketing communications (e.g., advertising). For example, individual

Figure 2.1 A Model of Health Service Relationships

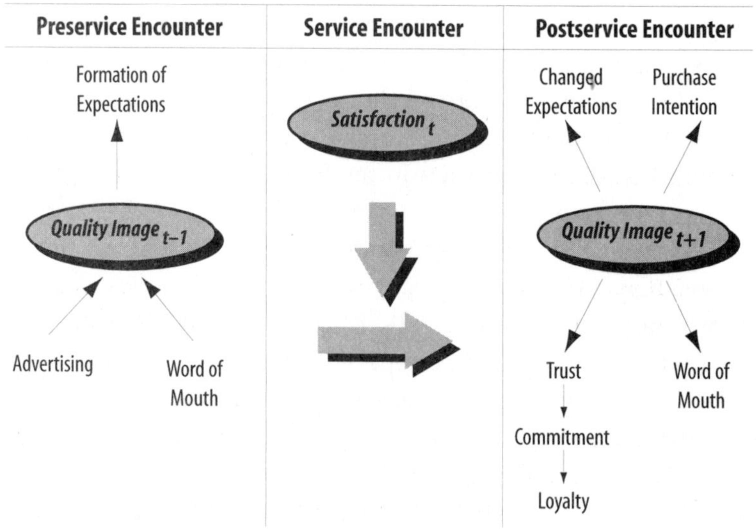

patients often seek information about health service organizations from friends, family, and coworkers prior to selecting a health service provider. Physicians may seek the advice of other physicians when considering joining a medical staff, seeking admitting privileges, affiliating with a managed care service, or targeting referral services. Even payers can have quality attitudes that may not be based on personal experience (within the context of organizational relationships). For example, an insurance firm may impose its perception of other hospitals in a particular geographic area or as part of a chain of health service organizations the first time it comes into contact with a specific health service organization. Fortunately, quality attitudes that are not based on personal experience are generally only weakly held. The primary outcome of Quality Image$_{t-1}$ is a set of expectations that will serve as a standard for comparing the perceived performance of a health service provider once the need for a service encounter arises.

This leads to the second section in the model presented in Figure 2.1. This section of the model is entitled Service Encounter and refers to the first time a customer personally interacts with a health service organization (time t). The *service encounter* is defined as the period of time during which a consumer directly interacts with a service (Shostack, 1985). The result of a service encounter is a judgment by the customer of either satisfaction or dissatisfaction. The judgment is the outcome of the patient's comparison of perceived service firm performance with the expectations he or she brought to the health service firm (i.e., Quality Image$_{t-1}$). When the perceived performance of the health service provider meets or exceeds the customer's expectations, the outcome is a satisfaction judgment. When the perceived performance of the health service provider fails to meet or exceed the customer's expectations, the outcome is a judgment of dissatisfaction.

The third and final section of the model depicted in Figure 2.1, titled Postservice Encounter, refers to the attitudes and actions a customer takes away from a service encounter (t+1). The primary outcome of a service encounter is a change in the quality attitude a customer holds toward a particular health service organization based on how satisfied he or she was with the service encounter. We will call this changed quality attitude Quality Image$_{t+1}$. Satisfaction strengthens positive quality attitudes—in other words, satisfaction judgments enhance the perception people have of an organization's quality image. Dissatisfaction, on the other hand, weakens the perception people have of the health service organization's quality image.

A changed quality image produces a number of results. First, people's expectations for the next service encounter are changed. A strong quality image can increase an individual's expectations for excellence in service firm performance in subsequent service encounters. We would also expect an increase in stated intentions for repurchase and positive word-of-mouth endorsements from customers who have strong quality attitudes based on satisfying personal experiences with a health service organization. Finally, positive interactions over time can lead to increased trust in and commitment to a health service organization, ultimately resulting in customer loyalty. Subsequent service encounters would serve either to strengthen or reduce customers' quality image of a health service organization, depending on their level of satisfaction with each subsequent service encounter.

In summary, the preceding section has presented a model of how relationships between health service organizations and their customers operate over time.

- Satisfaction with individual service encounters either strengthens or reduces the customer's perception of the organization's overall quality image.
- The customer's quality image of the health service organization serves as the basis for subsequent expectations; future repurchase intentions; word-of-mouth behaviors; and ultimately the trust, commitment, and loyalty a customer has toward the organization.

The next section identifies how managers can translate an understanding of how relationships develop between health service organizations and their customers into effective customer relations programs.

❧ DEVELOPING EFFECTIVE CUSTOMER RELATIONS PROGRAMS

The preceding discussion and model (see Figure 2.1) make clear the need for managers of health services to develop customer relations programs that focus on ensuring patient satisfaction and a positive quality image of the firm. The trick, of course, is knowing how to accomplish this end. Fortunately, the emerging services marketing literature provides some direction for consideration by managers of health service organizations.

This chapter takes the position that customer relations programs based on a market orientation and relationship marketing techniques can eventually form the basis for competitive advantage in today's dynamic health care industry. Figure 2.2 presents a seven-step framework for the development of customer relations programs in health services based on this premise. The proposed framework brings together recommendations from a number of sources in the emerging services and relationship marketing literatures; however, it relies particularly on the works of Quinn (1992), Kotler (1994), and Berry (1995). The remainder of this section discusses each step in the proposed framework for customer relations in greater detail.

Figure 2.2   A Framework for Customer Relations

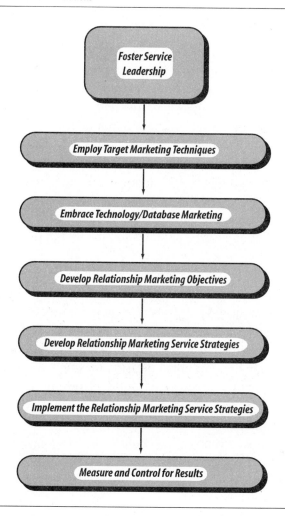

Foster Service Leadership

A useful place to begin the process of developing customer-centered customer relations programs that are consistent with relationship marketing theory is with the
health service organization's leadership. According to Heskett, Sasser, and Hart (1990),
leaders of breakthrough service companies that excel in developing a market-oriented
culture often employ strategic service visions. These authors suggest that a strategic
service vision is a comprehensive view of the business that forms the basis for organizational decision making. Heskett, Sasser, and Hart further identify four key elements

for successful strategic service visions: (1) target market segment identification; (2) a service concept that is defined not in terms of products or services but rather in terms of the results produced for customers; (3) an operating strategy that addresses organization, controls, and financial, marketing, and operating policies ensuring the delivery of the promised service concept; and (4) a service delivery system, which is the equivalent of the "plant" from which services are marketed and delivered. Thus, one way to foster effective service leadership is to ensure that the senior management of the health service organization develops a strategic service vision.

The second way in which health service firms can foster leadership is by identifying the organization's distinctive competency, namely, what the firm does best that is important to customers. Quinn (1992) emphasizes the importance of leadership that strategically focuses the organization on key knowledge and service competencies. In short, Quinn argues for organizational leaders of service firms to identify and develop critical skills to keep or make the organization the best in the world at specific activities from the customer's point of view.

For example, Sasser, Hart, and Heskett (1991) present a case concerning Shouldice Hospital Limited in Ontario, Canada. This hospital was able to develop a distinctive competency in the surgical repair of hernias based on reduction of pain, time to full recovery, and hospital-acquired infection rates. This organization was able to develop and maintain a competitive niche by concentrating on this single distinctive competency and engaging in organizational decision making to ensure its continued status as the best provider of this service in the world. For example, it required all of its physicians to receive extensive training in the superior surgical technique. It did not allow any form of entertainment that would encourage patients to stay in bed after the surgical procedure (e.g., televisions). Rather, the hospital strongly encouraged patients to ambulate almost immediately after surgery. Finally, it also provided instruction to other physicians serving to enhance its image as the premier source of care for the repair of uncomplicated hernias.

Berry (1995) similarly calls for nurturing service leadership and identifies a number of specific qualities in leaders that foster service achievement in organizations:

- A service vision and a view of service excellence as a key differentiating factor between competitive firms.
- A strong belief in others, stressing communications, coaching of subordinates, and a minimization of rules in the workplace.
- A love for the business they are in. The best business leaders love their businesses and approach them as a craft. This love, like enthusiasm, can be contagious.
- Personal integrity—doing the right thing even when it is inconvenient or expensive.

Thus, a third means of fostering service leadership in the organization is by identifying mechanisms that will bring about the recognized leadership qualities.

Berry (1995) provides guidance in this regard by identifying some mechanisms by which service leadership can be cultivated in organizations. He suggests using service leadership criteria in promoting people, stressing personal involvement in service improvement, emphasizing the importance of trusting employees—by assuming that they are honest and worthy of such trust—and encouraging leadership training, since leadership appears to be a learned skill.

In short, the primary benefits of service leadership involve (1) focusing the organization on those activities that will contribute most to the development and maintenance of strong relationships with customers and (2) bringing about an organizational culture that fosters and supports relationship marketing activities. Simply put, if the leadership of the organization does not foster service leadership and tangibly demonstrate a customer orientation toward its employees, it is unlikely that employees will consistently and effectively demonstrate a customer orientation toward the organization's external customers.

Employ Target Marketing Techniques

The second step of the proposed framework for relationship marketing is target marketing. Target marketing involves identifying and selecting a segment from the total pool of potential customers as the customer base of interest for the firm's marketing activities. Kotler (1994) states that target marketing involves three steps: market segmentation, market targeting, and market positioning.

Market segmentation is the act of identifying and profiling distinct groups of customers who might require separate products and/or marketing mixes (Kotler, 1994). In other words, marketers in a health service organization can use market segmentation to reduce the total population of people or organizations with access to its services and break it up into discrete, identifiable groups called market segments. In health care, patients might be segmented by injury versus illness, long-term versus episodic illness, primary versus secondary versus tertiary care needs, payment source, or demographic indices such as age or gender. Market segmentation based on organizational relationships might occur along lines such as organizational size, geographic region, growth potential, and so on.

Market targeting, the second step of target marketing, is the act of evaluating the attractiveness of each identified market segment and then selecting a particular market segment for the attention of marketing mix variables. For example, an outpatient clinic service might target Medicare patients, or an HMO might target one or more particularly large local employers. The appropriate selection of a market segment toward which to direct marketing activities is a critically important decision. According to Porter (1985), health services marketers should consider five factors that may threaten the attractiveness of market segments in market targeting: intense segment rivalry, new entrants, substitute products, growing bargaining power of buyers, and growing bargaining power of suppliers. The degree to which a market segment will constitute an attractive opportunity for a particular health services provider will largely depend on the presence of these threats relative to the specific market segment.

Finally, market positioning is the act of establishing and communicating the key distinctive benefits of the product/service (Kotler, 1994). In developing a positioning strategy, health services marketers generally wish to distinguish their products/services from competitive offerings. Kotler (1994) suggests that differences used for purposes of positioning are worth establishing only to the extent that they satisfy the following criteria:

- The difference must be important, or highly valued, to the customer.
- The difference must be substantial and clear in relation to competitor offerings.
- The difference must make the product/service clearly superior to substitute products/services.
- The difference must be communicable and visible to buyers.
- The difference must not be easily copied by competitors.
- The buyer must be able to pay for the difference.
- Introduction of the difference should yield profitable results.

Recognition as a provider of superior technical/functional quality of care and patient satisfaction is increasingly being recognized as an efficacious basis for positioning strategies. Quality and satisfaction are highly valued by customers, very difficult for the competition to replicate, and recognizable by customers when appropriately included as an emphasis of marketing communications.

Having identified differences in an organization's products/services that can serve as a basis for positioning, the market must next develop a positioning strategy. Treacy and Wiersema (1993) identify three strategies that can lead to successful differentiation and market leadership: (1) operational excellence, that is, providing customers with reliable products or services that are easily available at competitive prices; (2) customer intimacy, which involves getting to know customers intimately and being able to respond quickly to their individual needs; and (3) product leadership, that is, offering innovative products and services that exceed competitive offerings and enhance customer utility.

In terms of health service organizations, a number of bases for positioning can support the above strategies for differentiation. However, the model of health services relationships presented in Figure 2.1 implies that ultimately, customer quality and satisfaction must be addressed in positioning strategies. As mentioned above, quality has been a popular basis for differentiation efforts by health services firms. Health services marketers should recognize that quality has both technical (i.e., outcome-related) and functional (i.e., *how* care is delivered) dimensions, both of which are important in terms of health services marketing. Technical quality problems such as a highly publicized surgical error or an abnormally high hospital-acquired infection rate can devastate a health service organization's quality image. Similarly, customers may agree that one hospital has the best surgeons yet still choose a competitor because the bedside manner of the first hospital's physicians is simply not tolerable.

One way health service organizations can initially build and maintain a strong quality image that meets the criteria previously listed for successful positioning strategies is to focus on its employees in its marketing communications. Such a focus serves the dual purposes of presenting a message consistent with relationship marketing objectives and recognizing and rewarding the organization's internal customers (i.e., employees). The key to such a positioning strategy based on the health service organization's employees is to identify and communicate to the target market salient attributes of the personal interactions between customers and the organization's employees during the service encounter.

Fortunately, the attributes that are generally important in the development of marketing relationships in areas such as health care can be found in the literature. Obviously, employees' technical competence is important. However, the *way* in which they provide the service to customers is often even more critical. Kotler (1994, p. 303) identifies the following key attributes that customers often find significant in forming their perceptions of the quality of service received (based on the original work of Parasuraman, Zeithaml, and Berry, 1985):

- *Competence*: The employees possess the required skill and knowledge.
- *Courtesy*: The employees are friendly, respectful, and considerate.
- *Credibility*: The employees are trustworthy.
- *Reliability*: The employees perform the service with consistency and accuracy.
- *Responsiveness*: The employees respond quickly to customers' requests and problems.
- *Communication*: The employees make an effort to understand and communicate clearly with the customer.

A final consideration in employing target marketing techniques as part of a customer relations program involves the way in which the health service organization communicates its desired position to customers. Marketing communications, when properly developed and implemented, can be a powerful tool supporting a firm's positioning efforts. Gronroos (1990, p. 166) identifies seven guidelines for effectively managing marketing communications in services such as health care:

1. *Direct communication efforts to employees.* Target employees as internal customers in marketing communications. Targeting both internal and external customers helps ensure a consistent position in communicating to both parties participating in service encounters. Promoting the position of employees can serve the additional purpose of providing positive motivation.

2. *Capitalize on word-of-mouth endorsements.* Health services are driven largely by word-of-mouth communications in terms of reach and impact. Health services managers should be aware that they will likely occur whether or not marketers desire them. It is generally in the best interests of the health services organization to positively influence word-of-mouth communications to the greatest possible extent. Focusing on easily communicable attributes and testimonials is often useful in this regard.

3. *Provide tangible cues.* Health services are some of the most intangible of service products. However, these services can be made concrete through both advertising and managerial actions. For example, comparing a hospital room with a four-star hotel room in an advertisement can help customers visualize the health service experience, while making sure employees are neat and clean can enhance customers' perceptions of quality.

4. *Ensure communication continuity.* Common themes in all marketing communications can help establish and maintain a consistent, positive position in customers' minds.

5. *Promise what is possible.* As noted earlier, customer satisfaction is achieved when perceptions of service firm performance exceed expectations. Thus, if marketing communications serve to establish customer expectations that cannot be met or exceeded, by definition the result will be dissatisfied customers.

6. *Observe the long-term effects of communications.* Customers' expectations, perceptions, and tastes can change over time. A funny marketing communication is usually funny only the first few times it is heard. After a certain point it may even be perceived negatively. Ongoing research into the effectiveness of marketing communications over time is strongly recommended.

7. *Be aware of the communication effects of an absence of communication.* In stressful situations, customers often perceive lack of information as negative because they lose control of the situation. It is often better to share bad news with customers than to say nothing at all.

The point is that market-oriented communications and a positioning strategy based on quality and satisfaction should generally convey to customers that the health service organization provides excellent services that will meet their needs, cares about them as individuals, and will do whatever it takes to ensure their satisfaction every time they interact with it.

Embrace Technology/Database Marketing

A central theme throughout the proposed framework is that strong long-term relationships between customers and an organization depend on the maintenance of a positive quality image and customer satisfaction. However, quality and satisfaction are defined by the customer. Therefore, it is imperative that the customer relations program capture customer satisfaction judgments and quality image perceptions through ongoing marketing research. This information can form the foundation for a strong customer database in health services organizations.

Valva (1992) terms such information a customer information file (CIF). Health care is perhaps one of the easiest forms of service in which to establish a CIF, given the preponderance of information customers generally make available when they first establish a relationship with a provider. From a marketing perspective, however, the key to the CIF is to link information on demographics, medical service provision, medical outcomes, and customer satisfaction in a single source. CIFs can provide the basis for a plethora of marketing research investigations, both to gain insights into customer segments and to monitor the efficacy of relationship marketing efforts.

Develop Relationship Marketing and Customer Relations Program Objectives

Kotler (1994, p. 52) suggests that the ultimate test for relationship marketing programs is customer profitability, which he defines as follows: "A profitable customer is a person, household, or company that yields a revenue stream over time, exceeding by an acceptable amount the company cost stream of attracting, selling, and servicing that customer." Thus, an appropriate objective for relationship marketing programs should be profitable customers over the totality of the relationship between the customer and organization.

The customer relations program objectives should support the overall objectives of the relationship marketing program and should therefore be framed in such a way as to optimize customers' lifetime value. These objectives should also be measurable, in order to gauge performance relative to these standards. The following are examples of customer relations objectives that meet these criteria:

- Increase mean customer satisfaction ratings of the target market by 5 percent over the period of the next 12 months.
- Increase intention-to-repurchase ratings by 5 percent over the next 12 months.
- Increase the mean quality image rating by target customers by 10 percent over the next six-month reporting period.

The theory behind stating the objectives of a customer relations program in terms of quality, satisfaction, intention to repurchase, and loyalty outcomes relates to the previous argument that long-term customers are more profitable. Therefore, if we can increase the number of long-term customers served, the overall profitability of the organization's relationship with its customer base should improve.

One way to capture quality image information from target market customers over time to gauge how well the firm is achieving its objectives is through a service quality information system (SQIS). According to Berry (1995, p. 33) an SQIS *"uses multiple research approaches to systematically capture and disseminate service quality information to support decision making"* (italics in original). Health services managers are increasingly considering linking CIFs to managerial decision making through technology to increase the effectiveness of decision making in this regard.

Develop Relationship Marketing Service Strategies

The preceding section identified how relationship marketing objectives and customer relations program objectives can focus a firm on the provision of quality care and patient satisfaction. Strategies are essentially plans determining *how* a health services firm hopes to achieve these organizational objectives and so ultimately fulfill its mission. We know that the bulk of value added for customers of service firms relates to service quality and customer satisfaction (Berry, 1995; Quinn, 1992; Taylor, 1993). Therefore, health services firms need strategies that specifically focus on how service quality will be provided.

Berry (1995) states that the best service firms have a service strategy that (1) explicates the reason the organization exists and (2) captures the value customers perceive in the service product. Berry further identifies a number of characteristics of successful service strategies, for example: (1) quality service should play a central role in service strategies; (2) the service strategy should provide genuine value (i.e., provide the customer with more than he or she sacrifices in order to obtain the service product); (3) the company must live its service strategy in terms of the organization's belief system and leadership examples; and (4) the strategy should foster genuine achievement in the organization by challenging employees to improve skills and knowledge.

Berry (1995) asserts that identifying an appropriate service strategy boils down to matching marketing activities that will prove successful to target customers and activities that the firm is capable of providing exceedingly well. Berry (1995, p. 72) further identifies a four-step process for identifying a service strategy: (1) identify the most important service attributes for meeting and exceeding customers' expectations; (2) pinpoint the important service attributes on which the competition is most vulnerable; (3) accurately assess the strengths and weaknesses of the firm in efforts to determine both existing and potential service capabilities; and (4) develop a service strategy that addresses the most important and enduring needs of customers and capitalizes on competitors' vulnerabilities as well as the strengths of the firm itself.

An example of a service strategy for a hospital might look like the following: XYZ *Hospital's service strategy is to provide superior quality and value for customers through pain-free, convenient, and friendly care in the areas of pediatrics, internal medicine, and family practice*. This service strategy first recognizes quality and value as the most important service attributes necessary to exceed customers' expectations and then identifies areas where the competition may be weak. In this example these areas include pain management, convenience, and friendliness of the medical and support staffs. Second, the service strategy clearly identifies those areas where the hospital has a distinctive competency and can excel, namely, pediatrics, internal medicine, and family practice.

Service strategies should not be confused with mission statements. Mission statements define *why* a firm exists. For example, a not-for-profit hospital might have a mission to "...meet the health service needs of all members of the local community," while the mission statement of a for-profit hospital might aspire to "...increase shareholder wealth." Service strategies, on the other hand, relate to *how* the service component of the health care product is provided to customers.

A final consideration in developing relationship marketing service strategies is to ensure that the developed strategies are clearly communicated to internal customers (employees). It is important to remember that service is provided when a service provider and a customer interact. Therefore, if the employees who are called upon to implement the service strategy are unclear as to their specific roles, it is unlikely that they will provide the highest possible level of service. In the case of the hospital example above, employees will readily recognize that achieving service quality and value should be their highest priorities when engaging in service encounters with customers. The service strategy tells them that they will achieve these ends by providing pain-free, convenient, and friendly health services.

Implement the Relationship Marketing Service Strategies

The next step in the proposed framework for developing a customer relations program involves implementing the relationship marketing service strategies identified above. A number of critical issues should be considered in efforts to implement the derived relationship marketing service strategy, including the appropriate organizational structure, the use of technology, and the management of service providers (Berry, 1995, Quinn, 1992).

The organizational structure of a health services firm can serve either to facilitate or to attenuate the implementation of a relationship marketing service strategy. Quinn (1992) demonstrates that new organizational structures are emerging as the United States moves from a manufacturing- to a service-based economy. One lesson learned from these new organizational forms is that, generally, the more layers of management and the greater the bureaucracy, the harder it is to implement a relationship marketing service strategy. Flatter organizations simply tend to be more responsive to customers. Health service organizations must be able to provide what customers want, when they want it, and with a personal touch every time the customer comes through the organization's doors. Therefore, health service firms must foster organizational cultures and management systems that can respond quickly to changing customer wants and needs.

Berry (1995, pp. 121–122) suggests that organizational structures that facilitate the implementation of a relationship marketing service strategy share the following characteristics: (1) emphasis on continuous service improvement, (2) properly guided and coordinated service improvement initiatives, (3) adequate resources and technical support for service improvement initiatives, (4) solutions for service quality issues, (5) service delivery that meets or exceeds the expectations of customers every day, and (6) a mechanism for service recovery when initial attempts at service provision fail.

In terms of the role of technology in implementing relationship marketing service strategies, processes should be reengineered before organizations are redesigned. In other words, merely adding computers or otherwise embracing technology is not enough. Health services managers must understand the process by which health services are provided from the customers' point of view if these services are to be designed most efficiently and efficaciously. An excellent technique for developing an understanding of the process of how health services are provided is service blueprinting (see Shostack, 1992 for a discussion of how to conduct a service blueprint).

Technology, when properly designed and implemented, can empower employees to be better problem solvers for customers. Organizational structures should facilitate the ability of employees to respond to customers by solving their problems. A generally consistent source of irritation for customers will be multiple referrals within the organization in order to have questions answered or problems resolved. Customer relations personnel must be reasonably empowered to solve customer problems themselves if effective implementation of relationship marketing service strategies is to become a reality.

Measure and Control for Results

The final step in the proposed framework for customer relations programs involves conducting marketing research to evaluate how effectively the implemented relationship marketing service strategies are achieving relationship marketing objectives. As previously argued, outcome measures that health services marketers should consider capturing at this stage include quality, satisfaction, commitment, and trust. Survey items can be found in the following studies to measure each of the identified constructs: trust and commitment (Morgan and Hunt, 1994), satisfaction (Oliver, 1993b), and service quality (Parasuraman, Zeithaml, and Berry, 1988).*

Health services marketers are also encouraged to measure each of these constructs longitudinally. The model of health service relationships presented in Figure 2.1 demonstrates that the formation and maintenance of these relationships occurs over time, with previous outcomes of service encounters influencing subsequent customer expectations. Therefore, marketing research protocols designed to operationalize the model in Figure 2.1 should reflect the longitudinal characteristics of the presented model.

In summary, the preceding section has presented a proposed framework for customer relations programs that captures both a market orientation and relationship marketing imperatives. The proposed framework allows a health service organization to manage its relationships with its customers to competitive advantage. The next section explores many of the challenges that remain for health services marketers in implementing the relationship marketing paradigm into health services marketing practice.

❧ FUTURE DEVELOPMENTS IN CUSTOMER RELATIONS

This chapter argues that customer relations programs founded on the relationship marketing paradigm can provide health services organizations with a competitive

---

*Readers are cautioned that the appropriate operationalization of the service quality versus customer satisfaction constructs remains an unresolved controversy in the services marketing literature. Readers interested in a recent discussion of these issues are directed to Cronin and Taylor (1994); Parasuraman, Zeithaml, and Berry (1994); Oliver (1993a); and Iacobucci, Ostrom, and Grayson (1995).

advantage in today's dynamic environment. Given the newness of the paradigm, however, published research on relationship marketing is only beginning to emerge. It is therefore not surprising that a number of challenges remain for health services marketers.

First, the model of health service relationships presented in Figure 2.1 requires empirical validation. While individual parts of the model have been independently assessed, health services marketers have yet to test the proposed model comprehensively in health care practitioner settings.

Second, additional attention is required to operationalize the identified constructs appropriately. That is, the instruments that currently exist to measure quality, satisfaction, trust, and commitment could all be improved through additional marketing research.

Third, more work must be done to improve our understanding of how the identified constructs relate to one another. Additionally, the identification of relevant influences not captured in the model of health service relationships presented in Figure 2.1 bears consideration.

Fourth, better measures are required of the true lifetime value of customers with whom the organization has established long-term relationships. This issue appears particularly timely given the growing emphasis on controlling health care costs.

Fifth, health services marketers could benefit from user-friendly computer measurement instruments to operationalize the health service relationships model presented in Figure 2.1. Such software packages would necessarily have to capture the statistical complexities associated with longitudinal studies.

Finally, although this chapter calls for the reduction of bureaucracy in the provision of health services for purposes of competitive advantage, the way to achieve this end in highly regulated industries such as health care has yet to be determined. Government and health service industry leaders must seek mechanisms to increase the efficiency of health services delivery by decreasing associated bureaucracy.

ن CONCLUSION

This chapter has asserted that a market orientation and relationship marketing perspective can assist health services marketers in developing effective customer relations programs. It has presented a model of how relationships in health services are formed and progress, based on the weight of the evidence in the existing literature. It has also suggested and discussed a framework for developing customer relations programs based on the model of health service relationships. This chapter has taken the position that in the current health services environment of increasing competition in an atmosphere of increased accountability for resource allocations, relationship marketing practices will likely enhance health services marketing. An emphasis on developing a loyal, dedicated customer base appears the best prescription for long-term organizational success in the health care industry for the foreseeable future.

ಇ REFERENCES

Berry, Leonard L. and A. Parasuraman (1991), *Marketing Services: Competing Through Quality*. New York: The Free Press.

Cronin, J. Joseph, Jr., and Steven A. Taylor (1992), "Measuring Service Quality: A Reexamination and Extension," *Journal of Marketing*, 56 (July 1992), 55–68.

——— (1994), "SERVPERF Versus SERVQUAL: Reconciling Performance-Based and Perceptions-Minus-Expectations Measurement of Service Quality," *Journal of Marketing*, 58 (January), 125–131.

Fisk, Trevor A., Carmheil J. Brown, Kathleen Cannizzaro, and Barbara Naftal (1990), "Creating Patient Satisfaction and Loyalty," *Journal of Health Care Marketing*, 10 (2), 5–15.

Furse, David H., Michael R. Bucham, Robin L. Rose, and Richard W. Oliver (1994), "Leveraging the Value of Customer Satisfaction Information," *Journal of Health Care Marketing*, 14 (3), 16–20.

Hawkins, Del J., Roger J. Best, and Kenneth A. Coney (1995), *Consumer Behavior: Implications for Marketing Strategy*. Chicago: Irwin.

Henthorne, Beth Hogan, Tony L. Henthorne, and John D. Alcorn (1994), "Enhancing the Provider/Patient Relationship: The Case for Patient Advocacy Programs," *Journal of Health Care Marketing*, 14 (3), 52–55.

Heskett, James L., W. Earl Sasser, Jr., and Christopher W. L. Hart (1990), *Service Breakthroughs: Changing the Rules of the Game*. New York: The Free Press.

Iacobucci, Dawn, Amy Ostrom, and Kent Grayson (1995), "Distinguishing Service Quality and Customer Satisfaction: The Voice of the Consumer," *Journal of Consumer Psychology*, 4 (3), 277–303.

Kotler, Philip (1994), *Marketing Management*, 8th ed. Englewood Cliffs, NJ: Prentice Hall.

McAlexander, James H., Dennis O. Kaldenberg, and Harold F. Koenig (1994), "Service Quality Measurement," *Journal of Health Care Marketing*, 14 (3), 34–40.

Morgan, Robert M. and Shelby D. Hunt (1994), "The Commitment-Trust Theory of Relationship Marketing," *Journal of Marketing*, 58 (3), 20–38.

Oliver, Richard L. (1993a), "A Conceptual Model of Service Quality and Service Satisfaction: Compatible Goals, Different Constructs," in *Advances in Services Marketing and Management*, vol. 2, Teresa A. Swartz, David E. Bowen, and Stephen W. Brown (eds.). Greenwich, CT: JAI Press, 65–85.

——— (1993b), "Cognitive, Affective, and Attribute Bases of the Satisfaction Response," *Journal of Consumer Research*, 20 (3), 418–30.

Parasuraman, A., Valerie A. Zeithaml, and Leonard L. Berry (1985), "A Conceptual Model of Service Quality and Its Implications for Future Research," *Journal of Marketing*, 49 (Fall), 41–50.

——— (1988), "SERVQUAL: A Multiple-Item Scale for Measuring Consumer Perceptions of Service Quality," *Journal of Retailing*, 54 (1), 12–40.

——— (1994), "Reassessment of Expectations as a Comparison Standard in Measuring Service Quality," *Journal of Marketing*, 58 (January), 111–124.

Peter, J. Paul, and James H. Donnelly, Jr. (1995), *Marketing Management Knowledge and Skills*, 4th ed. Chicago: Irwin.

Porter, Michael E. (1985), Competitive Strategy. New York: The Free Press.

Reichheld, Frederick W., and W. Earl Sasser, Jr. (1990), "Zero Defections: Quality Comes to Services," *Harvard Business Review*, September–October 1990, 301–307.

Rust, Roland T, and Richard L. Oliver (1994), *Service Quality: New Directions in Theory and Practice*. London: Sage.

Sasser, W. Earl, Jr., Christopher W. L. Hart, and James L. Heskett (1991), *The Service Management Course*. New York: The Free Press.

Shostack, G. L. (1985), "Planning the Service Encounter," in *The Service Encounter*, J. A. Czepiel, M. R. Solomon, and Carol F. Suprenant (eds.). Lexington, MA: Lexington Books, 243–54.

——— (1992), "Understanding Services Through Blueprinting," in *Advances in Services Marketing and Management*, vol. 1, Teresa A. Swartz, David E. Bowen, and Stephen W. Brown (eds.). Greenwich, CT: JAI Press Inc., 75–90.

Taylor, Steven A. (1993), "The Roles of Service Quality, Consumer Satisfaction, and Value in Quinn's (1992) Paradigm of Services," *Journal of Marketing Theory and Practice*, 2 (1), 14–26.

——— (1994), "Distinguishing Service Quality from Patient Satisfaction in Developing Health Care Marketing Strategies," *Hospital & Health Services Administration*, 39 (2), 221–236.

Taylor, Steven A., and J. Joseph Cronin, Jr. (1994), "Modeling Patient Satisfaction and Service Quality," *Journal of Health Care Marketing*, 14 (1), 34–44.

Taylor, Steven A., and Thomas L Baker (1994), "An Assessment of the Relationship Between Service Quality and Customer Satisfaction in the Formation of Consumers' Purchase Intentions," *Journal of Retailing*, 70 (2), 163–178.

Treacy, Michael and Fred Wiersema (1993), "Customer Intimacy and Other Value Disciplines," *Harvard Business Review*, January–February 1993, 84–93.

Vavra, Terry G. (1992), *Aftermarketing: How to Keep Customers for Life Through Relationship Marketing.* New York: Irwin.

Wagner, Henry C., David Fleming, W. Glynn Mangold, and Raymond W. LaForge (1994), "Relationship Marketing in Health Care," *Journal of Health Care Marketing*, 14 (4), 42–47.

Williams, Stephen J. and Paul R. Torrens (1984), *Introduction to Health Services*, 2nd ed. New York: John Wiley & Sons.

Woodside, Arch G., Lisa L. Frey, and Robert Timothy Daly (1989), "Linking Service Quality, Customer Satisfaction, and Behavioral Intention," *Journal of Health Care Marketing*, 9 (4), 5–17.

Strategic Hospital Alliances:

Countervailing Responses to Restructuring Health Care Markets

3

Roice Luke, Virginia Commonwealth University
Peter C. Olden, University of Scranton
*James D. Bramble, Virginia Commonwealth University**

ᕒ OVERVIEW OF STRATEGIC HOSPITAL ALLIANCES

One of the hottest topics in the organizational literature and in boardrooms across the country is the use of strategic alliances to accomplish the market and financial objectives of collaborating organizations. This organizational form represents a significant break from the hierarchical, control-oriented structures that had become so commonplace throughout this century (Astley and Brahm, 1989). The strategic alliance brings together otherwise independent organizations to pursue shared strategic goals. Among a variety of claimed advantages, the strategic alliance offers flexibility and speed in responding to rapidly changing market conditions. It also provides a mechanism for building organizational mass and distinctive competencies, without requiring the partnering organizations to invest internally in unnecessary capacity

*Appreciation is expressed to the General Medical Corporation, Johnson & Johnson, EDS, and the Dupont Corporation for their generous support of the Williamson Institute research into strategic hospital alliances.

development or relinquish cherished organizational autonomies (Zuckerman, Kaluzny, and Ricketts, 1995; Badaracco, 1991; Powell, 1987).

Strategic alliances are emerging in many industries as a major organizational approach to achieving competitive advantage. And many have spread across market, political, even national boundaries. They range from informal arrangements among contractors and subcontractors within the residential construction industry—forming into what Eccles characterized as "quasi firms" (Eccles, 1981)—to joint ventures and networks linking multiple and diverse companies within the computer industry (Dess, Rasheed, McLaughlin, and Priem, 1995). In health care, strategic alliances join rival hospitals within local markets (Luke and Olden, 1995), bringing physicians into contracted service arrangements with hospitals (Murphy and Harding 1994), health care providers into insurer-created networks (Longest, 1990), and hospitals and integrated systems into novel outsourcing agreements with distributors and suppliers.

While much has been written about strategic alliances in health care (e.g., see Zuckerman et al., 1995), little is actually known about their distinctive organizational features. A possible exception is physician-hospital organizations, an area in which much attention has been given to alternative legal structures (Goldstein, 1995; Murphy and Harding, 1994). Information on hospital-hospital alliances has been especially lacking, despite the significant number of hospitals that have entered into strategic alliances with local rivals in recent years.

This chapter focuses specifically on strategic hospital alliances (SHAs), which are defined as *two or more hospitals in a given market that unite in order to generate critical competitive advantages and pursue their collective survival in the marketplace.*

Given the sheer number and strategic importance of the SHAs, it is essential to explore and analyze them fully. A natural starting point would be to develop a typology of these unique organizational forms (Longest, 1990). Unfortunately, most of the extant typologies of hospital systems were initially designed to measure either multihospital, as opposed to local system, combinations (e.g., see DeVries, 1978); physician-hospital arrangements (Goldstein, 1995); or more general models of strategic alliances among businesses, as reported in the business literature (e.g., see Dess et al., 1995; Provan, 1983).

This chapter presents a typology of SHAs as they have evolved in local markets across the country. In addition, it illustrates key dimensions of the typology by examining national distributions of SHAs. The chapter concludes by exploring some possible implications of the identified organizational forms for market and organizational strategies and for the viability of SHAs well into the next century.

The typology and presentations of data are based on an extended study and monitoring of local hospital systems and networks. Beginning in 1989, faculty at the Williamson Institute of the Medical College of Virginia, Campus of the Virginia Commonwealth

University, initiated a national database of local hospital systems—clusters of two or more hospitals in the same system located in and or around the same market. As the network model became more prominent in the early 1990s, these more loosely coupled arrangements were added to the database. The project also supported a series of site visits to major markets to capture the perspectives of executives in charge of the leading local systems. The site visits explored with those executives the strategic issues they and their rivals faced in their local markets. The typology presented in this chapter draws upon both the database and the collective experience of the faculty in monitoring SHAs in local markets around the country.

Background on SHAs

Luke and Olden (1995) report that by the middle of 1995, nearly 60 percent of urban, acute care general hospitals had become members of one or more strategic alignments with other hospitals, including relationships within urban areas and/or with hospitals in nearby rural areas. These alignments also included both system (owned, managed, leased) and network arrangements. For the urban members of these alignments only, this proportion represented an increase of about 30 percentage points since 1989 and 40 percentage points since 1982. (In 1989, the percentage of urban hospitals in clusters of two or more hospitals was 28, and in 1982 it was 19.) And in the major markets, defined as the 100 metropolitan statistical areas (MSAs) with populations of 450,000 or over, the proportion approached 70 percent. And new consolidations and affiliations are announced nearly every week.

The significance of this increase in strategic alignments among hospitals cannot be overstated. It can reasonably be expected that by the close of this century, over 80 percent of urban hospitals will have entered into strategic alignments with other hospitals in their local areas. Indeed, by the time this movement is completed, most markets will have been reduced to a very small number of provider systems—typically from two to four major players per market (Luke and Olden, 1995). The following chart, focusing specifically on SHAs, indicates the degree to which a few SHAs already dominate selected MSAs (Luke, Rossiter, Swisher, and Bramble, 1995):

MSA	No. of SHAs	Percentage of MSA Bed Capacity
Denver	4	100
Kansas City	4	94
Orlando	3	94
Cincinnati	5	93
St. Louis	4	88

MSA	No. of SHAs	Percentage of MSA Bed Capacity
Louisville	3	87
Houston	6	87
Milwaukee	3	86
San Diego	5	85
Salt Lake City	3	84
Jacksonville	2	84
San Francisco	4	79

Even in Chicago, a metropolitan area with over 70 acute care general hospitals, five SHAs control over 50 percent of the bed capacity, and ten control 75 percent. It is anticipated that within three to four years many unaffiliated hospitals in the Chicago area will join SHAs and some of the existing SHAs will consolidate. Similar patterns can be observed in the other major MSAs across the country.

In addition to urban market consolidation, rural providers are joining regional systems and networks. Their partners are being selected from among other rural providers or from major SHAs forming in nearby urban markets. While the percentages of rural hospitals in system or network arrangements are far less than for urban hospitals (the percentages for rural hospitals range from 20 to 40 percent, depending on how such arrangements are defined), they are rather high in some states. For example, in Utah, New Mexico, Arizona, Tennessee, Kentucky, Illinois, and Alabama, over 60 percent of the rural hospitals are already involved in some type of strategic alliance with other hospitals in the state (Luke et al., 1995).

Not only are the numbers of hospitals entering local systems and networks very large, but hospital-based alliances are taking the lead in consolidating other elements into integrated health care delivery systems. The jury is still out, however, on whether or not hospital companies will remain at the helm in system building. Growing evidence suggests that they may be encountering some stiff resistance. For example, physician-hospital organizations, a possible linchpin for hospital-initiated integrated systems, are experiencing difficulties in securing physician cooperation in many areas (Goldstein, 1995). Countering the hospital-based systems, managed care companies are aggressively forming their own networks, which often cut across the organizational boundaries of established SHAs. Such networks directly challenge SHA attempts to use single signatures to assure that all alliance partners are included in managed care contracts.

Also, the model emerging in the Los Angeles area, where a number of large physician groups have taken the lead in contracting with managed care organizations and assembling integrated delivery systems, represents an alternative to the leadership of

SHAs. Over time this model could achieve national significance, but only if certain somewhat improbable scenarios come to pass. To compete successfully with hospital- or insurance-based systems in the costly business of system building, physicians would have to join physician-initiated networks in significant numbers and gain greater access both to financial markets and to the kinds of organizational expertise needed to develop and manage integrated systems. While some national physician organizations have formed and experienced rapid growth in recent years (e.g., Phycor in Nashville and Coastal in Durham, NC) they would have to grow substantially to be strong enough to challenge the rather substantial positions already achieved by SHAs in many markets.

Determinants of SHA Growth.   What has precipitated the rapid growth in the numbers of SHAs? Many forces are bringing organizations together into alliance relationships, some of which have been identified in the general business literature. Two such factors appear especially important: the growth in new technologies, particularly information technologies, and the precipitous rise in global competition (Kanter, 1994; Badaracco, 1991). The new global competition has taught firms worldwide that they must find new ways to bring costs under control, raise the quality of their goods and services, and shorten dramatically the time required to bring new products to market. It has also taught them that the necessary human and other resources are often acquired at less cost or risk by venturing with other firms, even old rivals, rather than by investing internally in new capacity development.

In health care the threats are unique and specific to changes in the industry itself. Central to the increased use of alliances to achieve strategic objectives, especially among hospitals in local markets, is the rising threat of managed care.* Since 1982, managed care has risen from covering 3.9 percent to 16.5 percent of the insured population, and projections suggest that this trend will continue unabated for years to come. The growth in managed care has been much greater in the larger markets. By the end of 1994, managed care penetration in the 100 largest MSAs averaged 21.4 percent, compared with 14.1 percent in the remaining 221 MSAs across the country.

Prior to the late 1980s and early 1990s, hospitals participated in alliances with other hospitals in their local markets for a wide variety of reasons (e.g., see Luke and Begun, 1988; Shortell, 1988). But over the last five to ten years, the rationale has clearly shifted; hospitals are now forming alliances primarily to position themselves to compete more

---

*This conclusion is based upon a careful reading of the popular health care literature (e.g., see Scott, 1995), as well as numerous interviews conducted by phone and during site visits by the faculty of the Williamson Institute.

effectively for managed care contracts. Even those systems and networks formed in earlier years are restructuring in order to cope more effectively with the unique and powerful incentives of managed care.

Hospitals have found that by aligning with other hospitals in their local markets, they gain or hope to gain several advantages in a managed care environment. First, many hospital combinations provide their members with expanded spatial positions, thus enabling them to negotiate for contracts covering whole communities. Second, these combinations give them greater mass and leverage, providing them with increased power to "countervail" (Galbraith, 1952) the growing strength of managed care companies. This is a critical motivation, as hospitals would otherwise be far more vulnerable to managed care companies bent on trading off one hospital for another in negotiations based on price. Third, the alliances place the hospitals in the position of being system builders, rather than deferring to either insurance companies or physician groups for leadership in forming integrated systems.

As will be seen in a later section of this chapter, the focus on managed care effectively transforms SHAs into unique, firmlike entities. By uniting to compete for managed care contracts, and with continuing growth in managed care penetration, hospital members depend increasingly upon their alliances to channel to them the essential revenue streams they require to survive as institutions. The alliance thus assumes a kind of corporate or strategic role for all participating members. And the more this occurs, the greater the strains will be on the fragile structures that bind the otherwise independent hospital members.

& TYPOLOGY OF SHAs

No single typology will fulfill the needs of all analyses. And the design of each typology depends directly on its intended purposes. For example, if its purpose was to provide clearer distinctions among the emerging models for combining physicians into groups, the typology might emphasize legal and organizational structures. This emphasis would differentiate among such organizational types as group practices without walls (GPWWs), physician hospital organizations (PHOs), medical service organizations (MSOs), and medical foundations. This approach to classifying physician organizations is now widely used in the literature (Murphy and Harding, 1994).

The terms *strategic* and *alliance* together establish the purpose of the typology to be developed in this chapter. *Strategic* refers to what could arguably be one of the most significant and wrenching decisions an organization might be called upon to make—whether or not to compromise independence in strategy making in order to conform to the strategic interests of a broader collective. Generally, SHA partner members shared a high level of strategic purpose, whereas collaborators in other alliances are likely to be considerably less committed to collective strategies. The health care alliances in effect create new, larger competitors that function collectively as firms (a point developed further below).

Alliance has to do with organizational form, with whether or not to adopt loose arrangements or integrate more fully into tighter organizational structures. Loose coupling, it is claimed, provides advantages of flexibility and innovativeness, because the members continue to operate with a high degree of autonomy (Zuckerman and D'Aunno, 1990). It also offers only limited capacity to coordinate members' efforts, a significant limitation for alliances in which the members share a high degree of strategic purpose. Since both the strategy and alliance dimensions clearly identify very distinctive features of these organizational forms, they provide the basis for the typology of SHAs as developed in this chapter.

These two dimensions have already been applied by Luke et al. (1989) in constructing their typology of collective organizations in health care. Given its compatibility with the purposes of this chapter, their typology will be used as a starting point for developing a framework for classifying and analyzing SHAs. As can be seen in Figure 3.1, the concept of the firm is at the heart of Luke et al.'s typology. Using the two dimensions, strategic interdependency and tightness of coupling, they identify four types of hospital alliances: firms, virtual firms, latent firms, and nonfirms.* Significantly for the purposes

Figure 3.1   Typology of Hospital Alliances

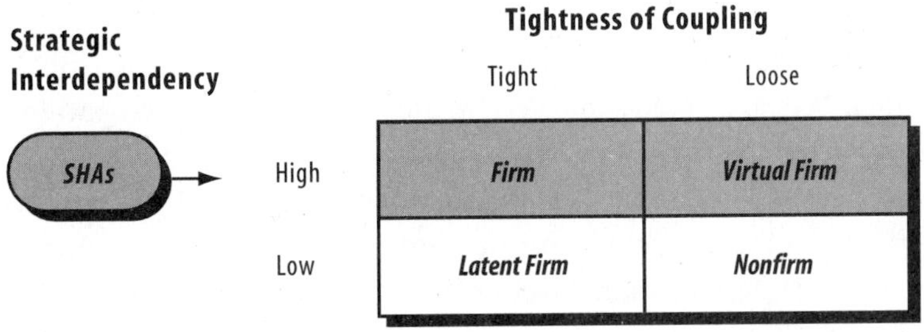

Source: Adapted from Luke et al., 1989.

---

*In their paper, Luke et al. (1989) used two terms—"quasi firm" and "network"—that are replaced in Figure 3.1 by the terms "virtual firm" and "nonfirm," respectively. With the exception of academic discussion, the term *quasi* is little used in common parlance when referring to strategic alliances. Further, the term *network* is now more commonly used as a synonym for the quasi firm. Thus, to conform to current usage and avoid confusion in the use of the term *network*, Figure 3.1 uses the new terms.

of this chapter, the four are differentiated by the degree to which the participating members are or are not highly strategically interdependent—firms and virtual firms represent high strategic interdependency among participating members, latent firms and nonfirms low strategic interdependency. These are briefly described below.

The first type, the firm, has long been conceived by economists as the primary competitive unit in markets (Coase, 1937). It is equivalent to the traditional, hierarchically structured organizational form. In the hospital industry, the concept of a firm may not apply as straightforwardly as in other sectors of the economy. The difference arises because hospitals have historically retained their own boards and operated with high levels of independence, regardless of whether they were members of multihospital systems or were freestanding. The hospitals' emphasis on autonomy has had important consequences for multihospital systems. Despite bringing hospitals under common ownership, these systems have done little to prevent members located in the same markets from competing with one another. Multihospital systems have had some success in exerting corporate or hierarchical control over their hospitals (Gray, 1986). But they have been distinctly ineffective in achieving a coordination of effort among geographically proximate hospitals (Shortell, 1988) regardless of ownership type—profit, not for profit, or Catholic. To some extent, such limitations are attributable to the constraints of antitrust oversight, but long-standing expectations of organizational autonomy also appear to have played an important role. Interestingly, a number of same-system and same-market hospitals have even merged with each other in order to surmount barriers to interhospital coordination.

In this chapter, therefore, all local hospital combinations, whether strictly system-based (owned, managed, or leased) or networks (partners come from different ownership groups) are counted as alliances. Returning to the typology, then, SHAs in which all hospital members are in the same system are referred to as *firms,* and those involving multiple ownerships or systems are termed *virtual firms.*

The other tightly coupled model type identified in Figure 3.1 is the *latent firm.* As explained by Luke et al. (1989), such firms are represented by system combinations that are, for the most part, insulated from market forces. They are thus not expected to function as competitive entities in a market environment. Providers that enjoy natural monopolies, such as public or highly specialized hospitals, might fall into this category. Lacking high strategic interdependencies among their members, such hospital combinations are not classified as SHAs.

Finally, Figure 3.1 identifies another loosely coupled organizational form that, in contrast to the virtual firm, is not considered strategic and is therefore labeled a *nonfirm.* These are especially important, since many alliances within this category are confused with the more strategically interdependent alliance types. Selected examples provided below illustrate more clearly the distinction between virtual firm and nonfirm alliances.

Most teaching affiliations fall into the category of nonfirms. Although they facilitate important manpower and referral exchanges, such affiliations are not strategic per se. They usually play a minor role in enhancing members' competitive advantages, channel slight revenue and only limited numbers of patients among partners, and contribute little to the ultimate survivability of the affiliated hospital members within their markets. In addition, most preferred provider organizations (PPOs) fall into the category of nonfirm alliances. They may assist their members in competing for managed care contracts but are not often counted upon to channel significant numbers of patients to their contracted members. Perhaps more important, they are not likely to be involved in members' crucial strategic decision-making processes as they seek to gain competitive advantages over their rivals. By contrast, SHAs exist largely to facilitate collective strategic decision making and strategic action on the part of their members and are designed to serve as a primary channel through which managed care contracts may be funneled.

Other types of nonfirm alliances include major outsourcing arrangements. An example would be a local hospital system, or even an HMO, that has contracted with a distributor to take over all of its system-level supplies distribution functions. This arrangement could include responsibility for any combination of the following: distribution to local warehouses; management of inventory and warehouses; redistribution of supplies to SHA hospitals, clinics, and other sites; handling and placement of supplies on the floor; and, possibly, monitoring of supply use. Such arrangements could be important from a cost control perspective but would not be expected to alter significantly the position of the contracting systems in their markets or determine their long-term viability. Certainly, they would not intermingle the strategic decision-making processes of the collaborating supplier and provider firms.

Most joint ventures are also of the nonfirm type. In a joint venture, two or more entities agree to engage in a business together, but without tying their overall businesses or strategic futures to one another. Two hospitals could, for example, enter into a shared effort to establish a line of primary care clinics. Such efforts could involve the outlay of significant resources and, as a result, could have a material impact on the economic position of the participating members. On the other hand, joint ventures in health care are rarely so important. Furthermore, they do not tie the collaborating firms into any kind of coordinated strategic actions beyond those of the joint venture itself.

Interestingly, outsourcing and joint venture alliances are among those most commonly highlighted in the general business literature on strategic alliances (e.g., see Dess et al., 1995; Kotabe and Swan, 1995). By contrast, alliances in which members are strategically highly interdependent, such as SHAs in the health care industry, have not been identified in that literature and have received only limited attention in the health care literature (e.g., see Zuckerman et al., 1995; Shortell et al., 1993). SHAs are potentially very much more strategic. They not only transform collaborating members into single firms, either through merger and acquisition or via the formation of loosely coupled virtual firms, but also dramatically alter the structures of health care markets by increasing the size and reducing the number of competitors in local markets.

One cautionary implication flows directly from the lack of analytic attention given to the SHAs, especially those that fall into the category of virtual firms. The lack of attention and, possibly, the relative newness of the virtual firm models mean that little more than anecdotal evidence is available to help determine whether or not they actually achieve the operational efficiencies or lasting strategic outcomes expected of them. To the extent there is a gap between expectation and performance, the loosely coupled organizational form could turn out to be a transitional model that serves more to facilitate initial partner choices than to accomplish the ultimate ends of system integration and competition.

It should be noted that performance is not necessarily tied to the degree to which an alliance has firmlike characteristics. Indeed, there are those who suggest that the more loosely coupled alliances may be the better performers (Zuckerman and Kaluzny, 1991), because the advantages of flexibility and innovation, which are enhanced by loose coupling, may offset those of coordination and control, the latter of which by definition are the strength of tighter coupling.

On the other hand, the advantages of loose coupling may well be inversely related to the level of turbulence in the environment. The more uncertain and threatening the environment, the more interorganizational coordination may need to be improved, especially in the area of collective strategic decision making. Nevertheless, the degree to which SHAs can be regarded as firms within a typology should be positively associated with both the level of strategic interdependency and the tightness of coupling among the collaborating hospital members.

Since this chapter is concerned with strategic rather than other alliance forms, its remaining sections will focus only on those that are firmlike, that is, the firms or virtual firms, as conceptualized in Figure 3.1. The next section introduces additional dimensions to the typology to enable the various types of SHAs forming in markets across the country to be further distinguished from one another.

?• EXPANDED TYPOLOGY

Since the foregoing discussion separated out alliances that are highly strategic from those that are not, it is important now to provide a basis for further differentiating among the highly strategic SHAs, which are themselves quite diverse. SHAs range from geographically expanded networks that extend into rural areas and/or cross multiple metropolitan boundaries to mergers between hospitals separated from one another by only a street. Some include one or more large teaching or hub hospitals surrounded by numerous smaller, community hospitals, whereas others comprise only two hospitals of any size or function. SHAs vary in their ownership mixes as well. Some are made up of hospitals belonging to a single system, others mix ownership types (e.g., profit, nonprofit, Catholic), and still others combine hospitals that come from the same ownership type (e.g., all Catholic) yet have different owners (e.g., distinct religious orders). Some have entered into complex affiliations in which there is a substantial mixing of assets and a reshuffling of internal powers, whereas others are grouped by the most meager of agreements, reflecting mere commitments to collaborate rather than formal decisions to enter into lasting partnerships.

In part, the diversity among SHAs is a product of the pace with which horizontal combinations have been pursued. Hospitals have been moving into local system arrangements for some time, but only recently have they rushed to choose sides. This development is also due to the limited options for partnering, especially after one or two alliances have already formed in an area. For these and other reasons, many unlikely partner combinations have been and continue to be created, producing some highly complex and in some cases unmanageable alliances. Along the way, of course, many would-be alliances fall victim to irreconcilable interorganizational conflicts, value incongruities, and misunderstandings, as well as to internal resistance on the part of powerful organizational members or the mere threat (if not the reality) of antitrust investigation.

Perhaps most important, SHAs differ in the degree to which they function as firms, that is, as entities united in their pursuit of shared strategic objectives. The two dimensions used in the typology actually provide important bases for distinguishing SHAs as firms. The more tightly coupled the SHAs, the greater the coordination among their hospitals and, therefore, the more firmlike they will be. Similarly, the more strategically interdependent their members are, the greater the probability that they will be committed to collective, as opposed to individual, strategic objectives and, regardless of the tightness of coupling, the more they can be expected to behave as single firms.

An elaborated typology is clearly needed to give further definition to the diversity of SHAs. To this end, this chapter expands the two dimensions—strategic interdependency and tightness of coupling—into two subdimensions, as shown in Figure 3.2. As indicated, strategic interdependency is directly related to the *importance* of the collective relationships among hospitals. Importance has two subdimensions that give meaning to strategic interdependency: (1) the relative *magnitude* of resources flowing through SHAs to collaborating hospitals and (2) the *criticality* of those resources in terms of their contribution to the hospitals' ultimate survival. Variance in either magnitude or criticality is

Figure 3.2   Expansion of Strategic Hospital Alliance Typology

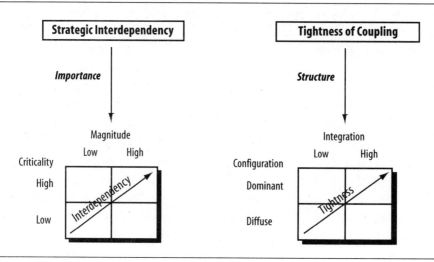

likely to contribute directly to the collaborating hospitals' degree of commitment to the collective goals of SHAs.

Tightness of coupling is directly related to the *structures* that unite the hospital partners within SHAs. Not only do SHAs need to coordinate clinical and operational functioning, but, possibly more important, they need to resolve power conflicts that could interfere with effective strategic decision making. Structure is therefore also conceived as having two subdimensions: (1) the *configuration*, or balance of power, that exists among the hospitals joined into SHAs and (2) the degree of *integration* among collaborating hospitals. Both configuration and integration are expected to affect directly the ability of SHAs to coordinate the efforts of member hospitals.

In sum, alliances can be distinguished both by levels of strategic interdependency and by the tightness with which they are coupled into unified strategic units. The four subdimensions—magnitude, criticality, configuration, and integration—are developed further in the following section.

Strategic Interdependency

Not all SHAs share the same degree of strategic interdependency and, therefore, the same commitment among members to their collective objectives. Many factors contribute to the degree of strategic interdependency. In their important work on the concept of interorganizational interdependency, Pfeffer and Salancik (1978) identify one factor in particular that should be closely tied to strategic rather than to other types of interdependency: the relative *importance* organizations ascribe to their exchange relationships with other organizations in their environments. Put simply, the more important the exchanged resources are to a given partner, the more dependent and vulnerable that partner will be. Also, the more dependent or vulnerable a partner is, the more it will seek alternative sources for the valued resources or attempt to build greater certainty into the exchange relationship (e.g., through merger).

The formation of SHAs, of course, represents a move on the part of hospitals to gain greater control over very important exchange relationships—in this case, between collaborating hospitals and managed care organizations. Managed care revenues and patients are supplied to SHAs in exchange for services provided by member hospitals. SHAs give collaborating hospitals both greater leverage as they negotiate with managed care organizations and more comprehensive service capacities, thus enabling them to compete more effectively for managed care contracts.

Magnitude. The relative magnitude of an exchange is viewed from the perspective of the collaborating hospitals. It is represented by the proportion of the resources (or managed care revenues) that are channeled through the SHAs. The higher the proportion of such revenues, the more committed the hospitals will be to the long-term success of their SHAs and, as a result, the more strategically interdependent they and the SHAs will be.

In her paper on vertical integration, Harrigan (1985) suggests that the magnitude of flows between vertically integrated organizations could be measured using two dimensions: the number of areas in which exchanges occur, which she referred to as *breadth*, and the proportionality of the total flow that occurred within each of those areas, which she referred to as *depth*. In the case of SHAs, a comprehensive breadth is assumed, simply because hospitals are defined as having come together to provide a full spectrum of services to contracted beneficiaries. Therefore, SHAs by design involve a broad range of exchanges among partnering hospitals. Exceptions might include tertiary and specialty members, whose breadth or number of areas might be limited by contract within an SHA. The more constrained the breadth, the more limited the strategic interdependency for such hospitals would be.

Even with the wide range of exchange assumed for most SHAs, the volume or proportion of a hospital's total exchange channeled through an SHA could vary significantly. Some hospitals might draw only a very small proportion of their total managed care revenues from their SHA, while others might depend heavily on their SHAs for the receipt of such revenues. Again, the degree of strategic interdependency will vary by the volume or magnitude of the flow involved in the exchange.

It should be noted that magnitude could be either *actual* or *expected*. At a given point in time, a hospital might derive only a small proportion of its revenues through its SHA but expect this percentage to increase steadily over time. Both actual and expected revenues thus contribute to the interdependencies that exist between hospitals and their SHAs. There could be situations, for example, in which actual penetration of managed care is low and future penetration is expected to increase little, at least in the short term. In such cases participating hospitals would have limited strategic interdependency with their SHA and, consequently, a low commitment to the SHA relative to their own strategic objectives.

Of course, if the resources involved in an exchange per se are not critical to the functioning or survival of collaborating organizations, their degree of strategic interdependency will be low, no matter what the magnitude of the flow might be. For example, if the exchange did not involve managed care revenues for patient services, but rather some other, less vital exchange for which there might be alternative sources (e.g., contracted management services), the relationship, no matter what the magnitude, might not produce high levels of strategic interdependency. Magnitude and criticality thus jointly determine the degree of strategic import attributed to an interorganizational relationship.

Criticality.   The other subdimension of importance is the criticality of the exchange. This represents the degree to which an organization perceives its ultimate survival as depending on its obtaining resources in an exchange. Of course, the more critical these resources are to their long-term viability, the greater will be the strategic interdependency among the exchanging organizations—assuming, of course, that the volume or magnitude of the exchange remains constant. If a dependent partner has multiple sources for a given resource (in which case the magnitude will likely be low), it will be less dependent on any single source, regardless of how critical to its survival that resource may be.

As has been argued, for SHAs the most important resource over time will be managed care contracts and revenues. SHAs have been defined as forming primarily to put participating hospitals in a better position to secure such contracts. Thus, as managed care penetration increases, these partnering hospitals will likely become increasingly dependent on their SHAs. In this case the rising penetration represents a growth in criticality; and the rise in the proportion of revenues coming through SHAs represents an increase in magnitude.

Many factors contribute to variances in expected criticality within alliance relationships generally. In the case of SHAs, however, given the current turbulence in health care markets, market forces should rank very high in their assessments of criticality. The diversity of threats that could exist in most markets has been conceptualized by Porter (1980) in his now well-recognized framework of competitive forces. As identified in Figure 3.3, the most important market threats come from five sources: rivals, buyers, sellers, potential entrants, and substitutes.

Clearly, SHAs face threats from each of these five areas, though the degree and particular source of threat vary significantly across markets. For instance, if the major employers in a market were to announce the formation of a buyer coalition or, even more significant, engage in the direct purchase of health service contracts, member hospitals might reasonably be expected to view their SHAs as more critical to their survival than they would otherwise have done. Alternatively, anticipated mergers between local managed care companies, the formation of rival SHAs, the entry of physician-based strategic alliances in the market, or acquisitions of hospitals or SHAs in their markets by major outside hospital companies could all increase significantly the criticality of a set of relationships embedded within affected SHAs. Criticality is therefore directly related to the degree of threat that participating hospitals perceive in their market environments, as indicated in Figure 3.3.

Figure 3.3   Market Threats—Illustrated Using the Porter Model

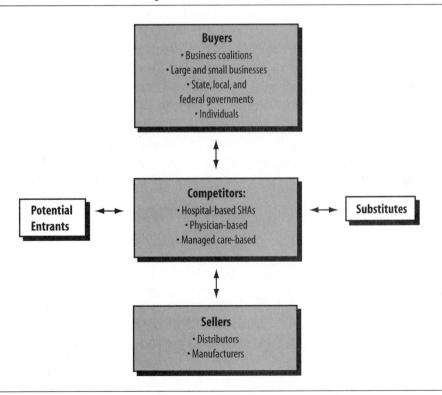

It should be clear by now that magnitude and criticality are essential and complementary dimensions of importance. Further, it should be apparent that both contribute directly to the strategic interdependency that exists between hospitals and their SHAs and, ultimately, these hospitals' level of commitment to the collective strategic objectives of their SHAs.

Tightness of Coupling

The second dimension for classifying SHAs is the tightness of coupling among participating hospitals. Relationships among hospitals within SHAs may be either very tight (e.g., members of the same system) or very loose (e.g., members of a contractually structured network) or somewhere in between (e.g., two local system clusters joined into an "operational" merger in which the two share common administration and intermingle assets but otherwise retain their autonomy as systems). As already discussed, SHAs are unique in their use of loose coupling to accomplish very high levels of shared strategic purpose. Thus, their major challenge is to balance the often opposing pressures for coordination and tighter organizational structures against the need to maintain autonomy and preserve independent action, flexibility, and innovation.

To expand the concept of coupling, as indicated in Figure 3.2, two dimensions are proposed for further differentiating among SHAs. The first, *integration*, includes all of the well-recognized organizational mechanisms—boards, administrative teams, committees, information systems, etc.—that might be needed to coordinate activities and functions across hospitals participating together in alliances (Gillies, Shortell, Anderson, Mitchell, and Morgan, 1993). The second, *configuration*, differentiates SHAs by the relative balance of power that exists across alliance partners. The point of configuration is that conflicts in power across alliance members and difficulties in making strategic decisions will vary according to individual members' size or influence within an alliance. In particular, the more a single member is able to shape the decision-making processes of an SHA, the more likely it is that the administrative mechanisms of that member will substitute for missing structural elements within the SHA.

Integration. Because of high strategic interdependencies, hospitals in SHAs will need to find creative ways to make and implement both strategic and operational decisions. In their search for structure, however, they will inevitably be pulled toward one or the other of two polar positions: full integration or complete dissolution (Luke et al., 1989). The breakup of an alliance could be the result of members' inability to work within the limitations of loose structures, especially when faced with uncertain and challenging environments. At the other end of the spectrum, different perceptions regarding the actual level of strategic threat or need for an alliance in the first place could also cause an alliance to unravel.

Convergence toward more hierarchical models is an alternative outcome of SHA struggles to find a workable structure. The push toward convergence will likely be accentuated in environments characterized by relatively high levels of threat and uncertainty. The trick here is for an alliance to hold the middle ground, maintaining the capacity to make the difficult strategic and operational decisions, while preserving valued organizational autonomies and maximizing the flexibility and innovativeness promised by more loosely coupled organizational forms.

Luke et al. (1989) identify two structural features that alliances seeking improved coordination will have to address. First, they will need to form effectively functioning strategic apexes, that is, governance and management structures capable of making and implementing important strategic decisions. Achieving these is primarily a question of allocating power among the members and between members and their SHAs. Second, they need to put in place the administrative mechanisms essential for implementing strategic decisions and generally coordinating their collective activities.

In their study of multihospital systems, Shortell et al. investigated in detail a large number of mechanisms that might be needed to improve interorganizational integration, which they examined at three levels: functional, clinical, and physician-hospital. They found that the systems studied achieved relatively low integration at the clinical level and only moderate integration at the functional and physician-hospital levels (e.g., see Gillies et al., 1993; Shortell, Gillies, Anderson, Mitchell, and Morgan, 1993). They argued that the need for clinical integration among hospitals and other provider partners is especially crucial in light of the great variety of clinical functions and interrelationships that exist within complex health systems. It is important to note that they studied a select group of advanced multihospital systems and did not examine the more loosely coupled forms, referred to in Figure 3.1 as virtual firms. Had they investigated the latter, they might have observed even less clinical integration across hospitals and other providers than they found within the systems (firms in the typology) they examined.

Most of the mechanisms identified for integrating across hospitals are what might be called *formal* or explicit mechanisms of control. These include governance and administrative structures, financing mechanisms and agreements, information and communication systems, reward and evaluative structures, and other such administrative devices. *Informal* mechanisms are also expected to play pivotal roles within alliances (Powell, 1990; Powell, 1987), given that most alliances by definition eschew formal structures. Informal mechanisms include such factors as expectations and patterns of reciprocity, trust, shared vision, value congruencies, and culture. They may be especially critical within strategic alliances, which rely less on authority and more on accommodation to achieve much-needed coordination across members. Informal mechanisms therefore often serve as the "glue" for strategic alliances, facilitating and sustaining negotiated relationships and often providing a first (sometimes the only) line of defense against alliance dissolution.

To achieve better internal integration, strategic alliances clearly need to pay attention to both formal and informal mechanisms. Unfortunately, alliances tend to focus too heavily on informal approaches, since these detract little from protected autonomies. Also, given the critical challenge of maintaining commitment as well as making difficult strategic decisions, formal mechanisms for achieving clinical and/or functional integration are often overlooked as leaders engage in seemingly neverending exercises of executive bonding. That is, so many obstacles complicate interorganizational coordination in strategic alliances that executives within them may rely too much on informal mechanisms to ensure a unity of effort among participating organizations.

Nevertheless, it is clear that both formal and informal mechanisms are essential for integrating the work of alliance members. Figure 3.1 implies that the more SHAs achieve either, the more firmlike they will become.

Configuration.   As suggested above, the configuration of a particular alliance might directly affect the degree to which formal or informal structures are needed to assure coordination and effective strategic decision making. If one member of an alliance could provide leadership on behalf of the whole, its own administrative structures might substitute for those structures that would otherwise be created within the alliance itself. For example, in a vertical alliance, the most downstream member, being the closest to the final customer, might naturally emerge as the strategic decision maker (Luke et al., 1989). As a result, somewhat less formal structuring might be needed to achieve strategic coordination among alliance members (indirect evidence for this assertion was found by Ghemawat, Porter, and Rawlinson, 1986).

In the horizontal alliances that are the focus of this chapter, issues of power and strategic decision making might more readily be resolved if one member dominated the alliance. The decision-making mechanisms of the dominant partner could then fill the power and administrative gaps, thus obviating the need to establish complex decision-making structures within the alliance itself. This does not mean that such mechanisms would not be needed, but that the administrative structures of dominant organizations might substitute for much of what otherwise would be required in alliances made up of more equally balanced partners. (Of course, in the special case of a single-system alliance, for example, all Columbia/HCA hospitals in the Houston MSA, the controlling multihospital system or possibly a division within the system could provide the structures for decision making on behalf of owned hospitals.) It is significant, as will be shown in a later section, that the majority of SHAs appear to have at least one dominant member. These SHAs are likely to face very different inter-organizational challenges than those whose member configurations are more equally balanced.

Figure 3.4 presents the configuration model types to be added to the typology. As shown, four models can be identified, two of which are characterized as *dominant* and two as *diffuse*. These terms reflect differences in the degree to which power might disproportionately be concentrated in the hands of a single alliance member (the dominant model) or distributed more evenly to two or more relatively equal partners (the diffuse model).

The dominant model is divided into two subtypes: one a single-ownership *firm* and the other a multi-ownership virtual firm in which one member clearly dominates the SHA, referred to as a *unimodal virtual firm* (unimodal in this case referring to the dominating player). Two model types are identified for the diffuse category. One is the *bimodal virtual firm*, a special case with an alliance of only two relatively equal partners; the other is a *multimodal virtual firm*, in which there are more than two partners but no one partner dominates the alliance (again, see Figure 3.4).

In sum, two general dimensions provide the foundation for distinguishing SHAs from other alliance forms: strategic interdependency and tightness of coupling. These dimensions are expanded by the addition of two subdimensions, each of which differentiates among identified SHAs. Strategic interdependency is seen to vary in direct proportion to both the magnitude and criticality of resources involved in exchanges between member hospitals and their SHAs. And tightness of coupling is related to the

Figure 3.4   SHA Configuration Model Types

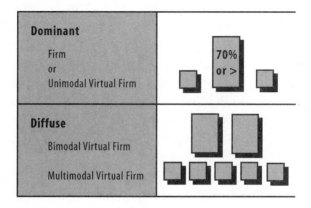

degree of integration achieved among members, as well as the unique configurations that result from the particular combinations of partners within SHAs.

૨ૐ SHA Distributions

This section presents distributions of SHAs, to the extent that the requisite data are available. Data are available showing the numbers of hospitals that are in either firms or virtual firms, as well as the numbers of those within the four configuration model types. Data are not available, however, that demonstrate either the criticality or the magnitude dimensions of strategic interdependency or the integration dimension of loose coupling.

First, it is important to see how many SHAs can be identified across the country and which of these fall into the firm and virtual firm categories. Recall that SHAs are deemed to exist when two or more hospitals generate critical competitive advantages and pursue their collective survival in the managed care marketplace. In the data, marketplaces are defined as the federally established MSAs.

A national database developed by the Williamson Institute at the Virginia Commonwealth University was used to identify urban-based SHAs from among various combinations of local systems and networks. This exercise involved several stages of effort. First, the system and network affiliations themselves had to be tracked over time. Second, since many hospitals may have entered into more than one system or network arrangement, these needed to be sorted out to determine which represented true strategic alignments and which did not. Third, these alignments then had to be sifted to determine which combinations amounted to SHAs. This last step was especially difficult to carry out with accuracy, both because system and network arrangements are continually changing and because many SHAs were at a relatively early stage in their formation. Each of these three steps was accomplished by monitoring published literature, conducting site visits, and making numerous calls to the local markets to seek clarifications from local executives on ongoing alliance formation within their markets. (Note that alliances that did not involve more than one urban member, for example, some urban/rural alliances, are not included in the analysis.)

Of the 2,743 nonfederal urban acute care general hospitals identified by September 1995, nearly 40 percent had not yet entered into any strategic alignment with another urban hospital. In other words, they had neither a system (again, based on ownership, management contract, lease arrangement, or sponsorship) nor a network partner in their local markets. A breakdown of the remaining 60 percent of hospitals that had at least one such relationship shows that 38 percent of urban hospitals had one relationship and 22 percent had more than one. Of those that had more than one system or network relationship, a number were in clusters that actually competed with one another. Obviously, therefore, those with multiple relationships will eventually be forced to choose one over another, as the process of partner selection in the local markets moves forward. Many other multiple relationships represented smaller strategic groupings that have already recombined into still larger alliances.

The various combinations of hospitals in the Oklahoma City MSA provide an excellent example of the multiple strategic relationships that can be observed among some hospitals locally. The three Columbia/HCA hospitals in Oklahoma City, which together constitute a system cluster (a cluster being two or more hospitals), have joined a local network, the Oklahoma Health Alliance, that was formed initially by the Baptist-led Oklahoma Health System. If it survives and reaches its potential, the Oklahoma Health Network should emerge as the strategic unit for both the Columbia/HCA and Baptist system clusters. The resulting combination has been classified in the database as a diffuse, bimodal virtual firm.

Many existing relationships appear to be in the early stages of SHA formation, as hospitals within them anticipate future negotiations leading to still larger alliance arrangements. Others represent combinations that are displacing older arrangements. In the Oklahoma City example, a few years ago an alliance called Arrowhead brought together two Columbia/HCA hospitals, two Catholic hospitals, and three other non-system hospitals (as well as other hospitals located elsewhere in the state). Since joining Arrowhead, the Columbia/HCA cluster has joined the Oklahoma Health Network and the Catholic hospitals have formed another network that competes directly with the Oklahoma Health Network. As a result, Arrowhead has ceased to be a meaningful strategic alignment. This example highlights the evolutionary character of the SHA formation process. The rapid pace of system formation and re-formation among hospitals is producing a number of temporary arrangements that will evolve with time into newer, more permanent alliance arrangements.

All such maneuvering blurs the boundaries of many emerging hospital systems and networks, at least in the short term, as the more lasting strategic alignments continue to evolve. And yet almost daily, the boundaries are clarified; strategic partners are selected; and more stable, firmlike entities are created.

In the data, virtual firms are deemed to exist when two or more ownerships (multiple systems and/or independent hospitals) are involved in given SHAs. Firms are defined as single-owner combinations. As mentioned above, with respect to the expanded typology, only the configuration categories are measurable at this time. The dominant models include all firm SHAs and all unimodal virtual firms, the latter defined as multiple ownership SHAs in which one partner controls 70 percent or more of an SHA's bed capacity. The two diffuse models include all remaining virtual firm SHAs. Those that have only two ownerships are defined as bimodal, those with three or more as multimodal.

Table 3.1 provides examples of the configuration model types. A good example of a firm-type SHA is the cluster of 14 Columbia/HCA hospitals in the Houston MSA. Columbia has no reported partners in that area outside its owned hospitals. The dominant/virtual firm model in Table 3.1 is illustrated by the BJC Healthcare Network located in St Louis. The BJC Network actually extends well beyond the St Louis area, with over 20 hospital partners located outside St Louis but within the states of Missouri and Illinois. Within the metropolitan area, however, only one non-BJC hospital is currently a member of the network. BJC thus controls over 90 percent of the total capacity in that SHA.

Four SHAs illustrate the bimodal and multimodal virtual firm models in the table. Alliances in Denver and Jacksonville, Florida, offer clear examples of the bimodal model. In Denver, Columbia/HCA, with three hospitals, is in the process of assuming a 50 percent interest in the HealthOne system, which itself has four hospital facilities. Columbia's hospitals represent approximately 40 percent of the total capacity of the combined systems, indicating that the capacities of the two systems are relatively equal. In Jacksonville, Florida, two Daughters of Charity hospitals have entered into an "operational" merger with three Baptist Health System hospitals, producing a major new competitor for a cluster of Columbia/HCA hospitals also located in that area.

Finally, combinations in Kansas City and Chicago illustrate the multimodal/virtual firm model. In Kansas City, the Health Midwest system has long been a strong player and has recently added five independent hospitals to its Kansas City network.

Table 3.1 SHA Examples Using the Typology

Dominant		
Firm		
• Col/HCA	Houston	15 Hosps
Unimodal Virtual Firm		
• BIC Reg HC Net	St. Louis	10 Hosps
Diffuse		
Bimodal Virtual Firm		
• Col/HCA/Hlth One	Denver	7 Hosps
• Bapt/D of Charity	Jacksonville	5 Hosps
Multimodal Virtual Firm		
• Health Midwest	Kansas City	15 Hosps
• Northwest'n Hlthcare	Chicago	6 Hosps

Health Midwest controls around 55 percent of the total bed capacity of its urban network. The Northwestern Health System in Chicago is an example of a highly diverse combination of players. A total of six hospitals participate in this system, two of which are themselves merged. Each player in the Northwestern Health System has an equal voting position on policy and strategy decision making. Actually, Northwestern is one of four major multimodal combinations located in the Chicago market. This pattern of hospitals coming together to form large, virtual firm SHAs is common in many large midwestern and northeastern MSAs.

Table 3.2 summarizes the percentages of urban hospitals that are in SHAs and shows the percentages of those in SHAs that belong to the firm and virtual firm model types respectively. It also includes the percentages of SHAs by model type. So far, over half (53 percent) of urban hospitals are in SHAs. Of those in SHAs, 55 percent are in firms, the remainder in virtual firms. A total of 440 SHAs have been identified thus far, 63 percent of them in firm models.

Table 3.3 breaks down the SHA hospitals and SHAs by the four configuration model types. The average number of hospitals per SHA is also shown. As can be seen, the percentage of hospitals that are members of virtual firm SHAs varies somewhat, with the multimodal model having the highest percentage (20 percent) and the bimodal model the lowest (10 percent). The percentages of SHAs, by contrast, are nearly identical across the three virtual firm models, with each in the 12 to 13 percent range. The differences in percentages of hospitals versus SHAs is clearly attributable to the relative sizes of the SHAs in each category. As indicated, the multimodal models are the largest on average (5.4 hospitals per SHA) and the bimodal and firm models the smallest (2.8 and 2.9 hospitals per SHA respectively).

Table 3.2   Percentage of Urban Hospitals and SHAs in Firms and Virtual Firms

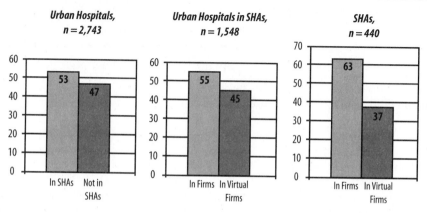

Table 3.3   Percentage of Urban Hospitals and SHAs and Number of Hospitals by Dominance Model

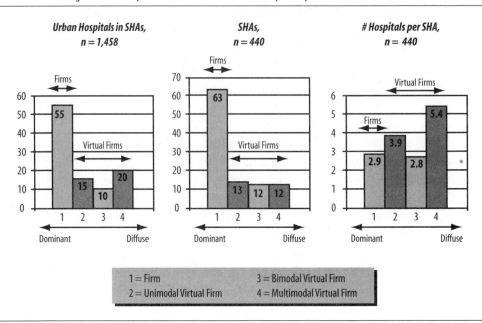

It is significant that according to the data, although the firm model is the most prevalent model type, a large number of hospitals have entered into the various virtual firm models. The largest percentage belong to the most diffuse model type, the multimodal virtual firm. As discussed earlier, it is not certain what the trends in model type will be in the short term. It is probable that some virtual firm SHAs will be transformed into firm models through mergers. Others will move in the opposite direction and break up, possibly reconfiguring into other SHAs. In addition, some of the firm models could partner with other systems and networks and/or with one or more unaligned hospitals in their area, resulting in a net increase in the numbers of virtual firm SHAs. It is reasonable to expect that if the markets remain turbulent for some years to come, especially with continued increases in managed care penetration, SHAs will shift toward tighter organizational forms to facilitate making the difficult strategic and operational decisions often required in highly competitive environments.

ᘒ IMPLICATIONS FOR ALLIANCES

A number of important implications can be derived from current trends in and patterns of SHA formation. These are perhaps best examined by exploring major decisions individual hospitals need to make, whether they are already in or are considering join-ing SHAs. Two decisions in particular should help to draw out some of the important implications:

1. *With which hospitals or SHA should a hospital affiliate?*
2. *How tightly coupled should the SHA be?*

The following sections discuss each of these questions in turn.

With Which Hospitals or SHA Should a Hospital Affiliate?

This question primarily addresses the issue of strategic interdependency, as identified in Figure 3.2. But given the unique requirements of loosely coupled organizations engaged in shared strategic effort, the likely comfort levels or compatibilities among potential partners must also be considered. This section explores both types of con-cerns as they relate to the choice of SHA partners.

Strategic interdependencies.   In entering an SHA, hospitals effectively place their long-term survival in the hands of other hospitals—including, sometimes, their closest rivals. As a result, they must to some degree be willing to sacrifice individual for col-lective strategic objectives. Few decisions for a hospital could be so important or have such far-reaching effects as choosing to become strategically interdependent by align-ing with other hospitals within an SHA.

Partner choices, of course, are limited by the number of other hospitals located in a given geographic area. Most markets contain only a small number of hospitals and, thus, few prospective partners with which to align. Seventy-seven percent of urban markets contain ten or fewer nonfederal, acute care general hospitals (Luke et al., 1995). And many of these are already in SHAs.

Also, in practice, not all of the available hospitals will constitute reasonable or fea-sible partners, thus reducing the number of real choices still further. It is essential, therefore, that hospitals carefully assess what few potential partners are available before making the critical decision to join an alliance. One consequence of a delayed decision, of course, is that desirable partners may pair off, leaving still fewer, possibly only suboptimal options. Choosing early has its drawbacks too, complicating even fur-ther the important decisions regarding alliance formation (e.g., partners chosen in one market context may become less desirable in light of changing market conditions).

Perhaps the most important criterion for the decision is the extent to which another hospital or a collective can help reduce strategic uncertainties in the environ-ment. Hospitals should therefore have a clear idea of what those uncertainties are and how they might best be addressed. They should also have a reasoned assessment of their own strategic capabilities and what additional capabilities they need (Badaracco, 1991). One important consideration is strategic purpose. A good partner for one purpose, say, to enter a joint venture in developing a women's pavilion, might not be so ideal if the purpose was to create a metropolitanwide network to compete for managed care contracts (in effect, to create an SHA).

The Porter (1980) model, introduced in Figure 3.3, provides an excellent framework for examining threats and uncertainties in markets. One of the most important forces identified by Porter is the threat of competitors. The degree of competitor threat is related to a number of factors, but particularly to the number of rivals in a market. Many hospital markets are oligopolistic, which means that only a small number of highly interactive rivals compete directly with one another. The choice of partners is especially important in oligopolistic markets. It represents not only a move to counteract the threats of existing rivals but also a defense against further consolidations among such rivals, which would create still fewer and more powerful competitors.

It should be remembered that when a hospital attempts to resolve uncertainties by aligning with other hospitals in a local market, the risks of violating antitrust regulations rise. Although many networks and mergers have passed antitrust scrutiny in recent years, there is still no guarantee that any given combination will not be challenged. Thus, the choice of partners among competitors must be considered far more closely than most alliance or other business decisions. The process is fraught with legal loopholes and pitfalls that must be fully considered at all stages of the partner selection process.

Strategic uncertainty arises not just in relationships among hospitals and associated SHAs but from a wide variety of other sources as well. As suggested earlier, managed care organizations, large employers, Medicare, and Medicaid all pose significant threats on the buyer side. A hospital must worry, for example, about whether such buyers will continue to purchase services from it or switch to other providers or SHAs. Consequently, it must align with other hospitals that can complement, not merely duplicate, the services and locations of a given hospital. If primary care is a critical requirement for competing for managed care, the logical partners might be those that have strong primary care or referral networks. Also, a potential partner with a unique location or a distinctive service capacity might be a more valuable partner than one that does not enjoy a strong market position. SHAs are mutually supportive entities from which all parties must benefit. Thus, in deciding with whom to align, hospitals must first see in their partners the resources and capabilities they need to counteract market threats. In return, they too must have resources and capabilities that are valued by potential partners.

Hospitals or their SHAs can also face threats from suppliers. Considering supply-side threats, hospitals might need to assess the contribution potential partners bring to building critical mass, their ability to exercise internal purchasing and utilization controls, or even their compatibilities with group purchasing companies. Alternatively, supplier relationships could contribute to a hospital's ability to control costs and thereby to compete on price for managed care contracts.

Also, as indicated in Porter's framework, hospitals or their SHAs face threats from potential entrants into their markets. Such threats could be a source of uncertainty for entire hospitals or, possibly, particular services such as physical therapy or cardiology. Although few entirely new hospitals are now being started and organized, there are still many prospective new entrants into the SHA markets, from outside companies attempting to acquire new hospitals or existing SHAs or cross-town hospitals planning to open up new, competitive services. In the early 1990s, Columbia/HCA became a source of strategic uncertainty for thousands of hospitals throughout the United States because it threatened (and continues to threaten) to enter many markets through acquisition. In sum, hospitals must choose partners and SHAs that enable them to reduce strategic threats, whether actual or anticipated, that might come from new entrants into their markets.

Substitute products and services create further strategic uncertainties that could lead hospitals to align with others in their markets. Collective strategies offer a powerful defense against threats from substitutes. A response to substitutes, for example, might be to align with hospitals that enhance the range or quality of services offered, which, if coordinated in the context of a larger local system, might make it more difficult for substitute offerings by rivals to gain a foothold in the market. For example, a rival's sports medicine clinic might serve as a substitute service for a hospital's own orthopedic and physical therapy services. If the hospital were to align itself with other hospitals in the community, together they might deepen the range of services offered over the total continuum of health services and thereby ward off the threats of substitutes. Such added capability might also give an important competitive advantage to hospitals competing for the increasingly important managed care contracts.

In summary, the choices of strategic partners will be shaped by the strategic interdependencies that exist among hospitals. The key point is that hospitals must make this critical decision—with whom to align—with a view to finding partners that will help them reduce strategic uncertainties. SHAs, however, can often add advantages that exceed the mere sum of partner strengths and weaknesses. Nevertheless, partners must add their individual capabilities and resources to make an SHA strong.

Strategic Congruency.   Aside from reducing strategic uncertainties, the choice of partners must also take other factors into account. The small number of candidates in most markets makes it imperative to select compatible partners. The need for this may be even greater for SHAs that adopt the more loosely structured organizational forms.

Kanter (1994) observed that the selection of partners should be based on three factors. (1) The partners, or potential partners, should serve to reduce market threats and uncertainties. (2) There should be good chemistry—personal rapport—between the CEOs of partner organizations. (3) Partners should be compatible with regard to such aspects as history and experience, philosophy and values, and strategy and future aspirations. The first, of course, has already been discussed. This section considers the role of congruencies in values and other factors related to perspective and outlook.

A number of authors have emphasized the importance of shared commitment not only for holding alliances together but also as a basis for partner selection (Zajac and D'Aunno, 1994; Zuckerman and Kaluzny, 1991). Commitment is equated with shared vision, values, expectations, risks, strategies, and resources. It is important to assess potential partners candidly with respect to how compatible their institutions, medical staffs, and CEOs are with the alliance's intended values, mission, and so on (Trout, 1991). In conducting such an assessment, a hospital should ask how centralized, open, and innovative the prospective partners might be. What is their vision for the future, and how do they value such areas as technology, financing, marketing, and quality? Finally, can they be expected to yield the appropriate amount of control and autonomy necessary to serve collective interests?

Kaluzny and Zuckerman (1992) note that alliances often seek homogeneity among members with respect to mission, organizational type, service type, ownership, and size. Homogeneity in such areas can be expected to improve coordination and to help resolve differences in strategic objectives.

Among the many considerations relating to organizational perspectives, many consider trust the fundamental ingredient in both choosing partners and maintaining the stability of alliances over time (Badaracco, 1991; Powell, 1987). Trust is the glue of alliances. Conversely, lack of trust precipitously raises the probability that the alliance will either dissolve or adopt tighter organizational structures to sustain fragile relationships, especially in the case of strategic alliances in which collaborators are highly interdependent and must be able to resolve inherent conflicts between individual and collective interests. Because of this, hospitals must fully evaluate possible partners in terms of that most important but intangible ingredient, trust.

How Tightly Coupled Should the SHA Be?

Once hospitals agree to align, they must decide what structures will be used to unite them. As discussed earlier, Gillies et al. (1993) conceptualized three types of integration: clinical, physician-system, and functional. Clinical integration coordinates the health care services of SHAs; physician-system integration joins the interests of medical staff and the SHA; and functional integration brings together the financial, human resource, information, marketing, and other key support activities of SHAs. Kanter (1994), in her study of alliances in many industries, identified five types of integration: strategic, tactical, operational, interpersonal, and cultural.

As seen in Figure 3.2, the coupling of hospitals in SHAs can be viewed from two dimensions of structure: configuration and integration. The configuration of an alliance is conceptually analogous to Gillies et al.'s physician-system integration and Kanter's strategic integration in that each pertains to the involvement of partners in the strategic decision making and governance of the combined organizations. The integration dimension introduced in Figure 3.2 is consistent with the clinical and functional forms of Gillies et al. and the tactical, operational, interpersonal, and cultural integration of Kanter. Implications of the configuration and integration dimensions are discussed below.

Configuration.   Although alliances are often conceived of as democratic organizations whose partners possess relatively equal power (Zajac and D'Aunno, 1994), in fact their power can vary quite considerably. Differences in power can be attributed to many factors, such as relative size, possession and control of critical resources, level of investment, and prestige (Alexander and Morlock, 1994; Pfeffer and Salancik, 1978). In the development of the typology in this chapter, relative power was conceptualized in terms of size and measured as the proportion of bed capacity controlled by a given member within an SHA. If a partner had a disproportionate size (defined as 70 percent or more of the total capacity), the SHA was said to have a dominant configuration. If not, it was labeled as having a diffuse configuration (see Figure 3.4).

Configuration and integration are closely interrelated as dimensions differentiating SHAs. As argued earlier, the management structures of dominant partners are likely to obviate the need for SHAs to develop their own integrative mechanisms, given the lead role such partners are expected to play in both operational and strategic decision making. But in cases where the partners share power more equally, it is less likely that any one of them will take the lead; organizational structures to ensure coordination and control would then need to be put in place.

Differences in how dominant versus diffuse SHA configurations might achieve a unity of effort among participating members can perhaps best be characterized using terms discussed by Thompson (1967). In his analysis of interorganizational relationships, Thompson identified three mechanisms that might be used to facilitate cooperation. Two of these appear to have particular applicability to interrelationships within SHAs: coopting and coalescing. Coopting, which involves extracting support—in this case from partners within SHAs—entails building commitment more than designing mechanisms of control. Coalescing, on the other hand, involves greater interplay among cooperating organizations as well as greater attention to the development of coordinating mechanisms. Coopting implies asymmetry, with one side, probably a stronger partner, seeking to generate commitment on the part of other partners. Coalescing, by contrast, implies greater equality, the need for greater commitment, and the sacrifice of treasured autonomy and independence in the interests of the whole.

Coopting strategies are likely to be better suited to the dominant SHA configuration, coalescing strategies to the diffuse. Given the asymmetry in power between the dominant and more dependent partner(s), the dominant models will require less elaborate and formal approaches to gain cooperation. Cooptation allows the dominant organization to sacrifice only limited amounts of autonomy while including and involving smaller partners in decision making, thereby securing their cooperation. The diffuse models require more involved approaches to achieving cooperation, since no one partner has enough power to drive decisions or secure commitments. In such cases, coalescing strategies may be more appropriate.

Integration.   While SHA configuration is determined by the relative power of each member, integration must be created and managed. Because hospitals will seek to retain as much autonomy as they can, they will naturally attempt to minimize the mechanisms for interorganizational control within SHAs. But the degree to which they resist or support integration will depend directly on the level of strategic interdependency.

Two factors in particular should condition the drive toward integration. The first one is market structure. In markets that are only moderately threatening, for example, hospitals may give priority to autonomy over further integration with an SHA. However, in threatening markets, that is, those in which strategic and operational decisions may need to be made rapidly and firmly, effective integration may be viewed with greater openness.

The effect of market threats on members' willingness to become more tightly integrated within SHAs can be expected to vary according to how dependent they are on their SHAs. The higher the proportion of managed care revenues derived from SHAs, the more willing SHA members will be to strengthen interorganizational integrative mechanisms.

The effect of market forces can also be expected to vary by how an SHA is configured. In a dominant model, the increased market threat may have little effect on the perceived need to integrate. Indeed, further integration could be seen as a possible impediment to the ability of the dominant partner to respond. Kanter (1994) asserts that control by one partner or the existence of a clear command center can reduce conflicts and make alliances more manageable.

In the diffuse models, on the other hand, the need to implement integrative mechanisms may be directly related to the perceived threats in the market. However, the tightening of interorganizational coupling could interfere with individual organizational flexibility and innovativeness, which, if diminished, could weaken the ability of diffusely configured SHAs to respond within rapidly changing market environments. For example, in markets experiencing large annual increases in managed care penetration, unencumbered partners could find creative ways to reduce capacity and shift resources. However, had the partners agreed to significant integration within their SHA, their ability as individual institutions to adapt strategically might be restricted. But if collective action is needed, the lack of integration in loosely coupled models could become a major disadvantage. This drawback would be especially evident if rival SHAs were more integrated and could move collectively and more quickly in response to market changes.

Integration among SHA members can be accomplished using a variety of mechanisms and systems. More formal integrative mechanisms include specific resource commitments (e.g., assets, staff time and expertise, program participation), established policies, rules and procedures, reward and sanction systems, information systems, and a wide variety of interorganizational committee and administrative structures (Zuckerman, Kaluzny, and Ricketts, 1995; Kanter, 1994; Kaluzny and Zuckerman, 1992; Trout, 1991; Zuckerman and Kaluzny, 1991; Zuckerman and D'Aunno, 1990). As discussed earlier, the more informal mechanisms—those mechanisms that shape perspectives, attitudes, and commitment—can also be important. Formal and informal structures can be mutually reinforcing. Commitment, for example, can be enhanced by contributed equity, time, staff, and service (Kanter, 1994). Also, mechanisms for increasing communications and resolving conflicts will likely also raise existing levels of commitment and trust among alliance members (Zajac and D'Aunno, 1994).

Trust, as has been pointed out, is an integral, informal mechanism for assuring coordination and support. Powell (1987) points out that trust is often grounded in historical exchanges among partners. If prior interactions among partners have been positive and reliable, future interrelationships should be sustained by greater levels of trust. Present actions also contribute to feelings of trust among alliance members. Fairness by the alliance boards and managers in dealing with individual members' concerns should enhance trust and commitment and thus reduce the need for implementing more formal mechanisms of control (Trout, 1991).

Zuckerman, Kaluzny, and Ricketts (1995) note that higher levels of trust among member hospital CEOs can contribute significantly to achieving the goal of system integration. However, such trust alone is often insufficient, especially given rates of CEO turnover (Zajac and D'Aunno, 1994). Trust among staff at levels below the CEO can play a major role in facilitating integration within SHAs. It is also important to remember that strategies and programs are executed at lower levels within member institutions and need the support and commitment of all member organizations to be well implemented. Yet in many cases lower-level staff are not well informed about strategy, especially alliance strategy, which is often tightly wrapped in secrecy among small cadres of collaborating hospital leaders.

Lower-level staff might not accept, understand or even be aware of the alliance's goals and vision, and may actually see these as interfering with their jobs and autonomy. Kanter (1994) emphasizes that this is especially true when member organizations employ strong, independent professionals whose goals and incentives differ from those of their organization. She describes a hospital alliance that could not achieve its goals, and eventually dissolved, because the heads of the member hospitals had agreed to a plan and vision that the respective staffs did not share or support. It should be apparent that organizations need to consider how to bring lower-level personnel on board when important collective strategies and programs need to be fully implemented.

As an alliance expands, its heterogeneity is likely to increase, and the difficulty of securing trust and commitment at lower levels within the partner organizations could increase. The same might also be true as SHAs evolve through developmental stages and as more and more individuals at different levels of partnering organizations become involved (Kanter, 1994). All such personnel might not share the same kinds of chemistry or personal rapport achieved by their CEOs. Differences in operational and managerial styles and differences in roles and cultures could be exacerbated, leading to greater and greater mistrust and disrespect.

& SUMMARY AND CONCLUSIONS

This chapter has presented a typology of one of the most distinctive and important organizational forms to have emerged in this century—the strategic hospital alliance. The SHA is especially unusual in the degree to which its partners become strategically interdependent. Hospitals joining SHAs face the very difficult challenge of trading long-standing autonomies for strategic gains in an environment in which survival is increasingly determined by success in capturing managed care contracts. In effect, the SHAs become the new competitors or firms in the marketplace, displacing the individual hospitals and other providers that historically had traded services for fees.

Given the distinctiveness of SHAs, it is important to differentiate them from other types of alliances and to identify differences among them as well. The typology presented attempts to achieve both of these objectives. First, it offers two dimensions that differentiate among the full range of interorganizational alliances. The first dimension, strategic interdependency, distinguishes among alliances according to how much their members' survival depends on their success. The second, tightness of coupling, recognizes the significant differences that exist among SHAs in terms of the structures that bind them together. (SHAs were defined to include all hospital alliances in which the members share high levels of strategic interdependency, regardless of the tightness of coupling that unites them.)

These dimensions reveal two general alliance types: firms and virtual firms. Firms represent all SHA combinations in which the hospitals are members of the same multihospital system (as defined by ownership, contract management, lease, or sponsorship relationships). Virtual firms represent those SHAs in which two or more systems and/or individual hospitals are joined, indicating diversity in ownership across SHA members. The national data show that 53 percent of all urban hospitals are already in identifiable SHAs; of those in SHAs, 55 percent are in firm models and the remainder are in virtual firms.

Each of the two major dimensions can be broken into two subdimensions. Strategic interdependency varies by the magnitude of exchange between the member hospitals and their SHAs (defined by the breadth and depth of flows of patients and revenues) and the criticality of the relationship between those hospitals and the SHAs (defined by the actual and/or expected level of threat in the markets). The greater the flows of revenues and patients between the hospitals and their SHAs and the greater the perceived threat in the marketplace, the more strategically interdependent the member hospitals will be, the more they will be committed to collective rather than individual strategic objectives, and the more firmlike the SHA will become.

Tightness of coupling is also related to two subdimensions, namely, the degree of integration and the configuration of partners within the alliance. Integration includes those formal and informal mechanisms SHAs introduce to assure unity of effort among their members. Configuration represents the degree to which a single member might dominate the SHA (because of its relative size within it). Four configurational models have been identified, representing differences in the distributions of power (based on relative size) within the SHA. Two are defined as dominant models: the firm (in which there is only one power center) and a version of the virtual firm—a unimodal model (measured by one partner having 70 percent or more of the total SHA bed capacity). Two others are defined as diffuse models: the bimodal virtual firm (only two partners, neither of which has a dominant position) and the multimodal virtual firm (three or more partners, none of which has a dominant position).

Configuration is important, given its interrelationship with integration. In those models in which one member dominates the SHA, there may be far less need to construct formal mechanisms of control to achieve coordination at either the strategic or operational levels of the SHA. This is because the structures already present within the dominant member organization may substitute for those that would otherwise be created to meet the SHA's needs. Over half the hospitals that are members of SHAs belong to the firm model; the remainder are distributed fairly evenly across the other three, virtual firm types.

It is essential that students of health care organization understand more fully the diversity of organizational forms emerging in the health care field. There can be little doubt that providers, payers, suppliers, and even buyers are restructuring themselves in some very interesting ways, all so as to gain greater control over the rapidly growing industry of health care. And the consequences will be far-reaching. Not only will the changes have a major impact on the cost, quality, and accessibility of care, they will in many cases simply be irreversible.

Interestingly, no one individual or group appears to be in the driver's seat, steering this important process to its inexorable conclusion. Rather, many players are involved at many levels. It is therefore incumbent on all of them to become as knowledgeable as they can about the forms and implications of change and thereby, at least in some small way, help build the health care systems of the 21st century.

❧ REFERENCES

Alexander, J. A. and Morlock, L. L. (1994). Power and politics in health services organizations. In S. M. Shortell and A. D. Kaluzny (eds.), *Health Care Management: Organization Design and Behavior.* (pp. 274–293). Albany, NY: Delmar.

Astley, W. G., and Brahm, R. A. (1989). Organizational designs for post–industrial strategies: The role of interorganizational collaboration. In C. C. Snow (ed.), *Strategy, Organization Design, and Human Resource Management.* (pp. 233–270). Greenwich, CT: Jai Press Inc.

Badaracco, J. (1991). *The Knowledge Link: How Firms Compete Through Strategic Alliances.* Boston: Harvard Business School Press.

Coase, R. (1937). The nature of the firm. *Economica, 4,* 386–405.

Dess, G. G., Rasheed, A. M. A., McLaughlin, K. J., and Priem, R. L. (1995). The new corporate architecture. *Academy of Management Executive, 9,* 7–20.

DeVries, R. A. (1978). Strength in Numbers. *Hospitals, 52,* 81–84.

Eccles, R. G. (1981). The quasi-firm in the construction industry. *Journal of Economic Behavior and Organization, 2,* 335–357.

Galbraith, J. K. (1952). *American Capitalism: The Concept of Countervailing Power.* Boston: Houghton Mifflin.

Ghemawat, P., Porter, M. E., and Rawlinson, R. A. (1986). Patterns of international coalition activity. In Michael E. Porter (ed.) *Competition in Global Industries* (pp. 345–365). Boston: Harvard Business School Press.

Gillies, R. R., Shortell, S. M., Anderson, D. A., Mitchell, J. B. and Morgan, K. L. (1993). Conceptualizing and measuring integration: Findings from the health systems integration study. *Hospital and Health Services Administration, 38,* 467–489.

Goldstein, D. (1995). Life after PHOs: MSOs take center stage. *Medical Interface: The Journal for the Managed Health Care Industry, 8,* 59–65.

Gray, B. H. (ed.). (1986). *For-Profit Enterprise in Health Care.* Washington, DC: National Academy Press.

Harrigan, K. R. (1985). *Strategic Flexibility: A Management Guide for Changing Times.* Lexington, MA: Lexington Books.

Kaluzny, A. D., and Zuckerman, H. S. (1992). Strategic Alliances: Two perspectives for understanding their effects on health services. *Hospital and Health Services Administration, 37,* 477–490.

Kanter, R. B. (1994). Collaborative advantage: The art of alliances. *Harvard Business Review, 72,* 96–108.

Kotabe, M., and Swan, K. S. (1995). The role of strategic alliances in high technology new product development. *Strategic Management Journal, 16,* 621–636.

Longest, B. B., (1990). Inter-organizational linkages in the health care sector. *Health Care Management Review, 15,* 17–28.

Luke, R. D., Begun, J. W., and Pointer, D. D. (1989). Quasi firms: Strategic interorganizational forms in the health care industry. *Academy of Management Review, 14,* 9–19.

Luke, R. D. and Begun J. W. (1988). Strategic orientations of small multihospital systems. *Health Services Research, 23,* 597–618.

Luke, R. D. and Olden, P. C. (1995). Foundations of market restructuring: Local hospital clusters and HMO infiltration. *Medical Interface, 8* (9), 71–75.

Luke, R. D., Rossiter, L. F., Swisher, K. N., and Bramble, J. D. (1995). *National Forum for the Study of Local Hospital Systems and Networks—1994–1995 Annual Report.* Richmond: Williamson Institute for Health Studies, Medical College of Virginia Campus of the Virginia Commonwealth University.

Murphy, T. M. and Harding, C. T. (1994). *Hospital-Physician Integration: Strategies for Success.* Chicago: American Hospital Publishing Inc.

Pfeffer, J., and Salancik, G. R. (1978). *The External Control of Organizations.* New York: Harper & Row.

Porter, M. E. (1980). *Competitive Strategy: Techniques for Analyzing Industries and Competitors.* New York: Free Press.

Powell, W. W. (1987). Hybrid organizational arrangements: New form or transitional development? *California Management Review, 30,* 67–87.

Powell, W. W. (1990). Neither market nor hierarchy: Network forms of organization. In B. M. Straw and L. L. Cummings (eds.), *Research in Organizational Behavior.* (pp. 295–336). Greenwich, CT: Jai Press Inc.

Provan, K. G. (1983). The federation as an interorganizational linkage network. *Academy of Management Review, 8,* 79–89.

Scott, L. (1995). U. of Minn. hospital seeks shelter from managed care. *Modern Healthcare, 45* (28), 20.

Shortell, S. M. (1988). The evolution of hospital systems: Unfulfilled promises and self-fulfilling prophesies. *Medical Care Review, 45,* 177–214.

Shortell, S. M., Gillies, R. R., Anderson, D. A., Mitchell, J. B., and Morgan, K. L. (1993). Creating organized delivery systems: The barriers and facilitators. *Hospital and Health Services Administration, 38,* 447–466.

Thompson, J. D. (1967). *Organizations in action.* New York: McGraw-Hill.

Trout, M. E. (1991). Managing alliances. *Frontiers of Health Services Management, 7,* 32–34.

Zajac, E. J., and D'Aunno, T. A. (1994). Managing strategic alliances. In S. M. Shortell and A. D. Kaluzny (eds.), *Health Care Management: Organization Design and Behavior.* (pp. 274–293). Albany, NY: Delmar.

Zuckerman, H. S., and D'Aunno, T. A. (1990). Hospital alliances: Cooperative strategy in a competitive environment. *Health Care Management Review, 15,* 21–30.

Zuckerman, H. S., and Kaluzny, A. D. (1991). Strategic alliances in health care: The challenges of cooperation. *Frontiers of Health Services Management, 7,* 3–23.

Zuckerman, H. S., Kaluzny, A. D., and Ricketts, T. C., III. (1995). Alliances in health care: What we know, what we think we know, and what we should know. *Health Care Management Review, 20,* 54–64.

Strategic Management

4

Peter M. Ginter, University of Alabama at Birmingham
Linda E. Swayne, University of North Carolina at Charlotte
W. Jack Duncan, University of Alabama at Birmingham

H ealth care managers may assume with confidence that during the last half of the 1990s they will have to guide their organizations through more change than at any previous time. Change has become so rapid, so complex, so turbulent, and so unpredictable that it is sometimes called simply *chaos* or *white water change*.[1] Health care managers will have to cope with this type of change and position their organizations to take advantage of emerging opportunities while avoiding external threats. Strategic management can help health care managers cope with both anticipated and white water change.

≈ THE NATURE OF STRATEGIC MANAGEMENT

Strategic management has become a major thrust guiding all types of contemporary organizations. In the United States more than 97 percent of the top 100 industrial companies and more than 92 percent of the top 1,000 industrial companies report the existence of corporate strategic planning efforts.[2] Business has embraced strategic management as a way to anticipate and cope with a variety of external forces beyond its operating control.

The environmental uncertainties and competitive pressures that have moved business organizations to adopt strategic management now beset health care organizations. Indeed, health care has become a complex business that uses many of the same processes and much of the same language as the most sophisticated business corporations.

The Benefits of Strategic Management

Strategic management is a philosophy or way of managing an organization; therefore, the benefits of strategic management are not always quantifiable. Strategic management ties the organization together with a common sense of purpose and shared values. It enables the organization to develop a clear self-concept, specific goals, and consistency in decision making. It is a unique perspective that requires managers to cease thinking solely in terms of internal operations and adopt what may be a fundamentally new attitude, an *external* orientation. Strategic management is basically optimistic in that it integrates "what is" with "what can be." It is the exciting future of effective health care management.

The Foundations of Strategic Management

The English word *strategy* comes from the Greek *strategos*, meaning "a general," which is in turn derived from roots that mean "army" and "lead."[3] The Greek verb *stratego* means "to plan the destruction of one's enemies through effective use of resources."[4] As a result, many of the terms commonly used in relation to strategy—"objectives," "mission," "strengths," "weaknesses"—were developed by the military.

Over the past 50 years, strategic management has been developed primarily in the business sector; the 1960s and 1970s were a time of major growth for strategic planning. Strategic management concepts have been applied in health care organizations only in the past 20 to 25 years. Prior to 1970, individual health care organizations had few incentives to employ strategic management because most of them were independent, freestanding, not-for-profit institutions, and health services reimbursement was on a cost-plus basis.

Although substantial *health policy* planning has been undertaken in the United States, *strategic planning* is specific to an individual organization. Strategic planning helps the organization respond to state and federal policy and planning efforts, as well as to a variety of other external forces. The major differences between strategic planning and other forms of health planning are that strategic planning

- is a market-driven and market-based approach;
- emphasizes qualitative rather than quantitative analysis;

- places the development of strategic plans under the direct control of the chief executive officer with delegation;
- requires the strategy to be clearly stated and persuasively communicated throughout the institution;
- creates final planning goals, objectives, and programs that must be vigorously implemented;
- requires middle management to be carefully prepared to engage in strategic planning;
- emphasizes data collection and analysis for the "nuts and bolts" of the health institution's business;
- must be integrated with other management functions; and
- places a strong focus on gaining and sustaining a competitive advantage.[5]

Strategic Thinking

For a number of reasons, health care organizations today place increasing emphasis on the scientific analysis of managerial decisions. First, rapid environmental change from diverse sources requires the manager to identify and monitor the systems that are likely to affect the organization. Second, the health care manager strives to achieve overall organizational effectiveness and avoid allowing the parochial interests of one organizational element to distort overall performance. Third, the strategic manager must act in an organizational environment that invariably involves conflicting organizational objectives.[6] In a strategic context this process is sometimes called *strategic thinking*.

Strategic thinkers built and continue to build the health care systems that will serve major metropolitan and rural areas during the next 50 years. Strategic thinkers are visionaries. They know what they want to become and what they want their organizations to be. Strategic thinkers look at assumptions, understand system interrelationships, create scenarios, and calculate the odds. They forecast external technological and demographic changes, as well as critical changes in the political and regulatory arenas. Planners, on the other hand, Figure out how to get where the strategic thinkers want to go. A planner gathers and evaluates data and tells the strategic thinker what it will take to achieve an objective.[7]

❧ WHAT IS STRATEGIC MANAGEMENT?

In understanding strategic management, it is useful to define *strategy* and *strategic planning*. Although these terms are often used interchangeably with strategic management, each has a distinct meaning.

Strategy and Strategic Planning

The term *strategy* has three related meanings or usages common in health care management. Consistency is the central theme linking the three usages of the term. First, a strategy may be viewed as a pattern that emerges in a stream of decisions concerning the positioning of the organization within its environment. In other words, when a sequence of decisions relating the organization to its environment exhibits a logical consistency over time, a strategy will have been formed.[8]

Second, in a broader context, as illustrated in Figure 4.1, strategy may be viewed as the "behavior" of the organization. The forces in the external environment influence

Figure 4.1   Strategy as a Behavior of the Organization

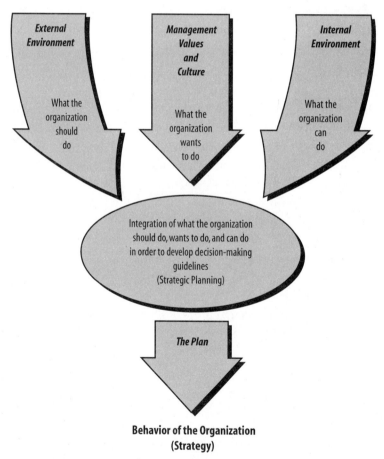

Source: Adapted from Fred Luthans, Richard M. Hodgetts, and Kenneth R. Thompson, *Social Issues in Business: Strategic and Public Policy Perspectives,* 5th ed. (New York: Macmillan Publishing Company, 1987), p. 12.

the strategic behaviors of the organization and suggest "what the organization *should* do." Strategic behavior is additionally influenced by the internal capabilities of the organization and represents "what the organization *can* do." The consistency of the behavior is "driven" by a set of common organizational values and goals. These values and goals are often the result of considerable analysis by top management and indicate "what the organization *wants* to do."

When management considers all of these forces and develops a series of consistent top-level decisions, the organization has a strategy. Only when there is consistency is there a strategy. When there is a formal planning process, decision consistency is born of extensive situational analysis.

Third, strategy may be viewed as a set of guidelines or a plan that will help assure consistency in decision making to move an organization from where it is today to a desired state some time in the future. Strategic plans indicate what types of decisions are appropriate or inappropriate for an organization. Strategy links management's understanding of the organization today with where it wants, can, and should be at some well-defined point in the future. The organizational process for identifying the desired future and developing decision guidelines is called *strategic planning*. Thus, the result of the strategic planning process is a plan or strategy.

Strategic Management

Although sometimes used interchangeably, the term *strategic management* is broader than strategy or strategic planning. *Strategic management* is an externally oriented philosophy of managing an organization that links strategic planning to operational decision making. Strategic management attempts to achieve a fit between the organization's external environment (political, regulatory, economic, technological, social, and competitive forces) and its internal situation (vision, values, culture, finance, organization, human resources, marketing, information systems, and so on).

Strategic management is based on the belief that organizations should continually monitor internal and external events and trends so that timely changes can be made. Strategic managers constantly relate the organization to its external environment, not just to assure compatibility and survival, but also to understand the environmental trends well enough to "create the future." Strategic managers successfully anticipate the future, positioning their organizations to be in the right place at the right time with the right products and services.

❧ THE CHARACTERISTICS OF STRATEGIC DECISIONS

Strategic management is, in large part, a decision-making activity. The strategy of an organization is the result of a series of managerial decisions. Although these decisions are often supported by a great deal of quantifiable data, strategic decisions are fundamentally judgmental. Generally, the more important the decision, the less quantifiable it is and the more we will have to rely on the opinions of others and our own best judgment.

The Attributes of Strategic Decisions

The mere fact that a decision is important to the success of an organization does not mean that it is necessarily a strategic decision. For a decision to be strategic it must meet all of the following characteristics. The decision must

- Be directed toward defining the organization's relationship to its environment.
- Take the organization as a whole as the unit of analysis.
- Be multifunctional in character, that is, it must depend on inputs from a variety of functional areas.
- Provide direction for, and constraints on, administrative and operational activities throughout the enterprise.
- Be important to the success of the enterprise.[9]

Types of Strategic Decisions

Considering the characteristics of strategic decisions, Robert C. Shirley has identified the following seven decision areas that are strategic in nature and accomplish the overall function of formulating the strategy:

- **Mission:** the fundamental purpose and broad aims of the organization.
- **Customer mix:** the specific target market(s) to be served by the organization.
- **Product mix:** the specific products or services to be offered by the organization in order to serve the needs of the target market.
- **Service area:** the geographic service area determined by the physical boundaries established for the organization's activities.
- **Goals and objectives:** the specific end results that the organization is seeking to accomplish.
- **Competitive advantage:** the means by which the organization seeks to differentiate itself from other organizations in the same industry or across industries.
- **Outside relationships:** relationships with government, suppliers, financing sources, and other major constituencies and interest groups.[10]

Once an organization has made decisions in these seven areas, it has defined the scope of its operations, mapped its future direction, and stated its overall relationship to its environment in terms of product/market scope, geographic boundaries, competition, and goals and objectives. In short, the organization has developed its strategy.

The Responsibility for Strategic Decisions

Strategic decision making is the responsibility of top management. The chief executive officer (CEO) of any health care organization is a strategic manager with the ultimate responsibility for positioning the organization for the future. If the CEO does not fully understand or support strategic management, it will not happen.

In the past, formulation of the strategy was primarily a staff activity. The planning staff would formulate the strategy and submit it for approval to top management. This process resulted in plans that were often unrealistic or did not fully consider the realities and resources of the divisions or functional departments. However, over the past decade, many large formal planning staffs have been dissolved as organizations learned that strategy development cannot take place in relative isolation. Today, the *coordination* and *facilitation* of strategic planning is typically designated as the responsibility of a key manager (often the CEO), whereas *development* of strategy has become a line job, with each manager responsible for the strategic implications of his or her decisions. The rationale underlying this approach is that no one is more in touch with the external environment (regulations, technology, competition, social change, and so on) than the line manager who must deal with it every day; however, someone must coordinate the organization's overall strategy and facilitate strategic thinking throughout the organization. As a result, the strategic planner acts as an extension of the CEO to ensure that an organized planning process is developed and used.[11] In organizations that have seriously adopted strategic management, all managers are strategic managers. As part of the job, every manager must be concerned with change and innovation. Each must ask critical questions: "Should we be doing this in the future?" "How should we be doing this?" "What new things should we be doing?"

🏵 A MODEL OF THE STRATEGIC MANAGEMENT PROCESS

A model of the strategic management process that illustrates and organizes the major components for health care organizations is presented in Figure 4.2. The model represents a clear and practical approach to understanding the setting (the external environment) for health care as well as the organization itself. As portrayed in the model, managers engage in several strategic processes—situational analysis,

Figure 4.2   The Strategic Management Process in Health Care Organizations

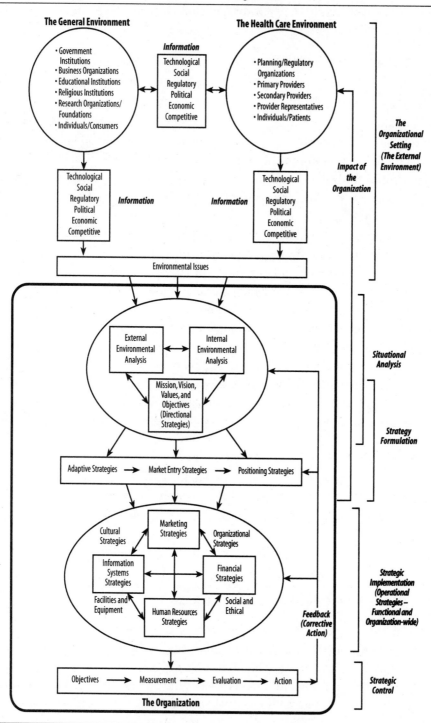

strategy formulation, strategic implementation, and strategic control—to position the organization best within the external environment and implement a strategy that will help assure success. Strategy is deliberate, carefully considered, and tightly reasoned.[12]

The Organizational Setting

The external environment exerts a powerful influence on the organization and may be referred to as the organizational setting. Conceptually, the setting may be viewed as being made up of the broader *general environment* and the more specific *health care environment* or health care industry. As indicated in the model, these environments affect each other as well as directly affecting the organization.

The General Environment. The general environment comprises all organizations and individuals outside the health care industry. Such organizations may include government institutions, business organizations, educational institutions, religious institutions, research organizations and foundations, and individuals and consumers.

Organizations and individuals in the general environment, acting alone or in concert with others, initiate and foster changes within society. These organizations and individuals generate technological, social, regulatory, political, economic, and competitive information that will in the long run affect many different industries (including health care), and perhaps the organization itself directly. Thus, external organizations, engaged in their own processes and pursuing their own missions, are developing new information that will affect other industries, organizations, and individuals.

The Health Care Environment. The health care environment concerns information generated within the health care industry. Obviously, this information more directly and immediately affects other health care organizations. The variety of organizations within health care defies easy categorization. However, the health care system generally may be grouped into the five segments shown in Figure 4.2.[13]

Organizations and individuals within the health care environment develop and employ new technologies, deal with changing social issues, address political change, develop and comply with regulations, compete with other health care organizations, and participate in the health care economy. Therefore, strategic managers should view the health care environment with the goal of understanding the nature of technological, social, regulatory, political, economic, and competitive changes. Focusing attention on these major areas of change (information flows) facilitates the early identification and analysis of industry-specific environmental issues that will affect the organization. This process is often referred to as "industry analysis." Industry analysis has been extremely important to health care managers as they chart the growth of integrated hospital systems and the changing nature of competition.

🖎 SITUATIONAL ANALYSIS

Analyzing and understanding the situation is accomplished by three separate processes: (1) external environmental analysis; (2) internal environmental analysis; and (3) the development of the organization's mission, vision, values, and objectives. It is the interaction and results of these processes that form the basis for the development of strategy.

External Environmental Analysis

To operate in today's changing environment, managers of health care organizations need a method for scanning external information that will affect the organization. This process is referred to as external environmental analysis. As information is accumulated and classified, managers must determine the *environmental issues* that are significant to the organization. They must also monitor these issues, collect additional information, evaluate their impact, and incorporate them into a strategy.

The Goals of Environmental Analysis.   Although the overall intent of environmental analysis is to position the organization within its environment, more specific goals may be identified. The specific goals of environmental analysis include the following:

1. To classify and order information flows generated by outside organizations.
2. To identify and analyze *current* important issues that will affect the organization.
3. To detect and analyze the weak signals of *emerging* issues that will affect the organization.
4. To speculate on the *likely* future issues that will have significant impact on the organization.
5. To provide organized information for the development of the organization's mission, vision, values, objectives, internal analysis, and strategy.
6. To foster strategic thinking throughout the organization.

The Process of Environmental Analysis.   There are a variety of approaches to conducting an environmental analysis. Regardless of the approach, four fundamental processes appear to be common to all environmental analysis efforts, as illustrated in Figure 4.3.

Figure 4.3   The Environmental Analysis Process

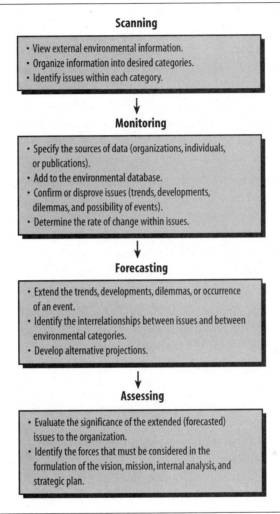

Scanning

- View external environmental information.
- Organize information into desired categories.
- Identify issues within each category.

↓

Monitoring

- Specify the sources of data (organizations, individuals, or publications).
- Add to the environmental database.
- Confirm or disprove issues (trends, developments, dilemmas, and possibility of events).
- Determine the rate of change within issues.

↓

Forecasting

- Extend the trends, developments, dilemmas, or occurrence of an event.
- Identify the interrelationships between issues and between environmental categories.
- Develop alternative projections.

↓

Assessing

- Evaluate the significance of the extended (forecasted) issues to the organization.
- Identify the forces that must be considered in the formulation of the vision, mission, internal analysis, and strategic plan.

The four processes include (1) scanning to identify signals of environmental change, (2) monitoring identified issues, (3) forecasting the future direction of the issues, and (4) assessing the organizational implications of the issues.[14]

External environmental analysis is the process by which an organization crosses the boundary between itself and the external environment in order to identify and understand changes (issues) that are taking place outside the organization. These changes will represent both *opportunities* and *threats* to the organization and may emanate from either the general environment or the health care environment. It is important for health care managers to understand the nature of these opportunities and threats well before they affect the organization. Opportunities and threats should influence the strategy adopted by the organization, that is, what the organization *should* do.

Selecting the Technique.   The intent of environmental analysis is to identify and understand the issues in the external environment. Figure 4.4 summarizes the primary focus as well as advantages and disadvantages of several environmental analysis techniques.

The technique selected for environmental analysis will depend on such factors as the size of the organization, the diversity of the products and services, and the complexity and size of the markets (service areas). Organizations that are relatively small, do not have a great deal of diversity, and have well-defined service areas may opt for simple techniques that may be carried out "in house," such as trend identification and extension, in-house nominal group technique or brainstorming, stakeholder analysis, critical success factor analysis, or Porter's structural analysis. Such organizations may include independent hospitals, HMOs, rural and community hospitals, large group practices, long-term care facilities, hospices, and county public health departments.

Health care organizations that are large, have diverse products and services, and have ill-defined or extensive service areas may want to use techniques that draw upon the knowledge of a wide range of experts. As a result, these organizations are more likely to set up Delphi panels and outside nominal and brainstorming groups. In addition, these organizations may have the resources to conduct dialectics concerning environmental issues, engage in scenario writing, and study the diffusion process. Such techniques are usually time-consuming, cost a good deal, and require extensive coordination. Organizations using these techniques may include national and regional for-profit health care chains, regional health systems, large federations and alliances, and state public health departments. (For an extensive review of these techniques see Ginter, Swayne, and Duncan *Strategic Management of Health Care Organizations 3e*, Malden, MA: Blackwell Publishers, 1998.)

Internal Environmental Analysis

The organization itself has an internal environment that represents the capabilities of the organization (what the organization *can* do). An understanding of the organization's capabilities requires an extensive, in-depth analysis of the internal functions, operations, structure, resources, and skills. An internal environmental analysis should reveal the *strengths* and *weaknesses* of the organization—its strategic capabilities. An understanding of the strengths and weaknesses provides a foundation for strategy formulation and is essential if a strategy is to be developed that optimizes and takes advantage of strengths and de-emphasizes and overcomes weaknesses. A process

Figure 4.4   Primary Focus, Advantages, and Disadvantages of Environmental Analysis Techniques

Technique	Primary Focus	Advantage	Disadvantage
Simple Trend Identification and Extension	Scanning Monitoring Forecasting Assessing	• Simple • Logical • Easy to communicate	• Needs a good deal of data in order to extend trend • Limited to existing trends • Does not foster creative thinking
Delphi Technique	Scanning Monitoring Forecasting Assessing	• Use of field experts • Avoids intimidation problems • Eliminates management's biases	• Members physically dispersed • No direct interaction of participants • May take a long time to complete
Nominal Group Technique	Scanning Monitoring Forecasting Assessing	• Gives everyone equal status and power	• Structure that may limit creativity
Brainstorming	Forecasting Assessing	• Fosters creativity • Develops many ideas, alternatives • Encourages communication	• No process for making decisions • Sometimes gets off track
Focus Groups	Forecasting Assessing	• Uses experts • Management/expert interaction	• Finding experts • No specific structure for reaching conclusion
Dialectic Inquiry	Forecasting Assessing	• Surfaces many subissues and factors • Allows conclusions to be reached on issues	• Does not provide a set of procedures for deciding what is important • Considers only a single issue at a time • Time-consuming
Stakeholder Analysis	Scanning Monitoring	• Considers major independent groups and individuals • Assures major needs and wants of outside organizations are taken into account	• May not consider emerging issues generated by other organizations • Does not consider the broader issues of the general environment
Critical Success Factor Analysis	Scanning Forecasting Assessing	• Identifies the factors for success • Directly links external factors with objectives and strategies	• Does not consider emerging trends or issues • Does not consider events in the broader general environment
Scenario Writing	Forecasting Assessing	• Portrays alternative futures • Considers interrelated external variables • Gives a complete picture of the future	• Requires generous assumptions • Always a question as to what to include
Porter's Industry Structure Analysis	Scanning Monitoring Forecasting Assessing	• Provides a structured analysis • Provides an extensive checklist of issues	• Does not consider the broader general environment • May be too structured to foster creative thinking
Diffusion Process	Scanning Monitoring	• Considers a broad range of issues • Emphasizes data collection • Systematic observation and plotting	• Not industry-specific • Little assessment

called an *internal audit* can be used to evaluate the various internal subsystems: (1) the clinical subsystem—physicians, nurses, respiratory therapists, and others directly involved in patient care, as well as groups providing direct support for patient care such as pharmacy, pathology, medical laboratories, and rehabilitation services—is the heart of the health care organization; (2) the marketing subsystem includes activities necessary to identify and deliver an adequate patient base for health care services; (3) the information systems subsystem collects and delivers information that is created both internally and externally; (4) the financial subsystem acquires and manages the financial resources needed for stability or growth; (5) the human resources subsystem consists of nonclinical personnel required to deliver health services effectively; (6) the general management subsystem includes the people, policies, and systems required to coordinate all functions; and (7) the physical facilities subsystem encompasses buildings, equipment, safety, housekeeping, and so on.

Estimating Strategic Capabilities.   Health care organizations must develop a means to assess internal strengths and weaknesses, but they can do this only in relation to the external environment. The task of identifying an organization's internal strengths and internal weaknesses is difficult, because strengths and weaknesses are both objective and subjective as well as absolute and relative. Some strengths possessed by a health care organization are clear by objective standards. For example, the mere presence of one organization in a particular location may provide it with a strategic strength that precludes any other organization from coming to that specific location. An example of an objective weakness is the health care organization that has used more debt financing for its facilities than its competitors.

At other times, a strategic strength or weakness may be subjective. Perhaps the administrator of a large hospital believes that her medical staff is superior to all others in the area. A look at the qualifications, specialties represented, and services provided, however, does not indicate any substantial differences among the competing hospitals. Despite this, the administrator "has a feeling" that "our staff is thought of as superior." Weaknesses can be subjective as well. The management team may regard the "philosophy" of the board of directors as more conservative than that of other organizations. As a result, they may characterize the board as "timid" when it comes to taking risks.

Sometimes organizational strengths and weaknesses are absolute, that is, almost everyone would agree that the strength or weakness identified is a strength or weakness. Finally, strengths and weaknesses may be relative. For example, one long-term care facility may have certain strengths, not in an absolute sense but relative to its competitors. One facility may have limited financial resources in comparison with national averages but considerably greater financial resources than any of its service area competitors.

Distinctive Competency and Comparative Advantage.   The process of understanding the opportunities and threats in the external environment and relating them to the organization's internal strengths and weaknesses enables strategic managers to determine the *distinctive competency* of the organization. Distinctive competency consists of a relatively small number of activities an organization is able to perform quite well. Health care managers need to think seriously about distinctive competency, especially as competition increases. What does our organization do better than anyone else? Depending on the environment, distinctive competency may or may not actually result in a *competitive advantage*, because other health care providers may possess similar attributes. Nevertheless, much of strategic management is a search for distinctive competency and ways to convert such competency into unique competitive advantages.

Mission, Vision, Values, and Objectives

The mission, vision, values, and objectives of an organization greatly affect which strategy it ultimately adopts. The organization's mission represents the consensus and articulation of its understanding of external opportunities and threats and internal strengths and weaknesses. It is a general statement of what distinguishes the organization from all others of its type and answers the questions, "Who are we?" and "What do we do?"

Components of Mission Statements.   There is no single way to develop and write mission statements. To capture the essence of an organization, its mission must highlight those elements that make it unique. Some of the more important components of mission statement include the following:

1. *Mission statements target customers and markets.* Frequently, the mission statement provides evidence of the kind of customers or patients the organization seeks to serve and the markets in which it intends to compete.
2. *Mission statements indicate the principal services delivered by the organization.* The mission should outline the primary services and products of the organization.
3. *Mission statements specify the geographical area (service area) within which the organization intends to concentrate.* This element is most frequently included when there is a regional aspect to the organization's service delivery.
4. *Mission statements identify the organization's philosophy.* Frequently, an organization's mission will include statements about unique beliefs, values, aspirations, and priorities.
5. *Mission statements include confirmation of the organization's preferred self-image.* The manner in which a health care organization views itself may constitute a uniqueness that should be included in the mission.

6. *Mission statements specify the organization's desired public image.* This component might manifest itself in statements such as the organization's desire to be a "good citizen" in the communities where operations are located or similar expressions of concern.

Not every one of the characteristics discussed can be included in a single mission statement; higher-performing organizations, however, generally have more comprehensive mission statements. Moreover, it appears that components such as organizational philosophy, self-concept, and desired public image are particularly associated with higher-performing organizations.

Characteristics of Effective Vision.   Vision, on the other hand, is that *view of the future* that management believes is optimal for the organization (hopefully based on an understanding of the external opportunities and threats and internal strengths and weaknesses) and is communicated throughout the organization. Vision profiles the future and constitutes what the organization *wants* to do.

A clear vision is simple. The driving forces of a vision should be basic directions and commitments, not complex analysis beyond the understanding of most employees. A vision is coherent when it "fits" with other statements, including mission and values. It is consistent when it is reflected in decision-making behavior throughout the organization. A vision "communicates" when it is shared and people believe in the importance of cooperation in creating the future that managers, employers, and other stakeholders desire.[15] Finally, to be meaningful, a vision must be flexible. The future is by definition uncertain. Therefore, the effective vision must remain open to change as the picture of the future changes and the strategic capabilities of the organization evolve over time.

Components of Vision Statement.   To outline the future effectively and facilitate the pursuit of organizational and individual excellence, visions should possess certain components:[16]

1. *Visions should be inspiring, not merely quantitative goals to be achieved in the next performance evaluation period.* In fact, visions are rarely stated in quantitative terms.

2. *Visions should be clear, challenging, and about excellence.* There must be no doubt in the manager's mind about the importance of the vision. If the "keeper of the vision" has doubts, those who follow will have even more.

3. *Vision must make sense in the relevant community, be flexible, and stand the test of time.* If the vision is pragmatically irrelevant, it will not inspire high performance.

4. *Visions must be stable but constantly challenged and changed when necessary.*

5. *Visions are beacons and controls when everything else seems up for grabs.* A vision is important to provide interested people with a sense of direction.

6. *Visions empower first our own people and then the clients, patients, or others we propose to serve.* The vision must first call forth the best efforts of our own people.

7. *Visions prepare for the future while honoring the past.* Effective visions always maintain a sense of where the organization has been and how its past influences where it can go.

8. *Visions come alive in details, not broad generalities.* Although inspirational visions are generally unconcerned with details, the accomplishment of the vision must eventually lead to tangible results.

Characteristics of Values. The values of an organization are the fundamental beliefs or "truths" that the organization holds dear. Values are the best indicator of the philosophy of the organization and specify what is important (honesty, integrity, customers, and so on) in the organization. Values are sometimes referred to as guiding principles.

Core values, beliefs, and philosophy seem to be clear during the early stages of an organization's development and become less clear as the organization matures.[17] Although values may certainly change over time, it is important, as with mission and vision statements, for organizations to reexamine their values, reaffirm them, change them, communicate them, and perhaps commit them to writing for all to see.

Strategic Objectives. The objectives of the organization broadly specify the major direction of the organization and link the mission to organizational action. Whereas well-developed missions are abstract and provide general direction, strategic objectives are specific and to the point. Strategic objectives should possess the following characteristics:

1. Objectives should be as *explicit* and as *measurable* as possible. Objectives should reflect organizational priorities so as to help managers make decisions with regard to the distribution of resources.[18]

2. Objectives should be *attainable*—challenging yet achievable. Objectives are motivational only if they are feasible.

3. Objectives should *relate to the key performance areas* identified by management. Because managers are often tempted to set more objectives than they can properly attend to, it is a good idea to restrict the number of strategic objectives to two or three for each key performance area.

4. Objectives should be *written.* There should be no confusion about what is to be accomplished, by what date, by whom, and with what resources.

As a practical matter, few things are more essential for effective management than carefully established and communicated objectives. In addition to all the other benefits, precise and understood objectives are effective motivators of performance. They focus the attention of employees on important factors, regulate how hard a person actually works, and increase an individual's resolve and persistence.[19]

ᴢ▲ Strategy Formulation

Decisions concerning the five types of strategies that make up the strategy formulation process—directional, adaptive, market entry, positioning, and operational—must be made sequentially; and each subsequent decision must define more specifically the activities of the organization. That is, directional strategies must be developed first, followed by adaptive strategies and then market entry strategies. Next, the products or services are introduced or reintroduced to the market in such a way as to be different from (or similar to) competitive products (positioning strategies); and finally, specific functional and organization-wide action plans are developed (operational strategies). The decision logic for strategy formulation is illustrated in Figure 4.5. Figure 4.6 summarizes the scope and role for the five strategy types.

Directional Strategies

Mission, vision, values, and objectives—the directional strategies—are a part of both situational analysis and strategy formulation. They are included in the strategy formulation process as well as in situational analysis because they are decision-making activities that set the broad direction for the organization. Directional strategies provide the basic philosophy of the organization.

Adaptive, Market Entry, and Positioning Alternatives

Figure 4.7 presents a comprehensive schematic or map of the hierarchy of strategic alternatives. Strategy development should be viewed as a process of evaluating and selecting from various alternatives. The map not only identifies the alternatives but also the sequential relationships among the strategies. Figure 4.8 presents a definition and example of the adaptive strategic alternatives.

These strategic decisions explicitly answer the questions, "What business(es) are we in?" "What business(es) should we be in?" "How are we going to compete?" At this point the broad organizational strategies have been selected. In addition, the strategic decisions previously outlined—mission, customer mix, product/service mix,

Figure 4.5   The Decision Logic of Strategy Formulation

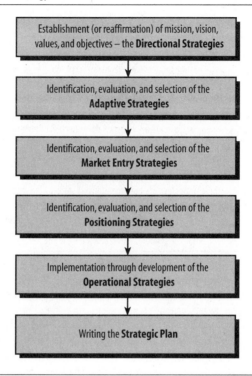

service areas, goals and objectives, competitive advantage, and outside relationships—will have been made.

Evaluation of the Strategic Alternatives

The methods for evaluating and selecting strategic alternatives are actually constructs or frameworks for helping managers think about the organization and its relative situation. These constructs allow health care managers to consciously balance organizational motives with community health needs. However, none of the methods provides a definitive answer to the question of appropriate strategy. None *makes* the strategic choice. Rather, the methods categorize and demonstrate the relationships inherent in the situation. The various methods help to structure the thought processes of decision makers.

Although the evaluation methods fine-tune the manager's perspective and organize thinking, ultimately the manager must make the decision. Managers need to

Figure 4.6   Scope and Role of Strategy Types in Strategy Formulation

Strategy	Scope and Role
Directional Strategies	The broadest strategies set the fundamental direction of the organization by establishing a mission for the organization (Who are we?) and providing a vision for the future (What should we be?). These strategies create an understanding of the philosophy or values and set benchmarks for success—objectives.
Adaptive Strategies	These strategies are more specific than directional strategies and provide the primary methods for achieving the vision of the organization. They delineate how the organization will expand, contract, or stabilize operations.
Market Entry Strategies	These strategies carry out expansion and stabilization strategies through purchase, cooperation, or internal development. They provide methods for access or entry to the market. Market entry strategies are not normally necessary for contraction strategies.
Positioning Strategies	These strategies position the organization vis-à-vis other organizations within the market. These strategies are market-oriented and best articulate the competitive advantage within the market. These strategies may be market-wide or directed to particular market segments.
Operational Strategies	The most specific strategies are developed for the functional areas (marketing, finance, information systems, human resources, and so on) and for the entire organization. Organization-wide strategies include culture, organization, facilities and equipment, ethics and social responsibility, and so on. In combination, these actions must accomplish the positioning, market entry, adaptive, and directional strategies.

understand the risks, make judgments, and commit the organization to some course of action. Thus, the evaluation methods cannot be used to obtain "answers" but rather to gain perspective and insight into a complex relationship between organization and environment. There is no right answer.

Evaluation of the Adaptive Strategies

The adaptive strategies specify how the organization will expand (diversification, vertical integration, market development, product development, or penetration), contract (divestiture, liquidation, harvesting, or retrenchment), or stabilize (enhancement or status quo) its operations. Adaptive strategies may be based on the organization's relative competitive advantage, financial strength, industry strength, and

Figure 4.7 Hierarchy of Strategic Decisions and Alternatives

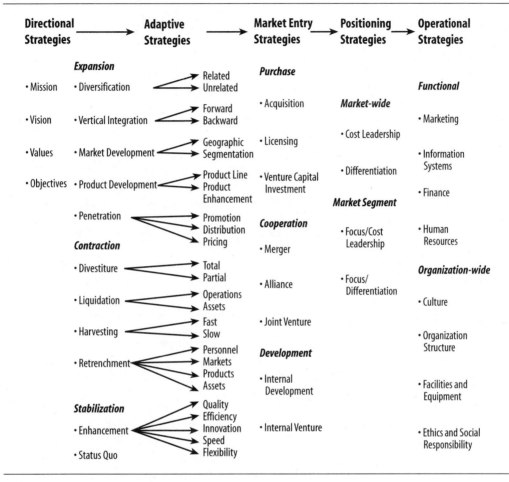

environmental stability. From an analysis of these factors a strategic posture may be determined. Figure 4.9 defines each of the four strategic postures based on these factors, and Figure 4.10 suggests the appropriate adaptive strategy for each strategic posture.

Evaluation of the Market Entry Strategies

Once an expansion or stabilization (enhancement) adaptive strategy is selected, one (or more) of the market entry strategies must be used to break into or capture more of the market. All of the expansion adaptive strategies require some activity to reach more

Figure 4.8   Definition and Examples of the Strategic Alternatives

Strategy	Definition	Example
Adaptive Strategies		
Related Diversification	Adding new related product or service categories, often requires the establishment of a new division.	Sun Healthcare, a long-term care chain, purchases Mediplex Group, specializing in subacute care. The principal reason for the purchase was to enter a growth market.
Unrelated Diversification	Adding new unrelated product or service categories, typically requires the establishment of a new division.	The University of Alabama Medical school owns a motel.
Forward Vertical Integration	Adding new members along the distribution channel (toward a later stage) for present products and services or controlling the flow of patients from one institution to another.	Merck & Company (pharmaceuticals) purchases Medco Containment Services (mail-order drug distributor).
Backward Vertical Integration	Adding new members along the distribution channel (toward an earlier stage) for present products and services or controlling the flow of patients from one institution to another.	San Angelo Texas Community Hospital moved into the wellness market by developing a fitness center open to those in the community aged 50 and over.
Market Development	Introducing present products or services into new geographic markets or to new segments within a present geographic market.	National Health Plans, a subsidiary of National Medical Enterprises, targets various regions of Californa for market expansion.
Product Development	Improving present products or services or extending the present product line.	San Pedro (California) Peninsula Hospital expanded its psychiatric program by establishing a therapy program for elderly patients who require little or no hospitalization.
Penetration	Seeking to increase market share for present products or services in present markets through marketing efforts (promotion, channels, price).	Integrated Medical Systems tries to increase its market share of automated communications between physicians' offices and health care delivery organizations through industry advertising.
Divestiture	Selling an operating business unit or division, which will typically continue in operation, to another organization.	Baxter International divests its $675 million diagnostics manufacturing business.
Liquidation	Selling all or part of the organization's assets (facilities, inventory, equipment, and so on) in order to obtain cash, and possibly to be used by the purchaser in a variety of ways and businesses.	MedCare HMO was liquidated by the state of Illinois.
Harvesting	Taking cash out while providing few new resources for a business in a declining market, sometimes referred to as "milking" the organization.	Many state health departments are planning harvest strategies for primary care services if comprehensive health care reform is passed. Health departments will slowly harvest these services as private providers assume patient loads.
Retrenchment	Reducing the scope of operations; redefining the target market; and selectively cutting personnel, products and services, or service area (geographic coverage).	National Medical Enterprises streamlines its psychiatric hospital division by cutting personnel and three regional divisional offices.
Enhancement	Seeking to improve operations within present product or service categories through quality, efficiency, innovation, speed, and flexibility.	AMI Brookwood initiates a complete reorganization to ensure that all activities revolve around the patient.

Figure 4.8 *Continued*

Strategy	Definition	Example
Status Quo	Seeking to maintain relative market share within a market.	VA hospitals call for steady state until specifics of health care reform are clearer.

Market Entry Strategies

Strategy	Definition	Example
Acquisition	Strategy to grow through the purchase of an existing organization, unit of an organization, or product/service.	HealthTrust—the hospital company—announces a $1 billion acqusition of Epic Healthcare Group.
Licensing	Acquisition of an asset (technology, market, equipment, etc.) through contract.	Medicaid waivers are licenses for providers (often health departments) to perform certain services for the Medicaid Agency.
Venture Capital Investment	Financial investment in an organization in order to participate in its growth.	Continental Equity Capital Corporation and Shamrock Investments provide venture capital to start Dynamic Health Systems, a rural hospital company.
Merger	Combination of two (or more) organizations through mutual agreement to form a single new organization.	Summit Health (California merges with OrNda (Tennessee) and American Healthcare Management (Pennsylvania).
Alliance	Formation of a formal partnership.	Rural Huntington (Indiana) Memorial Hospital signed a clinical affiliation agreement with urban Lutheran Hospital of Indiana (Fort Wayne) to share clinical services.
Joint Venture	Combination of the resources of two or more organizations to accomplish a designated task.	Tufts Associated Health Plans, Healthsource, and Health New England create a point-of-service network.
Internal Development	Products or services developed internally using the organization's own resources.	Swedish Covenant Hospital of Chicago develops a health and fitness center (37,000 square feet) in area from its cardiac rehabilitation program.
Internal Venture	Establishment of an independent entity within an organization to develop products or services.	Columbia University's College of Physicians and Surgeons establishes a center for alternative and complementary medicine.

Positioning Strategies

Strategy	Definition	Example
Cost Leadership	Low cost/price strategy directed toward the entire market allowing the organization to have greater profitability, or, if necessary, lower prices.	HEALTHSOUTH Rehabilitation Corporation is a cost and price leader in rehabilitation.
Differentiation	Development of unique product/service features directed toward entire market.	Holy Cross Medical Center of Mission Hills California opens a regional cancer center, where patients will receive treatments in private or semiprivate cabana-type rooms equipped with television, videocassette recorders, and audio equipment. Other support therapies include acupressure, art, yoga, and pain management.
Focus—Cost Leadership	Low cost/price strategy directed toward particular market segment.	Presbyterian Hospital of Charlotte, North Carolina, offers $35 mammograms. Presbyterian is targeting women over 35 years of age.
Focus—Differentiation	Development of unique product/service features directed toward particular market segment.	AMI's St. Francis Hospital in Memphis plans to convert 42 beds to subacute care, targeting patients not sick enough to stay in the hospital but not ready to go home.

Figure 4.9 Strategic Postures

Aggressive Posture

This posture is typical in an attractive industry with little environmental turbulence. The organization enjoys a definite competitive advantage, which it can protect with financial strength. The critical factor is the entry of new competitors. Organizations in this situation should take full advantage of opportunities, look for acquisition candidates in their own or related areas, increase market share, and concentrate resources on products having a definite competitive edge.

Competitive Posture

This posture is typical in an attractive industry. The organization enjoys a competitive advantage in a relatively unstable environment. The critical factor is financial strength. Organizations in this situation should acquire financial resources to increase marketing thrust, add to the sales force, extend or improve the product line, invest in productivity, reduce costs, protect competitive advantage in a declining market, and attempt to merge with a cash-rich organization.

Conservative Posture

This posture is typical in a stable market with low growth. Here, the organization focuses on financial stability. The critical factor is product competitiveness. Organizations in this situation should prune the product line, reduce costs, focus on improving cash flow, protect competitive products, develop new products, and gain entry into more attractive markets.

Defensive Posture

This posture is typical of an unattractive industry in which the organization lacks a competitive product and financial strength. The critical factor is competitiveness. Firms in this situation should prepare to retreat from the market, discontinue marginally profitable products, aggressively reduce costs, cut capacity, and defer or minimize investments.

Source: Alan J. Rowe, Richard D. Mason, Karl E. Dickel, and Neil H. Snyder, _Strategic Management: A Methodological Approach_, 3rd ed. (Reading, Massachusetts: Addison-Wesley Publishing Company, 1989), pp. 145–150. © 1989 by Addison-Wesley Publishing Company. Reprinted with permission of the publisher.

---

consumers with the products and services. Similarly, enhancement stabilization strategies indicate that the organization must undertake to "do better" what it is already doing, which requires market entry analysis. Contraction strategies are ways to leave a market either rapidly or slowly and therefore do not require a market entry strategy.

The market entry strategies include acquisition, licensing, venture capital investment, merger, alliance, joint venture, internal development, and internal venture. Any one (or several) of these strategies may be used to enter the market; however, mergers and alliances have received most of the media attention in the 1990s. Mergers and alliances are the principal cooperation strategies.

The specific market entry strategy or strategies considered appropriate depend on (1) the internal skills and resources of the organization and (2) the external conditions. These areas should be scrupulously evaluated in the selection of the appropriate market entry strategy.

**Internal Requirements.**   Each of the market entry strategies requires different internal skills and resources (Figure 4.11). Before selecting the appropriate market entry strategy,

Figure 4.10   Adaptive Strategic Alternatives for Strategic Postures

<table>
<tr>
<td>

Conservative

- Status Quo
- Unrelated Diversification
- Harvesting

</td>
<td>

Aggressive

- Related Diversification
- Market Development
- Product Development
- Vertical Integration

</td>
</tr>
<tr>
<td>

Defensive

- Divestiture
- Liquidation
- Retrenchment

</td>
<td>

Competitive

- Penetration
- Enhancement
- Product Development
- Market Development
- Status Quo

</td>
</tr>
</table>

Source: Adapted from Alan J. Rowe, Richard O. Mason, Karl E. Dickel, and Neil H. Snyder, *Strategic Management: A Methodological Approach*, 3rd ed. (Reading, Massachusetts: Addison-Wesley Publishing Company, 1989), p. 157.

a review of the internal strengths and weaknesses should be undertaken. If the required skills and resources are available, the appropriate market entry strategy may be selected. On the other hand, if they are not present, another alternative should be selected or a combination strategy of two or more phases should be adopted. The first phase would be directed at correcting the weakness prohibiting selection of the desired strategy, and the second phase would be the initiation of the desired market entry strategy.

External Conditions.   Next in the process of selecting a market entry strategy is the evaluation of the appropriate conditions. A review of the external environmental opportunities and threats and supporting documentation should provide information to determine which of the market entry strategies is most appropriate. Figure 4.12 lists representative external conditions appropriate for each of the market entry strategies.

Evaluation of the Positioning Strategies

After the market entry strategies have been selected, the products or services must be positioned within the market using the generic positioning strategies of cost leadership, differentiation, or focus. All of the expansion, contraction, and stabilization strategies

Figure 4.11 Internal Requirement for the Market Entry Strategies

Market Entry Strategy	Required Internal Skills and Resources
Acquisition	• Financial resources • Ability to manage new products and markets • Ability to merge organizational cultures and organizational structures • Rightsizing capability for combined organization
Licensing	• Financial resources(licensing fees) • Support organization to carry out license • Ability to integrate new product/market into present organization
Venture Capital Investment	• Capital to invest in speculative projects • Ability to evaluate and select opportunities with a high degree of success
Merger	• Management willing to relinquish or share control • Rightsizing capacity • Agreement to merge management • Complementary strengths • Ability to merge organizational cultures and organizational structures
Alliance	• Lack of competitive skills/facilities/expertise • Desire to create vertically integrated system • Need to control patient flow • Coordinative board/skills • Willing to relinquish share control
Joint Venture	• Lack of a distinctive competency • Additional resources/capabilities required
Internal Development	• Technical expertise • Marketing capability • Operational capacity • Research and development capability • Strong functional organization • Product/service management expertise
Internal Venture	• Entrepreneurial skills • Entrepreneurial organization • Ability to isolate venture from the rest of the organization • Technical expertise • Marketing capability • Operational capacity

Figure 4.12 External Conditions Appropriate for Market Entry Strategies

Market Entry Strategy	Appropriate External Conditions
Acquisition	• Growing market • Early stage of the product life cycle or long maturity stage • Attractive acquisition candidate • High-volume economies of scale (horizontal integration) • Distribution economies of scale (vertical integration)
Licensing	• High capital investment to enter market • High immediate demand for product/service • Early stages of the product life cycle
Venture Capital Investment	• Rapidly changing technology • Product/service in the early development stage
Merger	• Attractive merger candidate (synergistic effect) • High level of resources required to compete
Alliance	• Market demanding complete line of product/services • Market weak and continuum of services desirable • Mature stage of product life cycle
Joint Venture	• High capital requirements to obtain necessary skills/expertise • Long learning curve in obtaining necessary expertise
Internal Development	• High level of product control (quality) required • Early stages of the product life cycle
Internal Venture	• Product/service development stage • Rapid development/market entry required • New technical, marketing, production approach required

require explicit positioning and operational strategies. Products and services may be positioned market-wide or for a particular market segment. Cost leadership and differentiation are used as market-wide strategies or to focus on a special segment of the market.

The way in which a product or service is positioned depends not just on the organization's capability but also on the competitive situation. Therefore, the positioning strategies must be selected based on both internal requirements and external risks.

Internal Requirements.   Figure 4.13 presents the internal requirements for each of the positioning strategies. In order to use a cost leadership strategy, an organization

Figure 4.13   Internal Requirements for the Positioning Strategies

Generic Strategy	Skills and Resources	Organizational Requirements
Cost Leadership	• Sustained capital investment and access to capital • Process engineering skills • Intense supervision of labor • Products and services that are simple to produce in volume • Low-cost delivery system	• Tight cost control • Frequent, detailed control reports • Structured organization and responsibilities • Incentives based on meeting strict quantitative targets
Differentiation	• Strong marketing abilities • Product/service engineering • Creative flair • Strong capability in basic research • Reputation for quality or technological leadership • Long tradition in the industry or unique combination of skills • Strong cooperation from channels	• Strong coordination among functions in R&D, product/service development, and marketing • Subjective measurement and incentives instead of quantitative measures • Amenities to attract highly skilled labor, scientists, or creative people
Focus	• Combination of the preceding skills and resources directed at a particular strategic target	• Combination of the preceding organizational requirements directed at a particular strategic target

Source: Adapted from Michael E. Porter, *Competitive Strategy: Techniques for Analyzing Industries and Competitors* (New York: The Free Press, 1980), pp. 40-41.

must have or develop the ability to achieve a real *cost* advantage (not price) through state-of-the-art equipment and facilities and low-cost operations. This competitive advantage must be maintained through tight controls and emphasis on economies of scale. Differentiation, the ability to distinguish the product or service from other competitors, typically requires technical expertise, strong marketing, a high level of skill, and an emphasis on product development. A focus strategy is directed toward a particular segment of the market, but either cost leadership or differentiation may be used. Therefore, the skills required are the same for a market segment and market-wide strategies alike. It is important that organizations adopting a focus strategy stay in close communication with their market so that specialized needs may be fully addressed and changes in the segment carefully monitored.

External Conditions.   Each of the generic strategies has its own external risks that the organization must evaluate (Figure 4.14). Perhaps the biggest risk for cost leadership

Figure 4.14 External Risks Associated with Positioning Strategies

Generic Strategy	External Risks
Cost Leadership	• Technological change nullifies past investments or learning. • Industry newcomers or followers undertake low-cost learning, through imitation or through their ability to invest in state-of-the-art facilities. • Required product or marketing change cannot be seen because of the attention placed on cost. • Inflation in costs narrows the organization's ability to maintain sufficient price differential to offset competitors' brand images or other approaches to differentiation.
Differentiation	• The cost differential between low-cost competitors and the differentiated firm is too great for differentiation to hold brand loyalty; buyers therefore sacrifice some of the differentiated organization's features, services, or image for large cost savings. • Buyers' need for the differentiating factor diminishes, which can occur as buyers become more sophisticated. • Imitation narrows perceived differentiation, a common occurrence as the industry matures.
Focus	• Cost differential between broad-range competitors and the focused organization widens to eliminate the cost advantages of serving a narrow target or to offset the differentiation achieved by focus. • Differences in desired products or services between the strategic target and the market as a whole narrows. • Competitors find submarkets within the strategic target and outfocus the focuser. • Focuser grows the market enough to make it attractive to competitors that previously ignored it.

Source: Adapted from Michael E. Porter, *Competitive Strategy: Techniques for Analyzing Industries and Competitors* (New York: The Free Press, 1980), pp. 45–46.

is technological change. Process technological changes may allow competitors to achieve cost advantages. Product or service technological changes may result in a differentiation of the product that makes the cost leader's product less desirable. The most significant risks for the differentiator are that the emphasis on differentiation will push costs too high for the market or that the market will fail to see, understand, or appreciate the differentiation. There are risks, also, for the organization adopting a focus strategy. Often, the focuser is dependent on a small segment that may diminish in size, or on purchasers who may turn to the broader market for products or services. Movement toward market-wide products and services will occur if the differences in cost or differentiation become blurred.

& STRATEGIC IMPLEMENTATION

Once the organization has formulated its strategy (directional, adaptive, market entry, and positioning strategies), it must develop *operational strategies* to support (accomplish) it. Operational strategies comprise both strategies developed within the functional areas of the organization and organization-wide operational strategies. *Functional strategies* and supporting programs and budgets must be developed for key areas in the organization such as marketing, information systems, finance, and human resources. These functional areas are directly and independently affected by the strategy formulation process, yet functional strategies must be integrated before the organization can move toward realizing its mission.

In addition to the functional strategies, organizations often develop *organization-wide strategies*. These operational strategies include initiatives such as changing the organization's culture, reorganizing, upgrading facilities and equipment, and formulating social and community strategies. They generally affect the entire organization and cut across all functional areas.

& STRATEGIC CONTROL

The final stage of strategic management is strategic control. This process includes (1) the establishment of standards (objectives), (2) the measurement of performance, (3) the evaluation of organizational performance against the standards, and (4) corrective action, if necessary. In Figure 4.15 the steps of the strategic control model are compared with the general concept of control.

Establish Performance Standards

Planning and control are inherently intertwined. The development of directional strategies (mission, vision, values, and objectives) establishes the broadest standard for comparison with organizational performance. Similarly, the adaptive, market entry, and positioning strategies, developed through an analysis of the external and internal environments of the organization, must be supported by explicit operational objectives. These planning elements provide the starting point for strategic control.

Measure Organizational Performance and Compare

Internal factors, external factors, and performance factors exert pressure for change in organizations. Organizational performance factors are the clearest indicators of whether the strategy is performing well or poorly. As a result, negative organizational performance provides valuable information and an incentive to take corrective action.

Figure 4.15 The Concept of Control and a Framework for Strategic Control

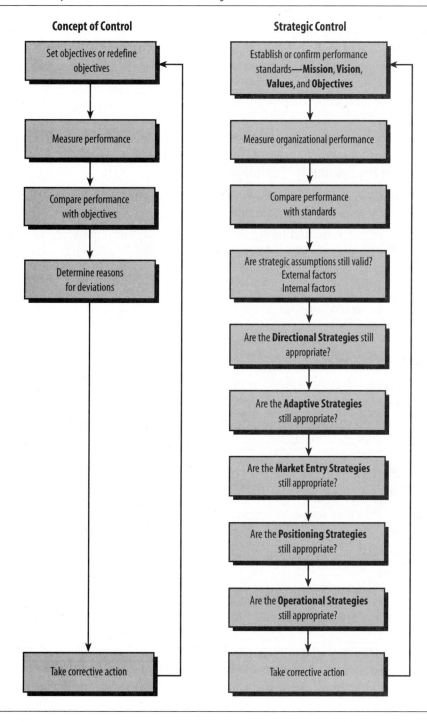

Qualitative and quantitative performance measures are commonly used to gauge the performance of an organization. For mission, vision, and values, performance measures are largely qualitative. Managers must match the actions of the organization to the templates provided by the mission, vision, and values statements, which is one reason they must be clearly stated and communicated throughout the organization. Five measures can provide a clear picture of performance for most organizations: market standing, innovative performance, productivity, liquidity and cash flow, and profitability.[20]

Determine the Reasons for Deviations

The fundamental question in strategic control, is "Why has the organization's performance not met the previously established performance standards?" In the model for strategic control presented in Figure 4.15, efforts to determine why the organization deviated from performance expectations are directed toward changes in three areas: the strategic assumptions (external and internal factors); the organizational strategy (directional, adaptive, market entry, or positioning strategies); or strategic implementation (operational strategies).

Take Corrective Action

The purpose of strategic control is to ensure that the organization has the appropriate strategies and is performing as expected. The strategic control process should identify any deviations in these areas so that management may take the necessary corrective action. In strategic control, revision is directed toward

- directional strategies–mission, vision, values, and objectives
- adaptive strategies–expansion, contraction, or stabilization
- market entry strategies–purchase, cooperation, or development
- positioning strategies–market-wide or market segmentation
- operational strategies–functional and organization-wide (implementation)

& Impact of the Organization

The final element of the strategic management model presented in Figure 4.2 is the impact of the organization on the external environment. Actions taken by the organization will affect the other organizations and individuals in the health care industry, as well as organizations and individuals in the general environment. Thus, implementation of a strategy may cause other organizations that are monitoring their environment (collecting competitive information) to react. Health care organizations are not only affected by the environment but also affect the environment through their behavior.

❧ OTHER DIMENSIONS OF STRATEGIC MANAGEMENT

Several additional dimensions of strategic management should be acknowledged and discussed. Strategic management is not always a structured, well-thought-out exercise. In reality, thought does not always precede action, perfect information concerning the environment and the organization is never available, and rationality and logic do not always prove superior to intuition and luck. Sometimes organizations "do" before they "know." For instance, intended strategies are often not the realized strategies. Sometimes managers are just able to "muddle through," or managers may have a broad master plan or logic underlying strategic decisions but can accomplish only incremental adjustments because of the complexity of the external and internal environments.

Defining strategies as patterns that emerge in a stream of decisions suggests that strategies may be viewed as the ex post facto result of decision-making behavior as well as a priori guidelines to decision making. Of course, a strategy does not always work out as planned (an *unrealized strategy*). In other cases an organization may end up with a strategy that was quite unexpected as a result of having been "swept away by events" (an *emergent strategy*).[21]

A strategy may be developed and subsequently realized. However, we must be realistic enough to understand that when we engage in strategic management, this theoretical ideal (strategy developed, then realized) may not and probably will not materialize. A great deal may go wrong. The possibilities include the following:

1. The strategy is reformulated during implementation as the organization gains new information and feeds that information back into the process, thus modifying the intentions en route (a function of strategic control).
2. The external environment is in a period of flux and strategists are unable to predict conditions accurately, as a result of which the organization may find itself unable to respond appropriately to a powerful external momentum.[22]
3. Organizations in the external environment implement their own strategies, blocking strategic initiative and forcing the activation of a contingency strategy or a period of "groping."

𝄢 Lessons for Health Care Managers

Strategic management is a complex and difficult task. The 1990s will place a higher premium on effective management and leadership than ever before. Yet no single approach may be adequate to understand social and organizational processes. The model and brief overview presented in this chapter were designed to provide the essential logic of the process involved in strategic management. However, the model must not be applied blindly or in the belief that "life always works that way." We must realize that our strategies, once introduced, are subject to a variety of forces both within and outside the organization. Sometimes we learn by doing.

𝄢 Notes

1. H. B. Gelatt, "Future Sense: Creating the Future," *The Futurist* 27, no. 5 (September–October 1993), pp. 9–13. See also P. M. Ginter, W. J. Duncan, and S. A. Capper, "Keeping Strategic Thinking in Strategic Planning," *Public Health* 106 (1992), pp. 253–269; W. J. Duncan, P. M. Ginter, and S. A. Capper, "Identifying Opportunities and Threats in Public Health," *European Journal of Public Health* 3 (1993), pp. 54–59; and J .M. Venable, Q. Li, P. M. Ginter, and W. J. Duncan, "The Use of Scenario Analysis in Local Public Health Departments: Alternative Futures of Strategic Planning," *Public Health Reports* 108, no. 6 (1994), pp. 701–710.

2. H. E. Klein and R. E. Linneman, "Environmental Assessment: An International Study of Corporate Practice," *The Journal of Business Strategy* 5 (1984), pp. 66–75. See also P. M. Ginter, W. J. Duncan, L. E. Swayne, and W. D. Richardson, "Analyzing the External Environment in Health Care," *Health Care Management Review* 16, no. 4 (Fall 1991), pp. 35–48.

3. J. Bracker, "The Historical Development of the Strategic Management Concept," *Academy of Management Review* 5, no. 2 (1980), pp. 219–224. See also D. Mercer, ed., *Managing the External Environment* (Newbury Park, CA: Sage Publishing, 1992), Section 2.

4. Ibid.

5. C. Clemenhagen and F. Champagne, "Medical Staff Involvement in Strategic Planning," *Hospital & Health Services Administration* 29, no. 4 (1984), pp. 79–94.

6. D. I. Cleland and W. R. King, *Systems Analysis and Project Management* (New York: McGraw-Hill, 1983), p. 17.

7. D. E. L. Johnson, "Strategic Thinking About Collaboration and Integration," *Health Care Strategic Management* 11, no. 3 (1993), pp. 2–3.

8. H. Mintzberg, "Patterns in Strategy Formulation," *Management Science* 24, no. 9 (1978), p. 935, and R. M. Grant, *Contemporary Strategy Analysis*, 2nd ed., (Cambridge, MA: Blackwell Publishers, 1995).

9. R. C. Shirley, "Limiting the Scope of Strategy: A Decision Based Approach," *Academy of Management Review* 7, no. 2 (1982), pp. 264–265.

10. Ibid., pp. 265–266.

11. D. L. Bates and J. E. Dillard, Jr., "Wanted: A Strategic Planner for the 1990s," *Journal of General Management* 18, no. 1 (1992), pp. 51–62.

12. B. D. Henderson, "The Origin of Strategy," *Harvard Business Review* 67, no. 6 (November–December 1989), p. 142. See also J. F. Moore, "Predators and Prey: A New Ecology of Competition," *Harvard Business Review* 73, no. 6 (November–December 1993), pp. 75–86.

13. B. B. Longest, Jr., *Management Practices for the Health Professional*, 4th ed. (Norwalk, CT: Appleton & Lange, 1990), pp. 12–18.

14. Liam Fahey and V. K. Narayanan, *Macroenvironmental Analysis for Strategic Management* (St. Paul: West Publishing Company, 1986).

15. D. K. Denton and B. L. Wisdom, "Sharing Vision," *Business Horizons* (July–August 1989), pp. 67–69. For the original and ongoing work on mission statements see J. A. Pearce II and F. David, "Corporate Mission Statements and the Bottom Line," *Academy of Management Executive* 1, no. 2 (May 1987), pp. 109–116; C. K. Gibson, D. J. Newton, and D. S. Cochran, "An Empirical Investigation of the Nature of Hospital Mission Statements," *Health Care Management Review* 15, no. 3 (Summer 1990), pp. 35–46; and W. J. Duncan, P. M. Ginter, and W. K. Kreidel, "A Sense of Direction in Public Organizations: An Analysis of Mission Statements in State Health Departments," *Administration & Society* 18, no. 3 (May 1994), pp. 11–24.

16. T. Peters, *Thriving on Chaos* (New York: A. A. Knopf, 1988), pp. 401–404.

17. J. C. Collins and J. I. Porras, "Organizational Vision and Visionary Organizations," *California Management Review* 34, no. 1 (1990), pp. 34–35.

18. For a discussion of organizational goals and objectives, see M. D. Richards, *Setting Strategic Goals and Objectives*, 2nd ed. (St. Paul: West Publishing, 1986).

19. E. A. Locke and G. P. Latham, *Goal Setting for Individuals, Groups, and Organizations* (Chicago: Science Research Associates, 1984).

20. P. F. Drucker, "If Earnings Aren't the Dial to Read," *The Wall Street Journal* (October 30, 1986), p. 15.

21. H. Mintzberg, "Patterns in Strategy Formulation," *Management Science* 24, no. 9 (1978), p. 945.

22. Op. cit. *Management Science* 24, no. 9, p. 946.

Tools of Health Care Management

II

Financial Accounting and Management in Health Service Organizations

5

Robert W. Broyles, University of Oklahoma
David J. Falcone, Univeristy of Oklahoma

❧ PURPOSE

This chapter has two purposes: (1) to clarify changes in the method of financing and delivering health services and (2) to describe the effects of the changes on the presentation of financial statements and fiscal management in health service organizations (HSOs). It focuses on those dimensions of accounting and financial management that are likely to endure for the foreseeable future and to be of greatest value to ensuring the viability of the HSO. For present purposes, HSOs refer to organized providers such as hospitals and group practices.

After describing some changes in the financial environment of HSOs, the chapter examines how financial reporting has been affected. It then turns to issues in HSO financial management and planning and control.

❧ THE FINANCIAL ENVIRONMENT

In the last 15 years perhaps the most dramatic change in the financial environment of the American hospital has been the implementation of the Medicare prospective payment system (PPS) and the adoption of similar mechanisms by other insurers. Unlike cost or charge-based reimbursement, under PPS the rate of compensation is fixed with respect to the costs of treatment and is determined by a price established for each diagnosis-related group (DRG). Therefore, the HSO absorbs a loss or makes a profit depending on whether costs of inpatient treatment are over or under the prospective price. Since the typical HSO must earn a net surplus, prospective pricing systems create imperatives to increase the proportion of cases assigned to profitable diagnostic groups; limit the volume and intensity of care per patient; improve the efficiency of operations; and, to the extent possible, control increases in the prices of resources.

The proliferation of alternative delivery systems, such as preferred provider organizations (PPOs) and health maintenance organizations (HMOs), and related competitive pressures have also increased the imperative to improve fiscal performance and financial management. The growth in alternative delivery systems has increasingly caused payment rates to be determined by capitation (i.e., a set payment per person regardless of cost), competitive bidding, and discounted prices. In these circumstances providers must be able to estimate costs accurately and ensure that actual expenses are less than the per capita rate of payment or the discounted price per service. The adoption of capitation systems similar to the Medicare pricing system by alternative delivery systems exerts pressures on providers to restrict the volume and intensity of service per enrollee; to improve the efficiency of operations; and, to the extent possible, control increases in factor prices.

Alternative delivery systems and prospective payment mechanisms also increase the importance of managing net working capital (current assets and liabilities) effectively. For example, the objective of managing accounts receivable is to minimize the amount of credit extended and compress the collection cycle, thus reducing the probability of bad debt, increasing cash receipts, and improving the net surplus. Similarly, the management of cash focuses on ensuring that reserves are neither inadequate nor excessive, thus minimizing the cost of being short of cash and the investment income that is forgone if balances are allowed to remain idle. Closely related to cash management is the need to manage the organization's investment portfolio. In this regard the objective is to maximize returns, subject to the risks management is prepared to assume. In short, the effective management of working capital must complement operational control if the HSO is to survive and flourish.

❧ CHANGES IN FINANCIAL STATEMENTS: AN OVERVIEW

Effective management of an organization's fiscal affairs requires a set of data that describe its financial position, changes in this position, and the effects of managerial decisions. Financial accounting is usually defined as the accumulation, adjustment, and presentation (in conformity with generally accepted principles) of financial information that depicts the fiscal position and financial results of the organization's operations. Traditionally, the financial reports of nonprofit organizations consisted of a balance sheet, a statement of changes in the financial position, an income statement, and a statement of changes in the fund balance.

Motivated in part by changes in the method of financing health services, the American Institute of Certified Public Accountants (AICPA), the Financial Accounting Standards Board (FASB), and the Healthcare Financial Management Association (HFMA) recommended a set of revisions to the format of financial statements (Bitter and Cassidy, 1990; Pelfrey, 1990). As indicated below, the changes are intended to ensure that the financial reports prepared by tax-exempt organizations are consistent with those of their proprietary counterparts.

The balance sheet is a statement of the organization's financial position that describes assets, liabilities, and the residual equity or fund balance. Historically, nonprofit organizations presented their assets, liabilities, and fund balances in conformity with the principles of fund accounting, thereby depicting their financial position in terms of unrestricted and restricted fund groups. The typical tax-exempt HSO prepared a separate balance sheet for the unrestricted fund group, the capital fund, the endowment fund, and the specific purpose fund.

The presentation of assets, liabilities, and residual equity in a single balance sheet is one of the most important changes recommended by the AICPA, FASB and HFMA. The condensed balance sheet shown in Figure 5.1 illustrates the recommended format for the presentation of restricted and general funds. As indicated in the exhibit, restricted donations, designated investments, and other assets subject to restrictions are presented as "assets restricted as to use." In addition, the fund balance of tax-exempt organizations, in which there are no investors with an ownership interest, is identified by the term "net assets," an item that reflects the sum of unrestricted net assets and net assets that are either temporarily or permanently restricted.

As recommended by the AICPA, the balance sheet presentation should be supported by schedules that list the balances of items representing assets with temporarily and permanently restricted use. The purpose of the Statement of Changes in Temporarily Restricted Net Assets is to show the amount of gifts and grants, list investment income derived from donor-restricted assets, and reclassify restricted resources to unrestricted net assets. Similarly, the Statement of Changes in Permanently Restricted Net Assets provides a detailed listing of endowment fund activity and gifts or bequests to the HSO.

The third component of the basic financial statement, the income statement, describes changes in financial position resulting from the organization's operations

Figure 5.1   Format for the Balance Sheet

Assets	$	Liabilities	$
Current		***Current***	
Cash	140,000	Accounts Payable	430,000
Accounts Receivable	1,250,000	Note Payable	230,000
Inventory	180,000	Currently Maturing Long-Term Debt	80,000
Prepaid Expenses	50,000	Accrued Expenses	420,000
Marketable Securities	10,000	Total Current Liabilities	1,160,000
		Long-Term	
Total	1,630,000	Bond Payable	1,300,000
Investments Restricted as to Use		Mortgage Payable	500,000
Depreciation Funds	1,450,000	Total Long-Term Liabilities	1,800,000
Construction Funds	1,150,000		
Permanently Restricted Assets	7,850,000	**Net Assets**	
Total Restricted Assets	10,450,000		
		Unrestricted	7,470,000
Property, Plant, and Equipment		Temporarily Restricted by Donors	1,000,000
Land	350,000	Permanently Restricted by Donors	7,850,000
Buildings	7,500,000	Total Net Assets	16,320,000
Equipment	3,340,000	Liabilities and Net Assets	19,280,000
less Accumulated Depreciation	(3,990,000)		
Net Property, Plant, and Equipment	7,200,000		
Total Assets	19,280,000		

and summarizes the revenues, expenses, and net surplus or loss for the period. Traditionally, the income statement of an HSO reported gross patient revenues, valued at established rates. Net patient revenue, representing actual or expected payments, was defined as the difference between gross patient revenues and deductions in revenue, an amount reflecting the sum of bad debts, charity care, contractual allowances (e.g., charges versus actual Medicare payments), and courtesy discounts.

The relevance of gross patient revenue to users of financial statements declined with the proliferation of PPSs and alternative delivery systems. The AICPA now defines revenue as the amount the insurer or patient is obligated to pay and, as shown in Figure 5.2, recommends that the HSO report only net patient revenue in the income statement. Bad debts resulting from an unwillingness to pay are regarded as an operating expense, whereas activity committed to charity care—the costs or volume of services provided to those who are unable to pay—is reported in notes to the financial statements.

Figure 5.2   Format for the Income Statement

	$
Operating Revenue	
Inpatient	5,200,000
Outpatient	2,100,000
Total Patient Revenue	7,300,000
Other Operating Revenue	190,000
Operating Revenue	7,490,000
Reclassification of Temporarily Restricted Donations	32,000
Operating Expenses	
Patient Care	4,700,000
Administrative	2,780,000
Total Operating Expenses	7,480,000
Operating Gain (loss)	42,000
Other Revenue (Expense)	
Unrestricted Donations	182,000
Investment Income	132,000
Gain on Disposal	37,000
Change in Net Assets Prior to Capital Reclassification	296,000
Capital Reclassification	
Temporarily Restricted Gifts	
Used to Purchase Equipment	250,000
Change in Net Assets	842,000
Unrestricted Net Assets	
Beginning of Year	6,628,000
End of Year	7,740,000

Several other changes in the format of the income statement are worthy of comment. First, rather than grouping expenses by object or natural classification (e.g., supplies), HSOs should report costs by function such as administrative, nursing, and ancillary services. Second, revisions in the format of the statement reduce the emphasis on results derived from operations and focus on the ending balance of the unrestricted net asset account. Third, contributions that are restricted by donors to operations—e.g., treatment of children with leukemia—are identified as a "reclassification," while the traditional listing of nonoperating revenue is replaced by the category "other revenue."

The recommendations of the AICPA, FASB, and HFMA also address the need to prepare a Statement of Cash Flows. When the direct method is used, the schedule lists the cash flows resulting from operating activity, restricted capital activity, financing activity, and investing activity. Cash flows derived from restricted capital include restricted donations and related investment income. Cash receipts or disbursements associated with financing activity include proceeds from issuing obligations and payments required by the provisions of outstanding debt instruments. The cash flows resulting from investing activity reflect the purchase or disposal of property, plant, and equipment.

The indirect method, used by the majority of HSOs, estimates cash flow by adjusting net revenue for items appearing in the income statement that do not represent a source or use of cash. To simplify, estimates of cash flow derived by applying the indirect method are given as the sum of the net surplus and noncash items such as depreciation expenses.

As mentioned, the revisions in the format of fiscal reports are intended to ensure that the financial statements of tax-exempt and proprietary organizations are compatible. Accordingly, widespread adoption of the recommended format is expected to facilitate comparison of the fiscal performance of proprietary versus tax-exempt organizations, an issue that is considered in the next section.

🐟 Financial Performance

Fiscal performance is usually evaluated in terms of the four dimensions summarized in Table 5.1. The first, profitability, refers to the facility's ability to earn more revenues than expenses and thereby contribute to unrestricted net assets. The profitability of the organization is usually measured by the operating margin, the return on equity, and the return on assets. Since the numerators measure the net realizable cash value of the operating surplus, the profitability ratios depict the amount of internally generated funding that might be used to retire existing debt or to acquire additional resources.

The second dimension, liquidity, focuses on the components of working capital and refers to the ability of the organization to honor currently maturing obligations. The current ratio indicates the amount of current assets for each dollar of an institution's current debt. The quick ratio and acid test are also used to measure the liquidity of the organization. The summary presented in Table 5.1 indicates that the numerator

Table 5.1   Measures of Fiscal Performance

Dimension and Ratio	Definition
Profitability	
Operating Margin	Operating Gain(Loss)/Operating Revenue
Return on Assets	$\dfrac{\text{Operating Gain (Loss) + Interest Expense}}{\text{Total Assets}}$
Liquidity	
Current Ratio	Current Assets/Current Liabilities
Quick Ratio	$\dfrac{\text{Cash + Net Receivables + Marketable Securities}}{\text{Current Liabilities}}$
Acid Test	$\dfrac{\text{Cash + Marketable Securities}}{\text{Current Liabilities}}$
Debt Structure	
Debt to Asset	Long-Term Debt/Net Fixed Assets
Times Interest Earned	$\dfrac{\text{Operating Gain (Loss) + Interest}}{\text{Interest}}$
Debt Service	$\dfrac{\text{Operating Gain + Depreciation + Interest}}{\text{Principal Payment + Interest}}$
Activity	
Current Asset	Operating Income/Current Assets
Fixed Asset	Operating Income/Net Fixed Assets
Total Assets	Operating Income/Total Assets
Inventory	Operating Income/Inventory

of the quick ratio is the sum of cash, marketable securities and the net realizable cash value of outstanding receivables, whereas the numerator of the acid test is the sum of cash and near cash (marketable securities). Accordingly, the quick ratio and the acid test are more stringent measures of liquidity than is the current ratio.

Debt structure, the third dimension of fiscal performance, measures not only the relative dependence of the HSO on external sources of credit to finance resources but also its ability to honor the terms of these obligations. Increases in the debt-to-equity or debt-to-asset ratio indicate a greater reliance on long-term obligations to finance resources and a potentially diminished capacity to honor interest and principal payments. The times-interest-earned ratio indicates the extent to which earnings might decline without impairing the ability of the organization to pay interest. The debt service ratio, which is more comprehensive than the times-interest-earned ratio, measures the magnitude of existing cash flows in relation to interest and repayment of principal. Since safety of principal and receipt of interest are important to debt holders, potential investors prefer high values of both ratios.

The intensity of using resources to provide patient care is measured by a set of activity ratios. As indicated in Table 5.1, ratios that depict the current, fixed, and total asset turnover measure the efficiency of employing each category of asset to provide care and generate patient income. In general, a high and rising value of each indicates that resources were used efficiently and that the intensity of asset use has increased.

Indicators of profitability, intensity of resource use, liquidity, and debt structure routinely form the basis for evaluating variation in the annual performance of the HSO or for comparing the organization with peer groups. However, the increase in the price of resources consumed by the typical HSO may compromise the reliability of the measures of fiscal performance and complicate their interpretation. In contrast to replacement costs or market value, the information presented in financial statements is based on the historic or original cost of acquiring assets, particularly inventory, property, plant, and equipment. The difference between historic and replacement costs tends to distort the set of financial ratios, a distortion that may conceal rather than reveal significant trends (Finkler, 1982).

To illustrate, consider the current ratio as an indicator of liquidity. A failure to adjust for increases in inventory prices understates the costs of replacing stock, suggesting that the current ratio misrepresents the liquidity of the HSO.

In a similar fashion, price changes are likely to distort ratios that measure performance in relation to noncurrent assets. As indicated by the summary presented in Table 5.1, the difference between replacement and historic cost results in an understatement of the value assigned to property, plant, and equipment. Other factors remaining constant, an understatement of property, plant, and equipment results in an inflated view of the intensity of using resources, as measured by the fixed and total asset turnover ratios, and of profitability, as indicated by the return-on-asset ratio. These observations suggest that the evaluation of fiscal performance based on unadjusted indicators might result in inaccurate impressions of the organization's fiscal performance, its ability to sustain operations at current levels, and the effects of implementing suboptimal decisions. Such inaccuracy could be reduced or eliminated by preparing financial statements based on replacement costs.

The problem of reporting financial information that depicts price changes might be resolved by resorting to one of several methods. The first solution is to adjust financial statements for changes in general purchasing power, as reflected by changes in the consumer price index or the gross national product implicit price deflator. Unfortunately, such adjustments fail to measure accurately changes in the prices of resources consumed by HSOs.

The second method of adjustment is to estimate the direct price of each item, based on current price lists or the judgments of professional appraisers. When possible, this method produces the most accurate adjustments. Alternatively, the current value of assets, independent of technological advances, might be based on reproduction costs, represented by the current costs of each component of a given item.

The third method of accommodating price changes is unit pricing, a variant on the use of direct prices that assigns values to assets for which no exact replacements exist. For example, current construction costs might be used to estimate the value of existing buildings. The details of calculating replacement cost, the presentation of related fiscal statements, and the evaluation of fiscal performance have been presented by Cleverly (1981, 1983) and by Friedman and Neumann (1979, 1980).

❧ FINANCIAL MANAGEMENT AND FISCAL PERFORMANCE: AN OVERVIEW

Financial management is the process of acquiring the funds the organization needs and ensuring that its resources are used effectively and efficiently. Financial managers thus rely on integrated approaches that improve profitability, liquidity, debt structure, and the intensity of asset use.

As indicated, PPSs and capitation methods require health service organizations to control the mix of services per diagnosis or per member; improve the efficiency of resource use; and, to the extent possible, limit increases in factor prices. Central to the problem of controlling operations and hence cost is an integrated system of planning, monitoring, and evaluating the use of labor, supplies, and equipment in providing health services. The provision of services simultaneously generates revenue and expenses. Periodic assessments are made of the variance in costs, revenues, and profitability. A variance is simply the difference between actual operations and the expected performance expressed in the budget. Evaluating favorable or unfavorable variances and measuring the portion of the variance that is controlled, to a significant extent, by an individual or group associated with the health service organization are fundamental components of an internal control system designed to improve profitability.

Frequently, the provision of service and the generation of revenue are accompanied by the extension of credit and an investment in the HSO's accounts receivable. As indicated, financial managers aim to limit the duration of the collection cycle and the amount of investment in outstanding receivables, thereby reducing bad debt expenses and opportunity costs. Hence, effective management of accounts receivable improves profitability, liquidity, the increment to unrestricted net assets, and the amount of internally generated funding that might be used to acquire additional assets or retire existing debt instruments.

Effective management of receivables is critical to ensure that the cash balance is neither excessive nor inadequate. As a consequence, methods of identifying the optimum cash balance are integral components of fiscal management that enable the HSO to minimize the costs of maintaining too little or too much cash.

To avoid opportunity costs or forgone investment income, the HSO should invest excess reserves in marketable securities. The financial manager should select those instruments that maximize returns, subject to the risks the organization is willing and able to assume. Depending on the level and composition of investment, returns on the portfolio can improve liquidity, profitability, and debt structure.

As with managing cash, the objective of managing inventory is to ensure that the level of investment is neither excessive nor inadequate in relation to productive activity. The monetary effects of maintaining too little inventory include not only lost patient revenue—resulting from shortages and disruptions in the process of providing care—but also the additional expenses incurred when supplies must be secured from nonroutine sources. The costs of maintaining too much inventory are represented by forgone returns, storage charges, and the cost of items that cannot be used or returned after specific periods of time.

The preparation of the capital budget is the final dimension of financial management that will be discussed in this chapter. A major function of the financial manager is to select those capital projects that are consistent with the strategic plan and promise to improve fiscal performance. A closely related but separate function is the selection of the least costly method of financing capital formation, a consideration that favorably influences debt structure, the ability of the organization to honor the provisions of debt instruments, liquidity, and profitability.

❧ Managing Working Capital

Working capital refers to the HSO's investment in current assets, whereas net working capital is the difference between current assets—such as accounts receivable, cash, marketable securities, and inventory—and current liabilities—such as accounts payable. Hence, an increase in net working capital improves liquidity as measured by the current ratio. Effective management of current assets reduces working capital needs and creates the financial latitude to improve profitability, the intensity of asset use, and debt structure.

The Management of Accounts Receivable

An investment in accounts receivable by the typical HSO is an operational necessity. Unfortunately, given the nature of demand for health care, a change in the terms of credit is unlikely to stimulate volume or improve profitability. Unlike other enterprises, HSOs incur all the costs but derive few, if any, of the benefits associated with the extension of credit.

The extension of credit results in several types of cost. The carrying cost of outstanding receivables is related to the time value of money and is calculated using the discounted cash flow method. Let C_t correspond to the realizable cash value of an outstanding account at the end of period t and i represent an appropriate interest or discount rate. The present value of the future cash flow is given by the ratio $C_t/(1+i)^t$. For example, if C is \$100, time 1 year, and the discount rate .06, the present value of the account is \$94.33. Opportunity cost might be defined as the difference between the time value of the cash invested in receivables and the income derived from an investment in an instrument that generates a return greater than i, the rate used to calculate time costs. Administrative or collection costs result from efforts to secure prompt payment and grow as an account ages. Further, as an account grows older, the probability of collection decreases, which further adds to bad debt.

McCormick (1993) argues that predictability and financing costs are categories of expense that should be considered when evaluating the costs of receivables. Predictability costs result when imprecise estimates of cash receipts precipitate the need to recast budgets, engage in crisis borrowing, and delay payments to vendors—outcomes that may compromise the HSO's credit rating. Finally, the organization's reliance on credit lines and other sources of funding required to smooth erratic cash flows generates financing costs.

The management of accounts receivable might be viewed as a process, consisting of five phases, that reduces the costs of extending credit and minimizes the organization's investment in receivables. First, during the preadmission phase, management should focus on elective or scheduled admissions, secure preadmission authorizations, and determine the expected financial responsibility, if any, of the patient and the insurer (Francis, 1985; Clarkin, 1990). The financial responsibility of the patient, resulting from copayment provisions and the expected use of uninsured services, represents the basis for establishing a preadmission charge in an amount equivalent to this anticipated obligation. Such an approach lowers the need to extend credit, the investment in receivables, and the costs described earlier. Alternatively, the preadmission assessment constitutes the basis for developing a payment plan for the patient, which compresses the collection cycle, lowers the probability of a bad debt, and improves profitability.

Second, the information provided during the admission phase concerning the patient's insurance status and ability to pay enables management to prepare routine forms and records. Hence, for scheduled admissions, in this second phase the patient should sign forms and other documents that might be required by the organization or insurers.

Third, during the delivery of care, whether provided on an inpatient or outpatient basis, the details of the care provided and the related charges for which the patient or insurer is responsible should be recorded promptly and accurately. Obviously, failure to do this extends the accounts receivable cycle.

The fourth phase occurs at discharge. If the mix of care provided and related revenues has been recorded promptly, a statement indicating the amounts owed by the insurer and the patient should be available at this time. Accordingly, the HSO should be prepared to accept payment from the patient and to submit a statement to the insurer on or immediately following the day of discharge. During the postdischarge phase, the focus of managing receivables is to ensure prompt payment, that is, to accelerate the transformation of receivables into cash.

Recently, the cash receipts derived from the extension of credit have been accelerated by the sale of outstanding accounts or the use of receivables as collateral to obtain a short-term loan (Kinkaid, 1993). At least three considerations suggest that selling outstanding accounts is preferable to borrowing. First, when accounts receivable are used as collateral, the lender may impose restrictive covenants that limit the organization's ability to issue additional debt or may otherwise limit its financial flexibility. Second, an HSO that uses receivables as collateral is responsible for ensuring prompt payment. This position implies that the organization assumes the risks and costs of collection. However, depending on the terms of a sale agreement, the HSO might transfer these costs and risks to the purchaser. Finally, the financial status of the HSO is of importance to the lender, since the outstanding accounts might form a portion of the bankruptcy estate in the event of failure.

Although selling receivables to finance working capital needs may benefit HSOs, the practice has several potential disadvantages that are worthy of note. First, due to legal issues concerning public insurers and the uncertainty of collecting from self-responsible patients, the sale of receivables is usually limited to claims against financially secure commercial insurers. In addition, the need to preserve the confidentiality of patient information frequently requires written consent to release data that will support the collection efforts of the purchaser. Finally, the HSO is required to provide representations and warranties that document the "clean claim" status of the receivables and to ensure that outstanding accounts are not subject to prior liens.

Health administrators rely on several indicators to measure the accounts receivable cycle and the effectiveness of management outstanding accounts. Traditionally, performance has been measured either by the accounts receivable turnover ratio (ART) or by the number of days charges in receivables (NODCIR). The numerator of ART is the amount of net patient revenue, while the denominator is defined as the net investment in accounts receivable. Accordingly, ART measures the rate at which receivables are collected. A relatively high or rising value indicates satisfactory management or an improvement in performance. Similarly, NODCIR is defined by the ratio of net receivables to daily net revenue, which thereby estimates the average lapse of time between the extension of credit and cash receipt. As with the evaluation of ART, a decline in the value of NODCIR indicates fewer days in the collection cycle, an outcome that results in lower credit extension costs.

Since ART and NODCIR are relatively crude measures of performance, most HSOs construct a distribution of outstanding accounts, grouped by type of payer and the number of days the receivable has been outstanding. The schedule usually lists the number, amount, and average value of receivables for each of the age categories. Since the probability that an account will be recognized as uncollectable increases over time, an increase in the proportion of outstanding receivables that are current indicates an improvement in performance and a decline in the costs of extending credit. The obverse is also true.

The Management of Cash

The management of accounts receivable and the administration of cash reserves are separate but interrelated functions. As indicated, one objective of financial management is to minimize the total costs of holding cash, an amount defined as the sum of long and short costs. Long costs result from maintaining excessive reserves and are usually measured by the returns that are forgone when cash remains idle. Other factors holding constant, long costs grow as the cash balance increases. Conversely, short costs are incurred when inadequate reserves are maintained, resulting in forgone discounts offered by vendors, interest expenses that accompany short-term borrowing, delays in paying creditors, and a deterioration in the organization's credit rating. Accordingly, short costs decline as the cash balance grows. These observations indicate that, other factors holding constant, total costs decline as the cash balance initially increases and, after a point, rise as reserves grow. In turn, the optimum cash balance is defined as the amount that minimizes the sum of long and short costs.

The cash balance is contingent on factors other than long and short costs. The random or nonrandom nature of receipts and disbursements is perhaps the most important determinant of the cash balance. A nonrandom cash transaction assumes only one value and is known with certainty. For example, during a reasonably short period of time, the timing and amount of cash that must be disbursed to employees or to entities that extend credit to the HSO are known with certainty. Conversely, the timing and magnitude of random transactions vary, suggesting that these cash flows pose problems for the maintenance of an optimal reserve.

Since virtually all organizations have nonrandom cash flows, it can be assumed that all transactions are known with certainty. An assessment of the optimum or desired cash balance under conditions of certainty can then form the basis for developing approaches that can be applied in conditions characterized by random behavior and uncertainty.

If the analysis is limited to nonrandom transactions, a net cash flow approach might be employed to determine the optimum, or desired, balance. Three estimates are required to implement the net cash flow approach. First, a schedule of cash receipts and disbursements must be prepared, reflecting the detail management requires. Once the schedule is prepared, the set of net cash flows (NCF) is determined by the algebraic difference between known inflows and outflows. The NCF is zero if receipts equal disbursements, negative if receipts are less than disbursements, and positive if receipts exceed disbursements. For each day in the planning period, receipts and disbursements need not be perfectly synchronized, even though both streams are known with certainty. Finally, management must establish the minimum cash balance (MCB), or the amount below which short costs are incurred. Compensatory balances that are required by lending institutions and management's preference for liquidity are among the most important factors that force the HSO to maintain a minimum cash balance.

Under conditions of certainty, the sum of the cash balance (CB) and the NCF represents the amount of cash available. Suppose that management is considering a set of strategies and that each option, CB_j, is a different cash balance. If $(CB_j + NCF) - MCB > 0$, the adoption of strategy CB_j results in excess funds and long costs represented by forgone investment income. Conversely, if $(CB_j + NCF) - MCB < 0$, the adoption of the strategy results in a shortage and a set of short costs represented by the interest expenses associated with cash borrowing or delays in paying creditors. On the other hand, if $(CB^* + NCF) - MCB = 0$, neither long nor short costs are incurred, and strategy CB^* is the desired cash balance.

An alternative to the net cash flow has been proposed by Baumol (1952). Baumol's model focuses on a situation in which the cash disbursements of the period are known and occur at a constant rate per day; it assumes that the disbursements of the period are financed either by short-term borrowing or the proceeds derived from disposing of marketable securities. Suppose that the cash disbursements of the period amount to D dollars and, in order to finance the outflow, a cash infusion of C dollars is obtained by short-term borrowing or the disposal of marketable securities. Suppose further that the costs of arranging the loan or disposing of securities are fixed and equal to b dollars per transaction. The cost of acquiring the cash infusion is the product of the cost per transaction, $\$b$, and the number of transactions, represented by the ratio D/C. Since the number of transactions and related costs decreases as C grows, management is induced to increase the amount of the periodic cash infusion.

Conversely, a short-term loan or the premature liquidation of marketable securities results in a cost represented by the opportunity rate of interest, i. If the cash infusion amounts to C dollars, an average balance of $C/2$ dollars is maintained as a reserve per cycle. Hence, the cost of sustaining an average balance of $C/2$ dollars is $i(C/2)$, suggesting that, as the value of C increases, the cost of holding cash grows. Unlike the cost of acquiring the cash infusion, the term $i(C/2)$ induces management to lower the value assigned to C.

It can be shown that

$$C = (2bD/i)^{1/2} \tag{1}$$

represents the optimal size of the cash infusion resulting from the loan or liquidation of marketable securities. To illustrate, suppose b is \$50 and disbursements, D, are \$100,000. If i is .10, the cash infusion is $[2(50)(100,000)/.1]^{1/2}$ or \$10,000. In summary of equation 1, a larger fixed cost, b, increases the cash infusion, while a higher opportunity rate of interest, i, lowers the value of C.

Since the typical HSO engages in random transactions, a separate approach is required to accommodate the problem of controlling the cash balance. The model developed by Miller and Orr (1966) assumes that the volatility of receipts and disbursements produces random variation in the daily cash balance that is constrained by an upper limit, h, a lower limit, l, and a return point, z. Variation in the net cash flow may result in a balance of h dollars, the upper control limit. A cash balance that is equivalent to the upper control limit induces management to invest h–z dollars, which reduces reserves to z. Similarly, variation in net flows may result in a cash balance that is equivalent to l, an outcome that induces management to secure a cash infusion of $z - l$ dollars and return the cash balance to the level specified by z.

The values of z and h minimize a cost function defined by the expected number of transactions, the fixed cost per transaction, the average daily balance, and the daily rate of interest earned on securities. If the transaction costs of acquiring or disposing of securities are independent of volume, z is given by

$$z = [3b\sigma^2/4i]^{1/3} \tag{2}$$

As before, b represents the fixed cost per transaction, while i refers to the daily rate of interest. The variance in the daily cash balance, σ^2, measures the degree of synchronization between receipts and disbursements.

To summarize, a large variance indicates a lack of synchronization; the obverse is also true. Assuming the cash balance exhibits no discernible trend, it can be shown that the value of the upper control limit, h, is given by $3z$ and the average cash balance is $4z/3$. The model indicates that the cash balance should grow as the value of σ^2 or b, the fixed cost per transaction, increases, while the investment in cash should decrease as the rate of interest, i, increases.

By way of illustration, suppose the minimum cash balance is \$50,000 and b is \$100. If i is .0004 and σ^2 is \$80,000, the value of z is given by

$$z = [(3)(100)(80,000)/4(.0004)]^{1/3}$$

or approximately \$2,466. The upper control limit, h, is 3(\$2,466) or \$7,398. Finally, the average cash balance is (4/3)(\$2,466), or \$3,288, and the total cash balance is the sum of \$50,000 and \$3,288, \$53,288.

The problem of managing the cash balance and the components of the net cash flow is complicated by the existence of the "float" of receipts. A negative float is usually associated with cash receipts and consists of a mail, a processing, and a clearing float. A mail float consists of the payments that have been mailed but not yet received by the HSO. The processing float represents the payments that have been received but not deposited or presented at the bank. The clearing float reflects the efficiency of the fiscal intermediary and consists of payments that have been deposited but have not yet cleared. Since a negative float comprises cash resources that are committed to the collection cycle and earn no return, one of the fiscal manager's objectives is to reduce the mail, processing, and clearing floats.

Unlike a negative float, a positive float is associated with cash disbursements and occurs when the bank balance exceeds the book balance. The most important component, the disbursement float, consists of cash disbursements that have been recorded by the organization but not yet cleared by the bank. In accordance with the goal of delaying payment, the objective of the fiscal manager is to increase the disbursement float.

Methods of reducing negative float include a lockbox system, sweep accounts, and electronic depository transfer checks. Designed to reduce mail float, lockbox systems require insurers and self-responsible patients to mail payments to a post office box from which checks are collected daily and deposited in the organization's account. Since bank fees are related to the number of transactions, the lockbox system is costly if many small checks are processed. A sweeping account enables the organization to reduce its checking account to a minimum level each day, thereby releasing funds for investment in income-earning securities or transfer to a central disbursement bank. A depository transfer check (DTC) might be used by multi-institutional arrangements to lower the clearing float. When participants in the arrangement are dispersed geographically, remittances are collected in a local depository bank and a central bank is notified of the amount. The central bank prepares a DTC, credits the amount to the organization's account, and electronically transmits the DTC to the local bank for deposit. The main advantage of the DTC is that clearing time is reduced from the two days required through the Federal Reserve to one day.

Constrained by the need to preserve its credit rating, the organization might slow cash disbursements by delaying payment until invoices are due. For example, vendors frequently offer terms of trade credit represented by 2/10/30, implying that the HSO is offered a 2% discount if payment occurs 10 days after the invoice date. In this case, payment should not occur before day 10. However, if the HSO does not pay within 10 days, it should wait to pay until day 30. The strategy of delaying payment should be limited to the credit period; creditors might ignore an occasional late payment, but a history of delinquency jeopardizes the organization's credit and may induce vendors to withdraw trade credit.

The fiscal effects of adopting one of the above cash management techniques might be approximated by calculating incremental benefits and costs. Typical costs include bank fees, salaries of employees, and occasionally capital equipment. The benefits are usually captured by the funds that are released and might be used to lower costs or generate short-term earnings. The net present value (NPV) of a given strategy might be determined by

$$NPV = [\Delta R - \Delta D][1 - T]/k \qquad (3)$$

where ΔR represents the change in before-tax receipts or revenues; ΔD corresponds to the increment in annual disbursements or costs; T is the marginal tax rate, if any; and k is the required rate of return, or the opportunity cost of capital. Obviously, if the change in receipts exceeds the increment to disbursements, the NPV of the technique is positive, and a decision to adopt the option would benefit the organization. Since NPV indicates the relative advantage derived from each option, its calculation forms the basis for ranking and evaluating the various strategies that might be adopted by management.

The Management of Marketable Securities

As indicated, surplus funds should be invested in securities that generate income, and a wide range of investment alternatives is available to the typical HSO. Each might be evaluated in terms of risk, maturity, marketability, and returns. In general, short-term instruments are characterized by a maturity of one year or less, a relatively low risk of default, and a correspondingly low rate of return. Given that the inflation rate might exceed the rate of return, an investment in short-term securities may expose the organization to the risk of a potential decline in purchasing power.

Short-Term Investments.   Treasury bills, certificates of deposit (CDs), and mutual funds are among the most important of the short-term investments. Treasury bills are obligations of the federal government that are characterized by little or no risk of default, a high degree of liquidity, and—contingent on market conditions—a reasonable rate of return. Treasury bills require a minimum investment of $10,000 and are available in maturities that range from 91 days to a year.

With maturities of 30 to 180 days, CDs are issued in large denominations by commercial banks. Although it is possible to withdraw funds prior to maturity, there are penalties for doing so. Further, since the bank promises to return interest and principal to the holder on the maturity date, CDs are negotiable instruments. Mutual funds accumulate capital from participants and use these funds to purchase short-term securities such as treasury bills, commercial paper, or CDs. A relatively high yield is available to participants who purchase shares or partial ownership in a mutual fund. The purchase of shares in a mutual fund requires an investment ranging from $1,000 to $5,000.

Long-Term Investments. *Bonds*: In addition to short-term alternatives, HSOs frequently acquire bonds issued by governments and corporations. Bonds are instruments of indebtedness characterized by several dimensions. First, bond issues are frequently quoted at prices that differ from par value. In general, the market price of an issue varies inversely with interest rates, thereby ensuring that the nominal yield is equivalent to the market yield of similar instruments. If the nominal rate of interest paid by the issuer of a given bond exceeds the market rate, the market price of the bond will exceed its par value by an amount that equates the effective yield with the current market yield. Accordingly, if the nominal rate of interest is greater than the current rate on issues of similar quality, the bond will sell at a premium. Conversely, the bond will sell at a discount if the nominal rate of interest is less than the market rate. In this case the price will exceed par value by an amount that equates the nominal yield with the current market yield.

A second characteristic of bond issues is the method by which the principal is paid. A term bond has a single maturity date on which the issuer is required to retire the entire obligation by repayment of the principal. A serial bond has multiple payment dates on which a portion of the obligation is due and payable.

Finally, bonds may be characterized in terms of the collateral pledged by the issuer. In the event of default, a secured bond entitles the holder to a legal claim to specified assets of the issuer. Conversely, issues that are unaccompanied by a legal claim on the assets of the issuer are known as unsecured bonds or debentures. The security of these bonds depends on the credit standing of the issuer and the promise to honor interest and principal payments in accordance with the provisions of the issue.

Stocks: Unlike bonds, shares of stock connote ownership and are a form of equity capital. The returns to stockholders are expressed in terms of dividend rather than interest payments. In contrast to bonds, stocks are not characterized by a fixed maturity date.

Corporations issue common and preferred stock, each conferring on the owner a set of rights and privileges. If dividends are declared, preferred stockholders must be paid prior to owners of common stock. Similarly, owners of preferred stock are entitled to exercise a prior claim on the firm's assets if liquidation occurs. Further, preferred stock is regarded as a fixed income security, since its dividends are usually expressed as a fixed percentage of par value.

Common stock also connotes ownership and entitles the owner to participate in the distribution of profits after all other obligations have been satisfied. Dividend payments to owners of common stock are less certain than those accruing to holders of preferred stock and are contingent on the firm's residual profitability. Although dividend payments can be substantial, the decision to invest in common stock is frequently based on anticipated returns that result from price appreciation and related capital gains. However, the potential volatility in security prices, dividends, and capital gains is the greatest disadvantage of investing in common stock.

Of particular importance to the investor in common stock is the method of distributing earnings per share, or profits divided by the number of outstanding shares of stock. Firms that adopt a regular dividend policy usually declare dividends quarterly and express the returns to the stockholder as the sum of a regular and an extra dividend per share. The regular dividend per share usually remains constant for several years, even though the earnings per share ratio varies. A regular dividend policy avoids changes in payments to owners that are related to the volatility in profitability. The "extra" portion of the dividend per share is usually distributed during the last quarter of the year and is identified as a separate increment to avoid the impression that the regular portion of the dividend will be increased.

In contrast to the regular dividend payment, some firms base dividends on a fixed payout ratio that indicates what percentage of each dollar of residual earnings will be distributed to owners of common stock. The dividend per share is calculated by the product of the earnings per share and the fixed payout ratio. Since the payout ratio is fixed, the dividend per share reflects variation in the earnings per share and the profitability of the firm.

It is very important to consider the risk associated with a given security when investing excess cash. With respect to debt instruments, interest rate risk refers to the variation in the price of a security that results from changes in market rates of interest. In general, prices of debt issues are inversely related to interest rates; a decision to dispose of the security after a rise in interest rates will likely result in a loss of principal. The organization might avoid interest rate risk by holding the instrument to maturity and redeeming it at par value. Default risk accompanies the debt instruments of business entities and refers to the possibility that the issuer will be unable to honor fixed obligations represented by interest and principal payments.

Investment Decisions.   The trade-off between returns and risk is fundamental to the evaluation of any investment alternative. Investors expect returns to increase with risk; and it is reasonable to maximize returns for a given level of risk or to minimize the risks associated with a given return. The relation of returns to risk is incorporated in the capital asset pricing model, a construct that indicates the return required from a given security. The return required from security j, represented by k_j, is

$$k_j = r_f + b_j(r_m - r_f) \tag{4}$$

In this case, r_f corresponds to the rate of return from a risk-free investment, such as a treasury bill, while r_m is the market rate of return, as measured by the average return on all securities included in the *Standard and Poor's Composite Index*.

The value of beta, b_j, measures the change in the returns from security j relative to those derived from the market index. If the value of beta exceeds one, the returns exhibit more variation than those in the market and the security is relatively riskier. Conversely, if the value of beta is less than one, the security exhibits little variation and is less risky than the market as a whole. As indicated, the capital asset pricing model captures the positive relation between risk and the required rate of return. As risk grows, as indicated by higher values of b_j, the required rate of return increases.

The required rate serves as a standard against which the expected returns from a given security are compared. Table 5.2 summarizes the indicators that measure the yield of bonds and other fixed income securities. The current yield measures the amount of interest income earned by each dollar invested in the issue; the yield to maturity reflects not only interest income but also the difference between the current market price and the maturity value of the security. Unlike the yield to maturity, the realized yield is based on the assumption that the organization will dispose of the security prior to the maturity date, implying that the amortization of the discount or premium is based on the expected sale price rather than par value. In this case, the expected sale price might be estimated by the present value of the stream of receipts, represented by interest and principal payments, that are available to the next owner. Like the internal rate of return, the effective bond yield is the discount rate that equates the current price with the stream of interest receipts and the par value or the expected selling price of the bond.

Once computed, the measure of the bond's yield is compared with the required rate. If expected returns are greater than or equal to the required rate, management is

Table 5.2   Measures of Fiscal Merit: Stocks and Bonds

Measure of Merit	Definition
Bonds	
Current Yield	iP/CP
Yield to Maturity	$\dfrac{iP + (PV - CP)/m}{(PV + CP)/2}$
Realized Yield	$\dfrac{iP + (SP - CP)/n}{(SP + CP)/2}$
Stocks	
Present Value	$\sum D_j/(1+k)^j + SP/(1+k)^j$
Expected Yield	$\dfrac{D + (SP - CP)/n}{(SP + CP)/2}$

Key:
i is the nominal rate of interest.
CP is the current market price of the security.
PV is the par value of the bond.
SP is the sale price expected prior to maturity.
D_j is the dividend expected in period j.
k is the required rate of return.
D is the average dividend expected by management.
m is the number of periods to maturity.
n is the number of periods management expects to hold security.

induced to purchase the instrument. Conversely, if the calculated yield is less than the required rate, the prudent fiscal decision is to abandon the bond.

Table 5.2 summarizes several indicators of the returns derived from an investment in common stock. The Table suggests that investment decisions might be based on a comparison of the current market price with the present value equivalent of dividend payments and expected sale proceeds. Obviously, if the current market price exceeds the present value equivalent of future returns, the security is not expected to generate the required rate and management should reject it as an investment. The obverse is also true. An alternative approach is to focus on the current dividends per share, D_o, and assume that these receipts will grow at a constant rate, g. If the required rate of return exceeds the growth rate, the maximum price the organization should pay for the security is given by the ratio $D_o/(k - g)$. Finally, as indicated in Table 5.2, the expected yield is based not only on the average dividend payments but also on the difference between the current and expected sale prices of a security that management expects to hold for *n* periods. When compared with the required rate of return or the yields available on comparable alternatives, these calculations form the basis for an investment decision concerning the stock.

The more general problem of managing a portfolio that consists of multiple securities requires the organization to specify its goals clearly. For the purposes of presentation, it is assumed that management policies are intended to (1) ensure the safety of principal and reduce risk; (2) earn the highest rate of return, subject to the risk the organization is prepared to assume; and (3) satisfy the institution's need for liquidity.

The risk accompanying a given security consists of diversifiable and nondiversifiable components. Nondiversifiable risk is a product of general market conditions and is applicable to all issues. Conversely, diversifiable risk is attributable to business or financial conditions that are specific to the issuer. If securities of which the portfolio is comprised reflect different business or financial considerations, returns are likely to covary negatively. As a consequence, the diversifiable component of risk declines as the number of different issues increases.

In addition, the portfolio should be made up of issues that satisfy the organization's need for liquidity. The marketability or liquidity of an issue might be evaluated in terms of the ease with which it can be sold without a loss of principal. The larger the amount that can be sold with little price variation, the more marketable the security. Further, the shorter the time required to transform the security into cash, the more liquid it is.

Since the prices of fixed income securities vary inversely with interest rates, the risks to which the HSO is exposed emanate from the possibility that the issue will be sold prior to maturity. Hence, management should ensure that the portfolio consists of securities that mature on different dates. Such an approach reduces the probability of selling the security prior to maturity and thereby lowers interest rate risk. In addition, the policy enables management to match maturity dates with projected cash needs.

The Management of Inventory

An inventory item is a current asset until it is used in a process resulting in patient care, at which time its cost becomes an operating expense. When accounting for supplies, management may employ either a periodic or a perpetual inventory system. Under a periodic inventory system, there is no attempt to record the number of units that are available on a day-to-day basis. Rather, the amount of actual stock is determined by a physical inventory. In addition to its simplicity, the periodic inventory system is relatively inexpensive. Since frequent counts are impractical, the amount of available inventory will be distorted until the next physical inventory is taken. In addition, since a periodic inventory system does not indicate what *ought* to be available, the potential for misappropriation is increased.

Under a perpetual inventory system, continuous records are maintained reflecting the receipt, issue, use, and availability of stock at any moment in time. Since the perpetual inventory system is relatively costly, the method should be applied only to inventory items that are critical to the life-saving function of the HSO or have a high annual rate of use or special storage requirements.

In addition to the differences between the perpetual and periodic systems, the values assigned to ending balances and supply expenses might be determined by one of several assumptions concerning the use or flow of inventory. Among the most common methods of inventory valuation are "last in, first out" (LIFO) and "first in, first out" (FIFO). The FIFO method assumes that items are issued in the order in which they are received, implying that inventory items remaining in stock are valued at the most recent invoice prices, while the supply expenses reported in the income statement reflect prices encountered during the more distant past. Conversely, the LIFO method assumes that items are issued from the most recently acquired stocks, suggesting that latest prices are used to value units used in operating activity. Hence, during periods of price inflation, the FIFO method tends to result in a lower supply expense, a larger net surplus and a greater investment in inventory than does the LIFO method. However, the LIFO method assigns a value to supply expenses that more closely approximates replacement costs than the FIFO method of valuation.

Two operating decisions are fundamental to the problem of managing inventory. First, managers must identify the reorder point, defined as the level of stock that signals a need to replenish inventory; second, they must assess the amount of stock that should be reordered. Both decisions focus on the need to minimize inventory costs, usually defined in terms of the costs of acquisition, the costs of possession, long costs, and short costs.

The costs of acquisition are incurred when inventory is replenished and are related to administrative functions such as securing bids, developing specifications, arranging payment, and inspecting shipments. The relation between the costs of acquisition, COA, and order size, Q, might be expressed in the form

$$COA = J(D_t/Q) \qquad (5)$$

where J is the cost per order and D_t is the demand for inventory during the period. If demand for inventory is known and invariant, an increase in the quantity ordered reduces the COA. Since the obverse is true, equation 5 indicates that the order size and the costs of acquisition are inversely related.

The costs of possession have two components and refer to expenses incurred after the acquisition of inventory. The first component is represented by the opportunity costs incurred when funds are committed to an investment in inventory. Under conditions of certainty, the lapse of time between ordering and receiving supplies is known and invariant, implying that $Q/2$ units will be held during the typical inventory cycle. If P is the purchase price and i the opportunity rate of return, opportunity costs are approximated by $iP(Q/2)$. The second component is related to the need to store, insure, and secure inventory. Letting G represent the storage costs per unit, total storage costs may be approximated by $G(Q/2)$. Hence, the cost of possession (COP) is simply the sum of opportunity and storage costs:

$$COP = iP(Q/2) + G(Q/2)$$

If K represents the carrying cost per unit (i.e., the sum of iP and G), the costs of possession are approximated by $K(Q/2)$. Unlike the costs of acquisition, the costs of holding inventory rise when Q increases.

It can be shown that the economic order quantity, EOQ, minimizes the costs of acquisition and possession. Given by

$$EOQ = (2JD_t/K)^{1/2} \tag{6}$$

the EOQ may be applied in conditions of both certainty and uncertainty. Suppose that the demand for inventory is 10,000 units, the cost per order is $5, and the carrying cost per unit is $10. Under conditions of certainty, the EOQ is 100 units, resulting in a total cost of $1,000. Other values remaining constant, assume that the demand for inventory is uncertain. If management erroneously expects to use 15,000 rather than 10,000 units, the EOQ is 123 units and total cost $1,021.50 rather than $1,000. In this case a substantial error (50%) in estimating demand increases the costs of possession and acquisition by 2.15% (i.e., 1,021.5/1,000). Thus, as long as the demand for inventory is estimated with reasonable precision, the EOQ is appropriate in both certain and uncertain conditions.

As indicated, the reorder point is the level of inventory that signals the need to replenish stock. In conditions of certainty, the daily use of inventory and the lead time are known and invariant. Hence, the reorder point is determined by the product of daily inventory use and the lead time. If the daily use of inventory is 20 units and the lead time is 10 days, the reorder point is 200 units.

In conditions of uncertainty, the organization is exposed to the risk of encountering a shortage during the lead time. To ensure that supplies are adequate, management should maintain a safety stock of items that result in high short costs or are critical to the life-saving function of the HSO. The safety stock is defined as the difference between the reorder point, R, and the average use of inventory during the lead time, AU, where R is greater than AU.

To determine the reorder point in conditions of uncertainty, the marginal costs of increasing the value of R by 1 unit must be compared with those resulting from a failure to add 1 unit to the reorder point. Since an additional unit likely remains in inventory, the additional cost of increasing the value of R by 1 unit is K. The cost of failing to add a unit to R, represented by ΔC, is given by product of the probability that use, U, will exceed the current value of R, $P(U > R)$, the short cost per unit, S_u, and the number of inventory cycles, D_t/Q. When the reorder point is relatively low, the costs of failing to add a unit to R are greater than K. As the value of R increases, the probability of a shortage decreases, implying that ΔC declines initially and approaches K from above. Eventually, increases in the value of R lower the probability of encountering a shortage, implying that, for high values of R, K is greater than ΔC. Accordingly, the optimum reorder point is defined by the condition

$$K = [1 - P(U < R)]S_u D_t/Q$$

After a slight rearrangement, it can be shown that

$$P(U < R) = 1 - KQ/S_u D_t \qquad (7)$$

When using equation 7 to determine the reorder point, it is necessary to find the EOQ and calculate the probability that the use of inventory during the lead time will be less than the reorder point. If demand during the lead time is distributed normally, let Z represent the standard normal deviate that is identified by the probability $P(U < R)$ and σ_u correspond to the standard deviation of use during the lead time. Employing this notation, the reorder point is

$$R = AU + Z\sigma_u$$

Hence, the reorder point is simply the sum of the average use during the lead time and the safety stock, represented by the product of Z and σ_u.

Recently, alternative approaches to determining the reorder point and the EOQ have been applied to the problem of managing inventory. Under a just-in-time (JIT) system, a principal vendor assumes primary responsibility for storage needs and makes frequent bulk deliveries that are intended to support the operational needs for inventory. The HSO assumes responsibility for preparing items for use and replenishing floor stock. The primary advantage of JIT is a decline in inventory and costs.

In a stockless program, virtually all of the organization's supplies are furnished by a principal vendor who not only assumes responsibility for storage but also prepares items for delivery to the operating units of the HSO. Accordingly, the vendor is an extension of the organization's material management program and, when a stockless program is adopted, the HSO is required to maintain the inventory levels necessary for emergency use.

ꝶ Planning and Controlling

In this section the focus shifts from the daily management of fiscal affairs to the general problem of developing organizational plans as expressed by the capital, operating, and cash budget. The operating budget, consisting of expected revenues, costs, and the net surplus, expresses the standard of performance against which actual activity is compared. The capital budget describes planned changes in the capital complement and methods of financing alterations. As such, the capital budget not only enables management to assess capital proposals, develop funding priorities, and evaluate alternative sources of funding but is also a partial expression of the strategic plan.

The Capital Budget

The importance of the capital budget and the process of capital rationing has increased as a result of recent changes in the financial environment of the health care industry. Focusing on the hospital sector as an example, the Medicare program initially based prospective prices on operating expenses and used the retrospective method to compensate the hospital for the costs of capital (i.e., depreciation, interest, and leases). Recently, however, these costs have been incorporated into the set of prospective prices. Since the number of discharges, the amount of related revenue, and cash receipts are volatile, the transfer of responsibility for paying these costs to HSOs increases the risks and the nominal rate of interest on the long-term debt instruments they issue. Accordingly, fiscal performance is contingent in part on the organization's evaluation of alternative funding sources and selection of capital projects.

The capital budget represents a framework that enables management to assess the fiscal impact of proposals to acquire plant and equipment, to dispose of capital assets, or to improve existing facilities. Therefore, the preparation of the capital budget consists of two essentially separate but interrelated phases. During the first, management identifies capital projects consistent with the organization's strategic plan and assembles the information required for subsequent evaluation. Given that it is not possible to fund all projects, the second phase focuses on the evaluation of capital projects and alternative sources of funding.

As described by Duncan, Ginter, and Swayne (1995), the strategic plan synthesizes what the organization is *able* to do, as indicated by an assessment of the internal environment; what the organization *ought* to do, as suggested by an evaluation of the external environment; and what the organization *wants* to do, an outcome produced by the vision of management. The strategic plan of the organization thus serves as a guideline for the identification of capital proposals and the initial selection of projects that will be considered for possible funding.

Capital proposals usually emanate from all levels of managerial responsibility in general and members of the medical staff in particular. Given the speed of changes in medical knowledge, administrators are usually not familiar with all technological improvements and are forced to rely on the advice of medical experts. However, administrators should evaluate recommendations in terms of their strategic positions and the potential impact of each proposal on fiscal performance.

The evaluation of capital projects might be facilitated by grouping proposals according to their primary benefits. For example, capital projects may reduce operating expenses or enhance net revenues horizontally or vertically. Proposals may increase income vertically by expanding the volume of existing services or horizontally through an investment that is unrelated to existing activities.

The taxonomy based on the primary benefit of the proposal might be extended to derive a measure of relative risk. In this regard, projects related to the introduction of a new product or service are usually accompanied by the greatest risk, since the demand for the service, operating costs, and related cash flows is relatively difficult to estimate. Similarly, projects that expand existing capacity are accompanied by medium to high risk, an outcome that is attributable to unanticipated variation in costs, revenues, and net cash flows. Alternatives that promise to reduce costs usually exert little, if any, influence on revenues and involve low to medium risk. Finally, proposals to replace existing capacity are frequently least risky, since these projects produce the most predictable cash flows.

In addition, it is useful to group proposals in terms of their economic or financial interdependence. Two proposals are complementary if the cash flow expected from the adoption of both exceeds the cash flows that would result from approving them individually. Projects are substitutes if the acceptance of one reduces the cash flows of another; they are mutually exclusive if the approval of one prevents the approval of the other. Finally, if the adoption of one alternative exerts no influence on the cash flows expected from another, the two proposals are independent. The classification of alternatives in terms of economic interrelationships enables management to assess groups of proposals that are independent of alternatives.

The assessment of proposals and the development of funding priorities should be based on a measure of fiscal merit and a standard of performance. Frequently, the standard of performance is the required rate of return, a concept that is based on the weighted cost of capital. The cost of capital is expressed as a percentage of available funds and is influenced by the relative dependence on debt, D, or equity, E. The common pool of funding is given by the sum of debt and equity. In the calculation of the weighted cost of capital, k_w, i represents the return required by debt holders; r_e corresponds to the return required on equity; α is the proportion of cost-based reimbursement, and θ is the marginal tax rate, if any:

$$k_w = [(1-\theta)(1-\alpha)iD]/(D+E) + r_eE/(D+E)$$

The first of the terms adjusts interest charges, iD, for the effects of the marginal tax rate and cost-based reimbursement. As indicated by the expression, the effective rate of interest decreases with greater dependence on cost-based reimbursement and a higher marginal tax rate.

The required rate of return is contingent on the relationship of the weighted cost of capital to debt structure. It is common to assume that the risks assumed by debt holders are less than those of equity owners and that the cost of debt, i, is less than return on equity, r_e. If the debt-to-equity ratio is relatively low, an increased dependence on debt results in a less costly mix of financing and a decline in the weighted cost of capital. However, if the debt-to-equity ratio continues to grow, the risks of default and the rate of interest increase, suggesting that the cost of debt will eventually exceed the return on equity. As a consequence, an excessive dependence on debt results in a higher weighted cost of capital. For present purposes, it is assumed that the institution maintains a debt structure that minimizes the weighted cost of capital. Accordingly, after adjusting for the relative risk of a given proposal, the weighted cost of capital represents the required rate of return and the standard of performance against which measures of fiscal merit are compared.

Table 5.3 lists the indicators that enable management to identify those proposals that are eligible for funding and to develop a funding priority. Let $R_1, \ldots, R_j, \ldots, R_n$ correspond to the net returns expected during periods $1, \ldots j, \ldots n$ respectively and C_o represent the initial investment associated with a given proposal. As indicated, the minimum acceptable rate of return is used to calculate the net present value (NPV) of the proposal.

To illustrate, suppose that k is 10%, the initial cost of a project is \$18,000, and net returns during its useful life are as follows:

Year	Net Returns ($)
1	8,000
2	10,000
3	6,000
4	4,000
5	2,000

The NPV of the project is given by

$$NPV = 8,000/(1.15) + 10,000/(1.15)^2 + \ldots + 2,000/(1.15)^5 - 18,000$$

or approximately \$3,744.

Table 5.3   Measuring the Fiscal Merit of Capital Proposals

Indicator	Definition	Retain	Funding Priority
Payback Period	$\dfrac{\text{Investment}}{\text{Annual Returns}}$	$PBP < MP$	
Accounting Rate of Return	$\dfrac{\text{Annual Profitability}}{\text{Average Investment}}$		
Net Present Value	$\sum R_j / (1+k)^j - C_0$		NPV_i / C_{io}
Internal Rate of Return	$\sum R_j / (1+r)^j = C_0$	$r > k$	r_i
Net Terminal Value	$S(n) - C(n)$ or $\sum R_j / (1+i_j)^{m-j} - C_0(1+i)^m$	$NTV > 0$	
Terminal Rate of Return	$r^* = [S(n)/C(n)]^{1/m} - 1$		r^*_i

If the NPV is positive, as in the illustration, the proposal should be retained for inclusion in the funding priority. Since larger projects may generate higher net present values that are attributable solely to scale factors, the relative attractiveness of projects should be based on the profitability index, PI_i, where the index i refers to a specific proposal.

Table 5.3 indicates that the internal rate of return is the discount rate that equates the stream of net returns with the initial capital outlay. If the internal rate of return, r, is greater than or equal to minimum acceptable rate, k, the proposal should be retained for inclusion in the funding priority. Since the internal rate of return is a relative measure of merit, values of r_i may be used to rank projects ordinally and develop funding priorities.

Unlike the internal rate of return and the NPV, the net terminal value (NTV) assumes that intermediate returns are reinvested at variable rates during the life of the project. When the NTV is used, it is assumed that $i_1, \ldots, i_j, \ldots, i_n$ are the rates of reinvesting returns $R_1, \ldots, R_j, \ldots, R_n$ respectively. If the planning horizon is m periods, the NTV measures the difference between the compounded value of receipts and the initial cost. Hence, if the NTV is positive, the proposal should be included in the funding priority. Similar to the internal rate of return, the terminal rate of return (TROR) is the discount rate that equates the compounded values of the stream of net returns and initial costs. Accordingly, the TROR, r^*, may be used to rank proposals, develop priorities and ration available funds. When combined with the NTV, the terminal rate of return also represents the basis for examining the sensitivity of investment decisions to variation in the set of reinvestment rates.

To illustrate, suppose that the initial cost of a project is $800 and that the following information is available:

Period	Returns	Reinvestment Rate
1	$1,000	10%
2	800	9%
3	700	8%

If the opportunity rate is 8%,

$$S_n = 1,000(1.10)^3 + 800(1.09)^2 + 700(1.08)$$

or $3,037.48 while

$$C_n = (1.08)^4 (800)$$

or $1,088.39. Hence, the NTV is $1,949.09, and the project should be retained for inclusion in the funding priority. The TROR is given by

$$TROR = (3037.48/1088.39)^{1/4}$$

or approximately 30%.

Planning and Controlling Operations

The emergence of alternative delivery systems, prospective payment, and increased restrictions on revenue-generating potential have increased the imperative to plan and control operations. Of particular importance are accurate estimates of the net surplus derived from capitation arrangements, PPSs, based on case mix, and discounted prices that are applied to components of direct patient care.

As indicated, the revenue budget reflects the amount of income management expects to derive from each payment mechanism. To simplify, let M_i depict the expected mix of patients–grouped by type of capitation arrangement, risk category, or DRG–and F_i represent the corresponding rate of compensation–expressed as a price per discharge or payment per member. The amount of revenue that management expects to derive from these systems is simply $\Sigma F_i M_i$. Similarly, let P_k and V_k represent the fee or negotiated price and volume of service k respectively. The corresponding projection of revenue is given by $\Sigma P_k V_k$.

As indicated, an assessment of the net surplus requires a full cost construction that corresponds to one of several units of payment. Focusing first on payment systems based on case mix, let M_i correspond to the portion of the population assigned to a given DRG, S_{ik} represent the use of service k by the typical patient assigned to the DRG, and fc_k represent the full cost of providing a unit of service k. In this case, using a hospital as an example, the mix of services includes stay-specific services, which are measured by the length of stay, units of ancillary service, and clinic visits.

Employing this notation, the full cost of providing care to patients assigned to the DRG, fc_i, is

$$fc_i = M_i \Sigma S_{ik} fc_k$$

while Σfc_i corresponds to the full costs of the services consumed by those whose care is financed by the set of prospective prices. Accordingly, a comparison of the full cost construction with the corresponding rate or level of compensation enables management to ensure that the net surplus derived from each profit center is adequate.

Similar to prospective pricing systems based on case mix, capitation arrangements transfer the responsibility for predicting and controlling costs from the insurer to the provider. To simplify, let M_j represent the portion of the membership assigned to risk category j, as defined by age and sex. Suppose further that the annual use of service k by the typical patient assigned to risk category j is represented by S_{jk}. The cost per member per month is determined by the use of each service/1,000 population, the number of enrollees, and the total annual cost. The annual volume of service k, V_k, required by the membership is given by $V_k = \Sigma M_j S_{jk}$, implying that annual costs might be measured by $\Sigma V_k fc_k$. The cost per member per month, CPMPM, might be derived by

$$CPMPM = Annual\ Costs/12/Number\ of\ Enrollees$$

Similar to the discussion of prospective payment based on case mix, the CPMPM requires an accurate measure of the full costs of each component of care.

Recently, HSOs have adopted several methods of measuring full costs, defined as the sum of direct and indirect expenses. For example, relative value units (RVUs) might be combined with the ratio of cost to charge (RCC) to estimate the cost of a given procedure, the care consumed by a patient assigned to a given DRG, or the provision of service to a population whose care is financed by per capita rates (Rezaee, 1993). The RCC approach assumes that the revenue and cost per unit are correlated positively. The full cost assigned to a responsibility center that generates revenue is given by the product of the RCC and the income that management expects to generate by providing an expected mix of care.

The costs assigned to the center are then allocated to individual procedures by relying on RVUs, a set of indicators that measure the relative resource consumption associated with each procedure. First, the weighted volume of service is obtained by $\sum RV_k V_k$, where RV_k is the relative value for service k and V_k is the volume of service k management expects to provide. Second, the cost per weighted unit is obtained by the ratio of costs to the weighted volume of service. Third, the full cost per unit of service is estimated by the product of the cost per weighted unit and the relative value of each procedure.

Unfortunately, conventional approaches produce imprecise estimates of full costs. In particular, the RCC approach is based on aggregated data and obscures the differences in costs produced by variation in the mix of care provided by HSO components. Viewed from the perspective of revenue, the RCC approach also obscures differences that result from variation in product mix and the "markups" that are applied to charges for services provided by an HSO component. Similarly, since RVUs are approximations of relative resource consumption, related cost estimates are likely to be correspondingly imprecise. Further, in the absence of frequent revision, RVUs fail to reflect changes in technology or the efficiency of resource use. As a consequence, the traditional approach, dominated by a dependence on RCCs and RVUs, is valid only for a specific mix of care and a given period of time.

In response to the need for greater accuracy, HSOs have adopted activity-based costing (ABC), microcosting, job order or procedure costing, and process costing as methods of deriving estimates of direct cost. Job order costing is a method of assembling the direct costs of labor, supplies, and equipment that are used on each occasion a well-defined procedure is provided. In general, job order costing should be applied only to those components of care for which the mix of resources is heterogeneous. If each unit requires a homogeneous mix of direct resources—consisting of labor, supplies, and equipment—process costing is an appropriate method of measuring direct costs. The direct costs of operating the process during a given time period are divided by the corresponding volume to obtain a measure of unit costs.

Microcosting is a method of determining the direct costs of each item in a detailed list of resources required to provide a given procedure. As such, the approach is relatively expensive but generates accurate cost data. A comprehensive application would require management to assemble the costs of all procedures. However, since the costs of implementation frequently are prohibitive, HSOs usually observe the 80/20 rule, which suggests that microcosting should be applied to the set of procedures that represent 80 percent of costs or revenues.

As indicated, full costs consist of direct costs and an equitable share of indirect costs. Conventional methods of assigning indirect costs usually rely on a single rate, which is based on the volume of service, hours of direct labor, or direct cost. For example, the indirect cost rate might indicate the amount of indirect expense that is assigned for each dollar of direct cost, hour of direct labor, or unit of service. Unfortunately, the conventional approach overstates the costs of high-volume services and understates the costs of low-volume services. As a consequence, reliance on conventional approaches to assign indirect costs results in biased estimates of full cost, an outcome that contributes to suboptimal decisions and fiscal performance.

Unlike conventional methods, activity-based systems focus on the full costs of the activities that must be performed to provide a procedure. The full costs of the procedure are measured by the accumulated costs of related activities. An activity is defined as a unit of work or function that is defined in micro or macro terms. A micro activity is performed within an HSO component (e.g., hospital department) and is managed daily. Macro activities are units of work or functions that are related to the accumulation of accurate cost and service data.

The implementation of ABC consists of several separate but interrelated phases. The first focuses on the identification of procedures or services for which a full cost construction is required. During the second, management identifies the activities or functions that must be performed when providing each of the procedures. In the third phase, management identifies and measures the mix of labor, supplies, and equipment consumed by each of the activities and determines the direct costs of each function. The fourth phase is based on an assessment of the factors that cause departmental and allocated overhead and involves the assignment of indirect costs to establish a way of measuring the full cost per unit of each procedure. In turn, this full cost can be used to determine the full cost of providing the services required by patients grouped by diagnostic nomenclature, or by those whose care is financed by capitation.

A simplified illustration of ABC is presented in Figure 5.3. It is assumed that the unit provides three services—A, B, and C—with corresponding volumes listed in the second row. The third row shows the supply costs per unit of service, amounts that represent the sum of the expenses assigned to the activities associated with each service. The hours of direct labor and equipment time are derived in a similar manner. The direct cost per unit of each service is simply the sum of supply expenses and the product of direct labor hours and the weighted wage rate of $20 per hour.

The precision of the indirect costs assigned to each procedure is a major benefit of activity-based systems, which rely on multiple rates to assign departmental and allocated overhead to services. For example, if each service requires the same amount of clerical services, the cost assigned to each unit is given by the ratio of clerical costs to total volume (i.e., $30,000/25,000 units). Similarly, the assignment of equipment and maintenance costs is based on the amount of equipment time required to provide a unit of each service. In particular, maintenance costs are assigned to each service by the product of equipment time and the amount of maintenance cost per hour, while the equipment cost assigned to each service is determined by the product of equipment time and equipment cost per hour. Finally, the illustration assumes that the cost of preparing and distributing supply items is the same for all items, implying that these costs might be allocated by applying the ratio of distribution costs per dollar of direct supply expense to the unit supply costs. In addition to those illustrated in Figure 5.3, other bases might be used to allocate departmental and allocated overhead. For example, the cost of preparing equipment to perform a given procedure might be determined by the product of the direct labor hours required per setup, the number of preparations, and the average wage rate. The ratio of these costs to the volume of the procedure yields the amount of cost assigned per unit of service.

In addition to the need for more precise methods of estimation, HSOs must ensure that the variance in profitability is favorable, an outcome that requires a comparison between actual and standard, or expected, costs. In turn, expected costs might be based on (1) basic standards that are invariant with respect to time; (2) theoretical or ideal standards that define the best performance possible, given the current operating environment; (3) currently attainable standards that express the expected performance after adjusting for factors such as idle time, routine maintenance, and breakdowns; or (4) standards that are based on previous performance, an approach that assumes operations were efficient in the past.

The standard of performance and the components that determine actual costs together constitute the basis for identifying a controllable variance. Recall that a controllable variance is defined as the difference between an actual and expected result attributable to factors that are controlled, to a significant extent, by an individual or group associated with the HSO.

Limited to differences between actual and standard direct costs, Table 5.4 summarizes the controllable variances that enable management to monitor and evaluate operations. To simplify the presentation, it is assumed that the HSO uses one resource to provide a single service to patients assigned to a given DRG or risk category. In the Table, M_a and M_s correspond to the actual and standard number of patients respectively; U_a and U_s represent the actual and expected use of service per case respectively; and R_a and R_s correspond to the actual and standard resource requirement per unit of service respectively. Finally, P_a and P_s are the actual and standard prices of the resource.

Figure 5.3 Activity-Based Costing

Service

	A	B	C	Total
Volume	15,000	8,000	2,000	25,000
Supply Cost Per Unit	$5	$10	$15	
Total Supply Cost	75,000	80,000	30,000	185,000
Direct Labor Hours	.1	.2	.3	
Equipment Time Per Service	.2	.4	.6	
Equipment Hours	3000	3200	1200	7400

Average Wage Rate: $20

Departmental Overhead:	Amount	Rate
Clerical	$30,000	$1.20
Equipment	$11,100	$1.50

Allocated Overhead:		
Maintenance	$5,920	$.80
Supply Distribution	$9,250	$.05

Service

	A	B	C
Direct Cost			
Supply	$5.00	$10.00	$15.00
Labor	2.00	4.00	6.00
Departmental Overhead			
Clerical	1.20	1.20	1.20
Equipment	.30	.60	.90
Allocated Overhead			
Maintenance	.16	.32	.48
Distribution	.25	.50	.75
Full Cost	8.91	16.32	24.33

As indicated, the portion of the variance in direct cost that results from the difference between the actual and expected number of patients, the volume of service per case, and their interactive effects is attributable to the admitting and prescribing decisions of the medical staff. Similarly, the portion of the variance in direct costs that can be traced to the difference between the actual and expected resource consumption per service is attributable to the efficiency of operations, a dimension that is the responsibility of line management. On the other hand, the portion that is

Table 5.4   The Variance in Direct Cost

Component	Definition	Responsibility
Variance	$M_a U_a R_a P_a - M_s U_s R_s P_s$	
Volume		
Cases	$(M_a - M_s) U_s R_s P_s$	Physicians
Volume/Case	$M_s (U_a - U_s) R_s P_s$	Physicians
Cases, Volume/Case	$(M_a - M_s)(U_a - U_s) R_s P_s$	Physicians
Efficiency	$M_s U_s (R_a - R_s) P_s$	Management
Factor Price	$M_s U_s R_s (P_a - P_s)$	Market, Fiscal Services
Joint		
Price, Resource Use	$(M_a U_a R_a - M_s U_s R_s)(P_a - P_s)$	Physicians, Management, Fiscal Services
Volume, Efficiency	$(M_a U_a - M_s U_s)(R_a - R_s) P_s$	Physicians, Management

related to the difference between actual and expected factor prices may reflect market forces or the performance of those assigned to fiscal services. Finally, the combined influence of differences between actual and expected operating efficiency, volume of care, and factor prices is the responsibility of fiscal services, the medical staff, and management, a situation that highlights the need to adopt an integrated approach to the problem of controlling costs and ensuring the fiscal viability of the HSO.

ea SUMMARY

This chapter has briefly reviewed rapidly changing fiscal stimuli in the environment of HSOs. For even the most heretofore protected HSO, such as the academic medical center, to survive, these environmental stimuli must be met with intelligent responses. Some of the financial management and planning tools for optimal adaptation to the environment, such as activity-based costing, are relatively new. However, the traditional methods can accommodate much of the change if applied diligently and sensitively.

We have discussed both new and older methods as they may be applied in the well-managed HSO. The discussion should make it clear that the (occasional) elegance of the methods does not obviate management decisions about where the HSO is, ought to be and really wants to be in the new era.

❧ SELECTED BIBLIOGRAPHY (GROUPED BY TOPIC)

Financial Accounting and Reporting

Bitter, ME, and JH Cassidy 1990 The new healthcare audit guide: its impact on hospitals and hospital reporting *Hospital Topics* 71(4):32

Cerrone, RA 1976 Reflect the true financial picture: prepare current value statements *Hospital Financial Management* 30(5):20

Cleverley WO 1983 Valuation:its impact on accounting measures of income and return on capital *Health Care Management Review* 8(2):51

Colbert RG 1990 The new health care audit and accounting guide *Topics in Health Care Financing* 16(4):14

Finkler, SA 1982 Ratio analysis: use with caution *Health Care Management Review* 7(2):65

Friedman LA and BR Neumann 1979 Replacement cost accounting: an alternative to price level indexes *Hospital and Health Services Administration* 24(4):9

Kovener RR 1990 New rules affect bad debt, charity care reporting *Healthcare Financial Management* 44(10):48

Neumann BR and LA Friedman 1980 Should financial statements disclose the cost of replacing hospital assets? *Health Care Management Review* 5(1):49

Pelfrey S 1990 How proposed financial statement rules would affect hospitals *Healthcare Financial Management* 44(2):54

Tillett JW and WR Titera 1990 What AICPA audit guide revisions mean for providers *Healthcare Financial Management* 44(7):52

Tripoli FJ 1975 Accounting for inflation in your financial statements *Hospital Financial Management* 29(12):25

Working Capital

Anderson ST 1988 Hospitals can improve cash flow by managing preauthorizations *Healthcare Financial Management* 42(12):56

Berling RJ and JT Geppi 1989 Hospitals can cut materials costs by managing the pipeline *Healthcare Financial Management* 43(4):19

Bort R and DR Schinderle 1994 Using EDI to improve the accounts payable department *Healthcare Financial Management* 48(1):78

Clarkin JF 1990 Managing accounts receivable: an overview *Topics in Health Care Financing* 17(1):6

Francis JM 1985 Reduction in accounts receivable begins before patient admission *Healthcare Financial Management* 39(11):60

Hauser RC and DE Edwards 1990 Cash budgeting leads to better cash management *Healthcare Financial Management* 44(2):77

Jupp DA 1987 Measuring and monitoring quality in accounts receivable *Healthcare Financial Management* 41(9):68

Kincaid TJ 1993 Selling accounts receivable to fund working capital *Healthcare Financial Management* 47(5):27

Ladewig TL and BA Hecht 1993 Achieving excellence in the management of accounts receivable *Healthcare Financial Management* 47(9):24

McCormick, EJ 1993 The hidden costs of accounts receivable *Healthcare Financial Management* 47(11):78

McFadden, DR 1989 How to gain maximum returns through cash management *Healthcare Financial Management* 43(10):44

Newton, RL 1993 Measuring accounts receivable performance: a comprehensive method *Healthcare Financial Management* 47(5):33

Puhala JM and MJ Barrett 1987 Patient accounting: vital for financial survival *Healthcare Financial Management* 41(9):25

Racca SR 1990 Health care financing note *Topics in Health Care Financing* 17(1):90

Rode D 1990 Gaining control of the uncontrollable in preadmissions *Healthcare Financial Management* 44(4):15

Sylvestre J and FR Urbancic 1994 Effective methods for cash flow analysis *Healthcare Financial Management* 48(7):62

Vogel LH Patient accounts management: it's what's up front that counts *Healthcare Financial Management* 41(9):42

Capital

Carroll JJ and Newbould GD 1986 NPV vs. IRR: with capital budgeting, which do you choose? *Healthcare Financial Management* 40(11):62

Cleverly WO 1987 Strategic financial planning: a balance sheet perspective *Hospital and Health Services Administration* 32(11):1

Cleverly WO and PC Nutt 1981 Credit evaluation of hospitals *Topics in Health Care Financing* 7(4):81

Gapenski LC 1989 A better approach to internal rate of return *Healthcare Financial Management* 43(4):93

Gapenski LC 1990 Using Monte Carlo simulation to make better capital investment decisions *Hospital and Health Services Administration* 35(2):207

Gapenski LC 1990 Risk factor helps determine debt maturity mix *Healthcare Financial Management* 44(11):82

Grossman M and F Goldman, SW Nesbitt and P Mobilia 1993 Determinants of interest rates on tax-exempt hospital bonds *Journal of Health Economics* 12:385

Newbould GD and JJ Carroll 1986 Inflation, risk, replacement, closure: concerns in capital budgeting *Healthcare Financial Management* 40(12):64

Sherman B 1990 How investors evaluate the creditworthiness of hospitals *Healthcare Financial Management* 44(3):25

Smith RG and JR Wheeler 1989 Accounting based risk measures for not-for-profit hospitals *Health Services Management Research* 2(3):221

The Operating Budget

Barry P 1993 The financial evolution of hospitals and the zero-base budget approach *Hospital Cost Management and Accounting* 5(7):1

Chandler WL 1986 Integrating case mix information into operating budgets *Healthcare Financial Management* 40(10):27

Cleverly WO 1987 Product costing for health care firms *Health Care Management Review* 12(4):39

Nackel JG, PJ Fenaroli and GM Kis 1987 Product line performance reporting: a key to cost management *Healthcare Financial Management* 41(11):54

Finkler SA 1985 Flexible budget variance analysis extended to patient acuity and DRGs *Health Care Management Review* 10(4):21

Goldschmidt Y and A Gafni 1990 A managerial approach to allocating indirect fixed costs in health care organizations *Health Care Management Review* 15(2):43

Gruenberg L, SS Wallack and CP Tompkins 1986 Pricing strategies for capitated delivery systems *Health Care Financing Review* annual supplement: 35

Hauser RC and DE Edwards 1990 Cash budgeting leads to better cash management *Healthcare Financial Management* 44(2):77

Kerschner MI and JM Rooney 1987 Utilizing cost accounting information for budgeting *Topics in Health Care Financing* 13(4):56

Thompson JD, RF Averill and RB Fetter 1979 Planning, budgeting and controlling–one look at the future:case-mix accounting *Health Services Research* 14(2):111

Management and Cost Accounting

Baptist AJ 1987 A general approach to costing procedures in ancillary departments *Topics in Health Care Financing* 13(4):32

Bennett JP 1985 Standard cost systems lead to efficiency and profitability *Healthcare Financial Management* 39(9):46

Bridges JM and P Jacobs 1986 Obtaining estimates of marginal cost by DRG *Healthcare Financial Management* 40(10):40

Broyles RW and MD Rosko 1987 The Medicare payment system: a conceptual approach to the problem of controlling profitability *Health Care Management Review* 12(3):35

Broyles RW and MD Rosko 1987 Full cost determination: an application of pricing and patient mix policies under DRGs *Health Care Management Review* 11(3):57

Chaffman BM and J Tallbott 1990 Activity-based costing in a service organization *CMA* 10(3):15

Chan YC 1993 Improving hospital cost accounting with activity-based costing *Health Care Management Review* 18(1):71

Cooper R 1990 The rise of activity-based costing–Part one: what is an activity-based cost system? *Journal of Cost Management* 1(2):45

Cooper R 1988 The rise of activity-based costing–Part three: how many cost drivers do you need and how do you select them? *Journal of Cost Management* 1(4):34

Glennie SC and PA Terhaar 1994 Activity-based costing *MGM Journal* July/August:89

Hogan AJ and RM Marshall 1990 How to improve allocation of support service costs *Healthcare Financial Management* 44(2):42

Lerner WM and WL Wellman 1985 Pricing hospital units of service using microcosting techniques *Hospital and Health Services Administration* 30(1):7

Messmer VC 1984 Standard cost accounting: methods that can be applied to DRG classifications *Healthcare Financial Management* 38(1):44

Razee Z 1993 Examining the effect of PPS on cost accounting systems *Healthcare Financial Management* (March) 58

Schimmel VE, C Alley and AM Heath 1987 Measuring costs: product line accounting versus ratio of cost to charges *Topics in Health Care Financing* 13(4):76

Suver JD, WF Jessee and WN Zelman 1986 Financial management and DRGs *Hospital and Health Services Administration* 31(1):75

Toso ME and A Farmer 1994 Using cost accounting data to develop capitation rates *Hospital Cost Management and Accounting* 6(1):1

Tselepis JN 1989 Refined cost accounting produces better information *Healthcare Financial Management* 43(5):27

Turney PB 1991 How activity-based costing helps reduce cost *Journal of Cost Management* 4(4):29

Health Economics

6

Vivian Valdmanis, University of Oklahoma

❧ INTRODUCTION

Health care expenditures in the United States currently constitute 14 percent of the country's gross domestic product (GDP) and are expected to continue to increase into the next century. Because of these vast expenditures, health care economics has emerged as a formalized study within the discipline of economics, which is formally defined as the study of how resources should be allocated. Focusing on health care economics in particular, this chapter examines how resources are allocated specifically within the health care sector as well as in the economy in general.

Economists generally contend that economic incentives drive behavior and that in the US economy these incentives have been structured to produce a drastic increase in health spending. If we accept this contention, the study of health care economics requires a thorough understanding of why and how these incentives behave, as well as how the health economy itself deviates from standard economic markets.

In standard economic markets, competition is waged in terms of prices. That is, the prices reflect both the face values that consumers are willing to pay for certain goods or services and the costs incurred to produce these goods. It is further assumed that consumers themselves possess the necessary information to make a coherent decision regarding whether to purchase a particular good. Health care economics, however, deviates from this type of price-valued market due to inherent market failures.

The market failures that currently exist within the health care market include asymmetric information, externalities, and the public/collective good nature found in health care. First, asymmetric information arises because the physician (or some other medical caregiver) possesses more information about a patient's condition than the individual patient. This asymmetry of information then leads to a principal-agency relation, in which one or more persons (defined as principals) engage another person or persons (agents) to perform some service on their behalf. Under a contract of this nature, the agent then assumes a certain portion of the decision-making authority (Jensen and Meckling, 1976). Following this definition, it may then be argued that information asymmetry may exist wherever either party has more information than the other. With this asymmetry, the physician may have an incentive to prescribe more medical care than the patient might deem necessary. Moreover, the presence of health care insurance also contributes to the incentives of both patients and physicians. Health care insurance lowers the out-of-pocket cost to the patient, leading him or her to purchase more care, which in turn leads the physician to perform additional medical care without worrying about the patient's ability to pay.

Next, externalities also arise in health care. More specifically, a third person is either positively or negatively affected by a transaction to which he or she is not a direct party. For example, medical care research benefits society as a whole, but society itself does not enter directly into the medical research process. Because of these externalities, the government maintains an interest in subsidizing medical research. In addition, the government is also involved in direct payments for medical care to certain populations, namely, the indigent and the elderly. The existence of both Medicaid (the program for the indigent) and Medicare (the program for the elderly) makes the government the largest single purchaser of health care services in the United States.

The purpose of this chapter is to present an overview of health care economics, which encompasses insurance, hospitals, physicians, nurses, and societal interest in health care and regulation.*

❧ Health Insurance

A major economic force in the US health care market is the prevalence of health insurance. The vast majority of the US population is now covered by either private or

---

*A glossary of economic definitions is given at the end of this chapter. Interested readers may refer to a microeconomics text for more details.

public health care insurance. As a result, the subsequent demand for health insurance actually represents a hidden demand for adequate medical care. In other words, health insurance also insures against financial ruin, especially in light of costly injury or illness.

In response to these insurance demands, most insurance literature is written based on the assumption that individuals are risk-averse (i.e., unwilling to accept financially risky situations). This assumption in turn emanates from the notion that individuals become risk-averse simply due to their desire to maintain their wealth and income.

With these concerns in mind, the individual is therefore willing to pay what is referred to as a "risk premium" (i.e., the amount paid) to avoid such financial risks. As a consequence, the more people dislike these risks, the greater the risk premiums become. In addition, the individual also enjoys a "welfare gain" if the price of insurance is less than the risk premium.

The actual premium, or price paid for insurance, is given where

$$\text{Premium} = E(B) - \text{deductible} + \text{Loading fee } (L).$$

$E(B)$ is the expected benefit amount, the deductible is the amount of health care that the patient must pay (before insurance coverage begins), while the loading fee is the price insurance companies charge for administrative costs. Moreover, $E(B)$ can be further broken down into the relation $E(B) = (1 - c)Pm * m$, where c is the coinsurance rate (the amount for which the patient is responsible), Pm is the price of medical care, and m is the average quantity of care. It is therefore in the individual's best interest to become insured only in cases where the types of care received are necessary (e.g., hospital days and physician services), since it is solely in these cases that the quantity of care demanded is less responsive to price.

Next, the insurance premium can be further defined as Premium $= (1 + L)$ $(1 - c)Pm * m -$ deductibles. If $L = 0$, then no administrative costs exist. If L increases, however, the coinsurance for which the individual is responsible must also increase in order to reduce the overall price of the insurance premium. One way to minimize these so-called loading fees is to provide group insurance. By providing the insurance to a large group, the insurance company can exploit economies of scale, whereby a reduction in adverse selection lowers the expected benefit payouts. The company reduces the incidence of an adverse selection by insuring a large group of individuals, who then proportionately lower the risks involved (i.e., reduce the risk per person).

When individuals choose a health insurance plan, they must confront two issues: moral hazards and selection bias. Moral hazards constitute an additional market failure characteristic of the health care market. It can be argued that since patients possess health care insurance, they consume more health care services than they would in the absence of health care insurance (because they pay a lower price). Hence, patients tend to overconsume health care services, a practice that may coincide with physicians' tendencies to overprescribe health care services. These two tendencies then cause costs to increase. Moreover, these behaviors stem from the aforementioned incentives.

As a result of the above tendencies to overconsume health care insurance, welfare loss of excess health insurance has been estimated at between $81.7 billion and $109.3 billion. Although it is true that consumers can obtain "free" medical care (in the absence of nonprice rationing), they will in fact use medical services up to the point where the last service performed has very low value (Feldman and Dowd, 1993). However, the marginal cost of these services remains unaffected by the insurance purchased, and may even increase if the insurance itself contributes to inflationary price increases that would arise in the supplier-induced demand situation presented above. The extra services thus consumed as a result of this "free" medical care have less value than their corresponding costs in terms of actual resources. Furthermore, it has also been suggested that because the demand for effective medical care is extremely inelastic, it should thus be the only type of care to be insured, which would in turn decrease the moral hazards involved.

Once the lump-sum premium has been paid (and any required deductible met), the only subsequent costs that influence the individual's subsequent decisions regarding any medical services are the so-called variable costs (i.e., the copayments). This type of insurance, in which the costs of the individual's office visits (and hospitals stays) for the procedures covered are lowered, is described as an indemnity type of insurance. Here, the main concern for indemnity insurance is that the freedom of choice of health care provider is maintained, but the moral hazard is conversely increased.

In light of the above circumstances, one way to combat the overuse of health care services by insured individuals is to implement a managed care system. Under this system, physicians are contracted by insurance companies to provide care for a fixed annual reimbursement, regardless of what the health care services provided actually cost. In other words, the financial risks of health care are passed on to the providers. As a result, the patient pays a small fee for visits to the contracted physician but incurs no further out-of-pocket costs. The providers, however, are then controlled through the capitated payment system, which curbs supplier-induced demand.

Managed care itself is described as an organizational approach intended to change physician behavior toward expenditure control while developing a more cost-effective style of care. Typical forms of managed care include health maintenance organizations (HMOs), which pay physicians on a capitated basis, and preferred provider organizations (PPOs) which negotiate with physicians and hospitals for a discounted fee. One feature of managed care, termed selective contracting, involves contracting with a panel of physicians and hospitals to limit fees while maintaining a conservative style of practice (Robinson, 1993). Under this system, the contract between the insurer (HMO or PPO) is therefore explicit, in contrast to the indemnity plans (free choice of provider), in which the contract is more implicitly written (Robinson, 1993). In addition to the above two features, other characteristics of managed care include a "gatekeeper" approach (in which the patient must first be seen by a primary care provider in order to be referred to a specialist); utilization review (or UR, in which the insurer reviews physicians' practices); and quality assurance (or QA, which consists of another insurance review to ensure that patients are being appropriately treated). Moreover, the managed care system also applies to hospitals, which may grant contractual discounts to the managed care insurer, which in turn reviews the managed care patients to ensure that methods of treatment are cost-effective.

One benefit of these managed care approaches is that they reduce both asymmetric information and the overuse of costly specialist care by insured patients. Asymmetric information may be reduced because the primary care provider intervenes in the process to provide details of the patient's health care needs, as well as outlining a treatment regimen.

To be sure, managed care is not a homogeneous enterprise but rather consists of several types of individual organizations. In the staff model HMO, physicians are actual employees of the HMO and treat only HMO patients. In the group model HMO, however, the insurer possesses an exclusive contract with a panel of providers and hospitals. In both of these cases, through a vertical integration approach, any possible conflicts that may arise between the HMO and its physicians are resolved through administrative mechanisms (Robinson, 1993).

A third HMO model is the independent practitioner association (IPA), through which the HMO contracts with individual physicians in a local area to provide services to the HMO's patients alongside the physician's other patients. A fourth major model is the PPO, in which all types of insurers contract with a panel of providers for reduced fees. Both IPAs and PPOs offer a stronger exit option, which then allows the physicians more latitude vis-à-vis the insurer than either their staff or group model counterparts (Robinson, 1993).

Although the above HMO arrangements are clearly effective cost reduction methods, the relationships between HMOs and physicians are not without their problems. To begin with, physicians have always enjoyed professional autonomy without any type of outside interference. Under managed care contracts, however, their autonomy is limited, and their objectives may be at odds with those of the managed care system.

In the supply and demand of health services, managed care attempts to restrict both quantity and price in an effort to reduce total costs and expenditures. Moreover,

HMOs can also decrease demand by steering the so-called taste of the individual away from highly priced specialist care. These efforts are appropriate when the primary care provider is a good substitute for the specialist (i.e., can provide quality care equivalent to that of the specialist). This substitution thus also reduces costs, since it is the less expensive provider who ultimately delivers patient care.

Within the above health care framework of supply and demand, the link between the workplace and health care insurance has become a major and distinctive feature of the US health care system (IOM, 1993). The interest employers possess in health care costs is not without reason: Employer expenditures on health care continue to occupy an ever-increasing portion of business receipts and labor compensation, and one that is expected to keep rising. Unfortunately, in terms of production costs, employers face higher labor costs, since the cost of labor includes both wages and fringe benefits. Employers, however, do obtain certain benefits by providing health care benefits to their workers. The most significant one is that the premiums paid for health insurance are excluded from both the employer's and employee's taxable income, thus making the provision of health insurance an attractive alternative to wage increases. A less appealing result of health benefits, however, is that these tax deductions translate into an estimated loss of tax revenues to the US government of approximately $40 billion per year (IOM, 1993). Moreover, this favorable tax treatment also affects risk takers, in that an individual may not wish to purchase health insurance with given risk preferences but may ultimately buy insurance because it is relatively cheaper.

With the above employment situation, the ownership form of health insurance companies in the United States also has implications. For example, the Blue Cross/Blue Shield companies are not-for-profit, tax-exempt organizations. One might therefore assume that the taxes paid by for-profit insurance companies would place them at a competitive disadvantage. Despite this, the "Blues" offer more coverage, albeit at a higher price, than do for-profit health insurance products, thus making the latter more price-competitive (especially for healthier individuals).

Two types of health insurance firms therefore coexist: The first type of firm offers greater coverage at a higher price, but without the burden of the premium tax. The second type of firm offers a less costly product, but along with the burden of the premium tax. As a consequence, if individuals were given the choice between insurance companies and their products, the resultant self-selection would cause one type of health insurer to have a healthier, less costly patient base (again implying a lower expected benefits payout), whereas health insurers with more generous coverage would tend to have a "sicker" patient base that would warrant higher premiums. Given that individuals are risk-averse, however, the "sicker" patients (or individuals who expect to have high health care expenditures) would logically be willing to pay a higher premium so that this type of market could work.

In light of the above two trends in patient bases, the health care market unfortunately cannot operate as smoothly as indicated, since some 33 to 37 million individuals in the United States are not covered by any type of health insurance whatsoever. If these individuals need hospitalization, they can receive hospital care only in emergency situations. Without insurance, these individuals cannot pay the hospital, so the hospital in turn charges a higher price to its insured patients (known as cross-subsidization). The resultant price charged by the hospital therefore consists of average costs instead of being based on marginal cost (as would be the case in a truly competitive market). This average pricing increases the expected benefit payout and therefore results in a higher premium—implying that individuals are paying not only for their own health insurance but also for the potential cross-subsidization (when they become hospitalized).

Whereas the problem of the uninsured has consistently been at the forefront of the debate on health care insurance in the past decade, it also constituted a major impetus in the development of the US government's only two health insurance programs—Medicare and Medicaid. Medicare, first implemented in 1966 as Title 18 under the Social Security Act, is an entitlement program that provides every individual (either US citizen or legal alien) over the age of 65 with health insurance benefits irrespective of financial status. The Medicare program comprises two basic portions: Part A and Part B. Part A consists of health care insurance and is mandatory for every person receiving Social Security benefits. In its original design, Medicare constituted an indemnity plan that paid first-day coverage similar to private health insurance plans which also reimbursed hospitals on a cost-plus basis. The actual costs of this coverage, however, significantly exceeded the costs predicted, partly because cost forecasts were made based on existing demand rather than unmet need. Since Medicare now provided health care at a lower price than private insurance, it also essentially increased individual income, allowing many individuals who had previously been too indigent to enter the health care market to do so. In economic terms, the total expenditures involved rose due to an increase in the quantity of services demanded as well as an increase in the demand itself. Since the price times the quantity equals total expenditures, this increase in quantity necessarily led to greater total expenditures, ceteris paribus. Hence, to be accurate, predictions regarding increased use of services must take into account not only existing demand but also potential demand.

In 1982 the reimbursement terms for hospital care were altered from a retrospective to a prospective approach. Simply put, this prospective payment system (PPS) reimbursed hospitals according to a predesignated formula based not only on the patient's diagnosis but also on other individual characteristics (e.g., age, number of comorbidities, etc.). If the costs for treating the patient happened to be less than reimbursement, the hospital could keep the difference. If the costs exceeded the prospective payment, however, the hospital would then absorb the losses. As a result, the Medicare program faced a different pricing mechanism reflecting the individual patient's resource use rather than the average resource use by all patients in the hospital. Medicare's PPS thus provides an annually updated, prospective, case-based payment for each type of hospital discharge, as defined through diagnostic-related groups, (DRGs).

Three features are important in understanding the effects of PPS: First, PPS employs case-based rates that involve financial risks for institutions operating with losses as well as the possibility of retaining any savings from enhanced efficiency and reduced care intensity. Second, PPS involves a movement toward national rates that creates greater financial stringency for higher-cost hospitals after PPS adjustments. Third, the PPS design inherently creates disincentives to encourage more admissions (Gold et al., 1993). These incentives, however, apply solely to hospitals, not to the physicians who order the hospitalizations.

Since the PPS was implemented in 1982, 40 percent of all hospital patient care has been Medicare-financed (Eckholm, 1993). As a result, from 1983 to 1990 PPS reduced the historical growth of Medicare Part A by 20 percent (one-third of which is attributable to declining admissions). A corresponding growth in case-mix severity over this period indicates that only the more seriously ill patients were hospitalized, which in turn implies a reduction in moral hazards. Nonetheless, it has been argued that PPS could be even more effective if it equalized pressure (rather than rates) among hospitals, thus implying a need for hospital-specific rates (Aaron, 1992).

In addition to PPS, capital payments have also been incorporated into the Medicare system, making hospitals dependent on Medicare coverage for both capital and operating payments. Here, it should be noted that firms tend to overconsume a cheaper input into their production function (known as the Averch-Johnson effect), so that Medicare's de facto financing of capital gives hospitals an incentive to overpurchase sophisticated technology. And these excessive purchases have been a significant factor in determining overall health care costs. On the other hand, capital pass-throughs have also been limited under PPS.

The incentives proposed by the government to contain Medicare costs are not surprising, given that Medicare alone accounts for 9 percent of all federal spending. Cost restraints, however, are not the government's only objective. For example, to promote the private sector to engage in both social and public goods production, the federal government provides "disproportionate share" and "indirect teaching cost" monies. Under the principle of disproportionate share, the government allocates an additional payment for each hospital that, as so designated, "1). serves a significantly disproportionate number of low-income patients; or 2). is located in an urban area, has more than 100 beds, and can demonstrate that more than 30% of its revenues are derived from state and local government payments for indigent care provided to patients not covered by

Medicare or Medicaid" (Soc. Sec. Act 1886 (d) (5) (i)). With these allocations, the government thus gave private hospitals incentives to provide care for the poor. Moreover, providing these resources may mitigate a given hospital's financial risk, along with its need to increase cross-subsidization, which has become more difficult with the advent of managed care and increasing efforts by private insurers to contain costs.

In a similar vein, the government also allocates payments to hospitals to cover the indirect costs of medical education, that is, the increased operating costs associated with approved intern and resident programs (*Medicare and Medicaid Guide*, 1995). By financing these indirect educational costs, the government thus diminishes the financial risk for teaching hospitals by reducing their related responsibilities for these expenses. This risk reduction benefits hospitals in at least two ways: First, it allows them to accumulate capital for expanding hospital services. Second, it enables them not to pass costs on to other patients (which might otherwise raise prices and possibly result in loss of market share to nonteaching hospitals).

In addition to paying hospital costs, Medicare, through its Part B program, also provides reimbursements for physician care. This Part B portion is underwritten through premiums paid by the Medicare beneficiary. Here, the payment is made in the form of a fee for services based on local physicians' usual, customary, and reasonable charges. Moreover, the government negotiates the price that it is willing to pay for the entirety of the physician's Medicare caseload. This negotiation (referred to as accepting assignment) typically accounts for 80 percent of allowable physician fees.

Any physician who then accepts assignment agrees to the fee schedule Medicare sets up and commits not to charge more than that amount. If physicians accept assignment (by accepting these lower fees), they are then compensated by the fact that these payments are guaranteed.

The federal government itself attempted to change the way physicians were reimbursed (under Part B) to a more prospective system, consisting of a single payment to all hospitalized Medicare patients, to be split among each of the physicians involved in the treatment of a given patient. This type of reimbursement scheme proved untenable, however, since each individual physician's contribution to the health care of one patient could not be readily measured. Moreover, since no outcome basis could be agreed upon, discord would most likely erupt among these physicians—to the ultimate detriment of the government and the patient as well. Medicare, therefore, uses the resource-based relative value scale (RBRVS), which was implemented to enhance efficiency incentives by establishing fees more closely aligned with those of real costs.

The RBRVS scale attempted to correct the perceived imbalance toward surgical and technical procedures relative to the number of visits and consultations that prevailed within the existing payment system, as well as to redistribute payment schedules from procedure-oriented specialists to primary care physicians. This type of payment schedule can also be used to provide incentives for graduating medical students to enter the field of primary care, which is presumed to be growing in proportion to the growth in managed care.

In addition to introducing medical insurance for the elderly in 1966, within the same year the federal government also implemented Medicaid legislation (Title 19), providing health insurance for low-income groups. This legislation is financed on a matching fund basis, whereby individual states allocate funds for their individual Medicaid program, which the federal government then matches. The states design and operate the Medicaid program under federal guidelines. Since benefits are not uniform across the United States, however, some states have more generous benefits and less stringent eligibility requirements than others. The federal government offsets this nonuniformity by providing additional resources to poorer states, to prevent massive migration (from poorer states to richer states) by people seeking more generous benefits.

The federal government collaborates with state governments in the poorer states to provide physicians and hospitals with incentives to care for the poor. Although these incentives lower the financial risk to physicians of treating patients, those physicians involved are typically reimbursed less for Medicaid patients than they would be for non-Medicaid patients. These lesser reimbursements may be problematic, because in some cases Medicaid patients have more health care problems (due to poverty), making them more expensive to treat. Another problem of the Medicaid program at this point is the types of care that are covered. With coverage existing for hospital rather than preventive care, Medicaid beneficiaries often opt for treatment in more expensive settings, where their out-of-pocket costs are significantly less.

The sources of revenue for Medicare and Medicaid also differ. Medicare is paid for through a Medicare trust fund, which is a separate government account funded by additions to each worker's current social security tax (Phelps, 1992). Medicaid, on the other hand, is paid for through the general tax fund by individuals' income taxes. Controlling the costs of these programs is, therefore, in the best interest of all taxpayers, who must subsidize medical insurance for both the elderly and the poor. In addition to proposed cuts in spending, Congress is also increasingly using managed care to better accommodate these two programs' beneficiaries.

Another difference between Medicare and Medicaid is that Medicaid pays for long-term care, which Medicare does not cover. To become eligible for Medicaid coverage for long-term care, an individual must "spend down" his or her assets and income (thus implying that an individual's deductible is actually his or her wealth). This system in turn implies that, although Medicaid coverage is available, the program does not provide insurance against financial losses.

In summary, health insurance plays a unique role in the health care market. Such a role not only affects expenditures but also attempts to provide incentives to both patients and providers. Moreover, the problems encountered with health insurance in the past have been characterized by market failures (such as moral hazards and biased selection), as well as the federal and state governments' involvement in stipulated health care insurance provisions. Finally, it has also been demonstrated that health care insurance is actually provided not to ensure health but to prevent financial losses. Consequently, the policy challenge for the health care insurance market is to devise plans that provide effective coverage without increasing costs as they have done in the past.

❧ HOSPITALS

Hospital expenditures account for the largest portion of US health care dollars, while also providing an organizational format that delivers inpatient as well as outpatient care. In essence, hospitals provide resources—both labor and capital—so that physicians can give their patients the necessary care. It should be noted, however, that within the United States, physicians traditionally are not formal employees of their hospitals; these hospitals, therefore, do not have a formal chain of command (or basic authority) over physicians' behavior. Rather, they permit physicians to admit their patients and use their resources for treatment. This relationship is symbiotic, in that the hospitals depend upon physicians for patients, whereas physicians rely on hospitals for the resources necessary to deliver patient care.

In order to carry out the aforementioned revenue-generating tasks, physicians in turn demand services from the hospital, namely, capital equipment and labor. In this respect physicians may be able to take advantage of hospital administrators through asymmetric information—for example, physicians know what types of services are necessary for effective medical treatment that hospital administrators may not know. In contrast, when resources were plentiful (before cost containment measures were implemented), hospitals invested in all of the capital (and sophisticated complementary labor) that physicians demanded. At that time, there was little conflict between the hospitals' and physicians' objectives. Hospitals practiced what is called "non-price competition," a type of market response that evolved because patients did not have to expend significant out-of-pocket resources for care, while the insurance companies (and the government) covered the costs (including the Medicare capital cost pass-through described above). Without any type of real-world price constraint, the hospitals' and the physicians' objectives were both met, including the maintenance of a technological advantage (along with the related perceptions of high-quality care).

Given these technological advantages, the next battle among hospitals was waged on the basis of the array of services and technology available per hospital. The high level of technology and services enabled both hospitals and physicians to maximize their incomes. What resulted, however, was a prohibitively expensive medical system that has been marked by both excess capacity and underutilization, high levels of intensity, and a high rate of procedures performed (Rasell, 1995).

In his classic 1975 article (cited in Ashby and Lisk, 1992), William Dowling proposed a general model of 11 cost-influencing variables that determine expenditure levels in hospitals:

1. number of cases treated
2. length of stay
3. complexity of case mix
4. intensity of services
5. scope of services
6. amenity levels
7. quality level
8. efficiency
9. input prices
10. investments in human and plant resources
11. teaching programs

In addition, intensity itself can be further separated into five smaller components:

1. changes in employee skill mix
2. productivity
3. patient case-mix complexity
4. intensity of services
5. non-labor factors

The above model shows why the inpatient case mix rose significantly after PPS was introduced, since low-complexity cases were transferred to outpatient settings, thus increasing the average complexity of the remaining inpatients (Ashby and Lisk, 1992). To compensate for this increased case-mix complexity, hospitals had to employ more professionally trained labor, which delivered higher-quality care, but unfortunately at an increased cost. The hospitals then responded to these higher costs by charging their insured patients higher prices. The chain of events continued, with insurance companies then paying these higher prices, finally leading to the spiraling costs observed between hospitals and insurance companies.

Another reason nonprice competition thrived in the US health care market is the predominance of the not-for-profit ownership form. The United States contains 3,026 private, not-for-profit hospitals, compared with 641 private, for-profit hospitals and 1,675 public (including federal, state, and local government) hospitals. Instead of having to distribute earnings to private shareholders, the private, not-for-profit hospitals actually use their excess revenues to increase their internal investments. Since net revenues are then reinvested into the hospital, they can then maximize hospital services by providing (1) a wide array of sophisticated services, (2) research, and (3) teaching. These features make the hospital increasingly attractive to highly specialized physicians. Because not-for-profit hospitals are now able to increase their internal investments, their average costs also increase. These hospitals, however, justify such increases (as in quality).

Economists have proposed several theoretical models to describe these not-for-profit hospitals, which are summarized in Table 6.1. It is interesting to note that all of these models lack the typical notions of price competition and efficiency.

It is questionable whether or not the not-for-profit sector can contain costs, and it remains equally unclear whether the for-profit sector can minimize its costs either. Private, for-profit hospitals are typically owned by large multihospital chain corporations.

Table 6.1 A Summary of Theoretical Hospital Models*

Newhouse (1970)	Utility Maximizing Model, in which the hospital decision makers optimize quantity and quality.
Lee (1971)	Conspicuous Consumption Model, in which the hospitals purchase inputs based on other hospitals' input decisions.
Pauly-Redisch (1973)	Physician Cooperative Model, in which physicians as de facto hospital decision makers maximize average physician incomes.
Harris (1971)	Hospital as two organizations, in which the hospital is represented by administration and the medical services are represented by physians.
Weisbrod (1975)	Non-Profit Hospital Model, in which non-profit hospitals exist to fill an unmet need in the for-profit sector.
Hansmann (1980)	Contract Failure Model, in which the non-profit hospital exists because it is difficult to quantify the nature and quality of the medical service delivered.
Bays (1983)	Interest Group Model, in which physicians prefer non-profit hospitals because they can exercise cotrol and not compete with shareholders.

* Folland, S., A. Goodman, and M. Stano. *The Economics of Health and Health Care.* New York: MacMillan Publishing 1993.

In addition to providing health care services to patients, they must also provide returns for their investors. Hence, the type of investment decisions they make must be aimed at maximizing shareholder wealth. By examining Dowling's 11 proposed sources of hospital expenditure, the for-profit hospitals can then curb their costs by limiting their case-mix complexity, scope of services, and teaching programs. Moreover, they can limit the provision of high-cost/low-profitability services (e.g., trauma centers, burn units, and neonatal units).

In addition to both the for-profit and not-for-profit health care sectors, the government is also directly involved in hospital care through its ownership of some hospitals. The federal government primarily owns the Veterans Administration hospitals, which provide medical services to veterans free of charge. State and local governments also own public hospitals, which provide the bulk of charity care for the uninsured and indigent as well as research activities and teaching opportunities for medical trainees.

From an economic standpoint, hospital care cannot be considered a purely public good (i.e., nonrivalrous or nonexcludable).* As a result, such care does not require direct government production (for example, like national defense). Nonetheless, certain characteristics of hospital care make it a "collective good." For example, in the case of uninsured and indigent patients, denying care in a hospital would be both ethically untenable and unacceptable to many Americans. These patients' failure to pay for their care, however, is unrelated to their consumption of health care services, resulting in market failure. Since private hospitals in the United States are not obligated to care for such patients (except in emergency medical situations) but do have the resources to provide effective care, they may not accept the financial ramifications brought about by this market failure. Accordingly, the government then enters the market to provide this care: In other words, if hospital care was completely in the domain of the private sector, not enough hospital care would be provided, so the public sector is then required to fill the gap. The government's direct ownership of hospitals thus allows it to exert hierarchical power over its administration in terms of budgeting, increasing payments, and staffing costs (including physicians).

Because of the three types of ownership, much debate has arisen over the precise role property rights play in hospital efficiency. Property rights in this context would entail the owner's right to decide on the proper use of the hospital's resources (and the right to keep the residual), as well as the right to sell any of the hospital's wealth. Hence, one would expect for-profit hospitals to be the most efficient of the three

---

*Nonrivalry and nonexcludability mean that the consumption of that good/service is equal for every member of society.

ownership forms, but this expectation has not been borne out in the empirical literature (Folland, 1993). The particular form of ownership seems not to be a significant determinant of hospital efficiency.

As a result of the above situations, changes have now been implemented in the US hospital system, one of which entails altering the existing relationship between hospitals and physicians. Whereas in past years physicians could hold multiple staffing privileges in several hospitals, forcing all of them to succumb to their demands for sophisticated equipment and labor and thus exacerbating the proliferation of overcapitalization and excessive service duplication (Pauly, 1980; Lee, 1971; Newhouse, 1970), many hospitals are now granting these privileges only to physicians who agree not to accept privileges at other hospitals. Since the physician's patient load is no longer split among several competing hospitals under such an agreement, hospitals can now make investment decisions more efficiently based on the expectation of treating more patients, thereby reducing (at least in part) excess capacity.

Another way in which the hospital-physician relationship has been altered is by hospitals' purchase of physician groups. These purchases allows hospitals to exert a more formal influence over physicians and further induce them to adopt behaviors leading to more effective management of the hospital itself. This change may be particularly relevant given that Medicare's efforts to contain costs have focused on hospitals rather than on physicians. If hospitals are forced to constrain expenditures because of this more stringent reimbursement methodology, they are less able to meet physicians' demands. By bringing physicians directly into the hospital decision-making process, however, hospitals give them an incentive to appreciate the need for cost-cutting approaches in hospitals to forestall financial exigency. It is this tie between physicians and hospitals that may ultimately help deal with managed care, third-party payers, which are likewise constraining costs. Ultimately, physicians and hospitals need to work together to achieve more competitive pricing in the face of both an increased patient load and greater market share.

Aside from the above physician-hospital objective, there are other policy considerations. For example, some policymakers question the not-for-profit status (and tax exemptions) of certain hospitals that do not always provide community services (e.g., charity care and other public health services). Alternatively, private business policy may then determine that freestanding community hospitals are often at a disadvantage not only for purchasing large-scale medical supplies but also for contracting with managed care systems. Some of these hospitals have adopted a private market response, buying out other community hospitals within the area, or even consolidating with other hospitals to make them more competitive with for-profit hospital chains.

A current trend in the hospital industry is the increasing number of hospital mergers. The definition of a hospital merger is the "combination of previously independent hospitals formed by either the disssolution of one hospital and its absorption by another or the creation of a new hospital from the dissolution of all participating hospitals" (American Hospital Association, 1992). The benefits of hospital mergers include the ability of the merged hospital to attract investment, establish a management base for health technology, and consolidate services in order to

- increase market share
- expand clinical services
- hire additional technical staff
- improve efficiency
- reduce overbedding and overstaffing (Alexander et al., 1996)

Another benefit of hospital mergers is that the new institutions can capture managed care patients by providing lower-cost care as a result of reduced personnel, overhead, and marketing and advertising costs as well as developing affiliations with medical centers (Kassirer, 1996). With the current emphasis on managed care in the United States, hospitals may soon no longer be the central providers of health care; mergers afford them a chance to diversify the products and services they offer. Mergers appear to be popular; in 1994, for example, 674 hospitals merged (Kassirer, 1996).

In addition to taking the above measures, both state and local governments are also reacting to political demands for lower taxes by selling their public hospitals to private hospital chains. Whether these changes will lower hospital costs overall, however, remains to be seen. One concern is that once the public hospital is sold, indigent patients will then have to be treated in these private hospitals. If these patients are uninsured, increases in Medicaid payments (if not disproportionate-share payments) are to be expected. In essence, such hospital sales thus reflect a shift in the health care burden from local governments to both the federal and state levels.

Despite this shift, however, some evidence exists indicating that hospitals are being forced to become price takers rather than price makers. If this is the case, inroads have been made into reducing hospital inefficiencies, excess capacity, and costs in general. Further inroads could be attained by curbing hospitals' ability to cross-subsidize, thereby undermining their past pricing practices (based on average costs).

ॐ Medical Labor

Physicians

Physicians currently play several roles in the US health care market. To begin with, they constitute inputs into the health care process, both as entrepreneurs and as an intermediate good (namely, the physician service). Moreover, physicians can also be regarded as firms. As such, physicians both hire and control resources. Logically, then, since firms aim to maximize their profits, so do physicians aim to maximize their outcomes (in terms of both health care and revenues). The most fitting description of the physician would then be as the patient's agent within the health care process.

From this point of view, the physician-patient relationship is the most fundamental in the health care system/medical care nexus. This relationship contains features that make it fit within the principal-agency theory. Here, one main feature of the principal-agency model is the presence of asymmetrical information, since in this case the agent (the physician) knows much more about medical treatments than the principal (the layperson patient). The standard theory of agency, as applied to any market characterized by asymmetrical information, assumes that both the principal's and agent's preferences for treatment are independent of each other (Mooney and Ryan, 1993). Mooney and Ryan also point out, however, that it is assumed in health care that the physician's and patient's preferences are in fact interdependent. In other words, both the physician and patient desire positive health care outcomes.

In a perfect world, the physician works in the patient's best interest (Feldstein, 1994). However, this concept in itself assumes that the physician knows what the patient's best interest is and can quantify or define it in some manner. If this is the case, both the physician and patient can agree on an outcome, and the agency issue may then be moot. In medicine, however, such outcomes may not be so easily defined. Since actual improvements in health may be difficult to measure, overall outcomes may instead be defined in terms of a process. Such a definition has its own difficulties, however. It has been argued here that physicians have tended to overuse diagnostic (or therapeutic) tools due to a "technologic imperative" (which in economic terms means that they expand the use of services until the marginal benefit of the last procedure performed equals zero). This approach may in turn be motivated by several premises: "do no harm," "everything that can be done will be done for the patient," or even a fear of medical malpractice suits, which will inevitably lead to an inefficient approach.

The foregoing process definition does *not* imply, however, that the physician is necessarily not acting as a perfect agent of the patient; it merely indicates that the patient may not (or cannot) grasp the value of the medical treatment provided vis-à-vis that treatment's costs. From one perspective it reduces the risks to both physician and patient because it diminishes the chances that something was overlooked. From another perspective, however, the patient (as the principal) does not gather the requisite information to influence the overall treatment regimen.

A physician who fails to understand fully the patient's best interest may substitute his or her own preferences, perhaps including a greater desire for more health care, for those of the patient. Such a substitution should not be confused, however, with inability to fulfill the patient's wishes (e.g., euthanasia) due to legal limitations.

In addition to the above implications, the financial arrangement between patient and physician entails additional principal-agency implications. The patient mitigates financial risk by purchasing insurance, whereby the insurance company then pays the physicians (based on the charges for the care provided) on a fee-for-service basis for all services covered. Moral hazards and asymmetrical information have produced both market failures and health care costs. One possible way to forestall these phenomena might be to increase control over the physicians themselves via managed care. As stated above, managed care aims to make the physician more efficient in his or her overall practice. Physicians have traditionally enjoyed professional autonomy in medical decision making without any type of outside interference. Under managed care contracts, however, physicians' autonomy is limited, and their objectives may be at odds with those of the overall managed care system. As more insurers move toward a managed care approach, however, physicians may have even less power to determine the types of care that can be ordered, especially in cases of either excessive costs or experimental treatments. Physicians may also lose some of their financing power, in essence becoming price takers rather than price makers. The philosophy of providing all available treatment may thus become a thing of the past.

The decision to become a physician itself falls under the economic theory of human capital investments. Professional studies involve a long, costly period of training; the financial burden is most extreme for medical students, whose post-graduate studies can last from seven to over twelve years (including medical school). The economic issues involved in deciding to become a physician can thus be broken down into two general areas: opportunity costs and time preference for income. An individual faces opportunity costs whenever he or she forgoes one opportunity for another. In this case the medical student forgoes immediate income from another career to become a physician. By postponing earnings, the individual demonstrates a preference for higher future earnings over lower present earnings (the time preference for income). To assess fully this economic rationale for pursuing a medical degree, the individual must therefore measure present earning power against the future rate of return, that is, a physician's income, which is higher than that of other comparable professions. The earnings potential, however, is not without limits.

Another way to review this investment concept is by the labor-leisure trade-off. For example, leisure is considered a "normal good," so as the price of leisure increases, the quantity demanded should correspondingly decrease. (The price of leisure is defined as the forgone wages an individual could have earned by working.) An increase in income should therefore result in a commensurate increase in the demand for leisure. According to this theory, at some point a physician will no longer be willing to work for more money. Hence, it has been argued that alterations of the nominal tax (or wage) rate will not necessarily directly affect the labor supply of physicians themselves.

In light of these trade-offs, it has also been argued that physicians do enjoy some degree of monopoly power, since the licensure of physicians is controlled via the medical education system (in terms of both the curriculum and the number of students who are admitted).

In addition to the above considerations, the decision to specialize further increases training time. Specialists, however, are able to command even higher revenues upon completion of their training, especially if their reimbursements are tied to board certification (along with other licensure and credentials). The higher fees they then charge for their specialist services are somewhat mitigated by the lower search costs incurred by the patients themselves. In other words, patients (as well as third-party payers) do not have to investigate a specialist to determine his or her level of competency but instead rely on the government requirements of licensure and certification.

The specialist also plays an interesting role in the marketplace itself. Once the decision to specialize (and in what particular area to specialize) has been made, the next question is where to locate. Location decisions are based on spatial competition and the expected demand for the specialty services. Given these considerations, the optimal solution is to find the most desirable location to create enough demand to sustain the specialist's target income.

This phenomenon occurs particularly when specialists spread into small towns, but they will not do so until the total physician-to-population ratios become sufficiently high to make the small towns effective competitors for them. Similarly, specialists respond to this effective demand by locating in regions where the physician-to-population ratio can logically afford to expand. Location decisions are therefore based on the potential for economic returns. Other factors that go into location decisions include regional amenities, professional support from colleagues, and access to technologically sophisticated medical equipment. It is these other factors that help to explain why physicians (especially specialists) tend to locate in (or near) urban areas.

In addition to locating in certain areas solely for economic reasons, physicians also vary by region in their medical practices. Detsky (1995) suggests three reasons why medical practices may vary by region or location: (1) differences in health care systems, (2) physicians' practice styles, and (3) patients' characteristics. For example, patients in a region characterized by fees charged for service (where patients have autonomy in their choice of provider) may undergo a high number of procedures, since the physician has an economic incentive to perform them. Conversely, patients in managed care settings with more limited access to a wide variety of treatment options may have fewer procedures. Since physicians tend to practice similarly by region, the question has also been raised whether their patients are being penalized for living in one area versus another. No definitive findings, however, have yet emerged linking practice variations to medical outcomes.

Nurses

After physicians, the most often analyzed labor pool in the health care market is that of nurses. Since labor costs make up the majority of hospital costs and nurses represent the largest category of workers in the hospital, their role in the health care process is highly relevant from an economic standpoint.

The largest debate concerning nurses is whether or not there is actually a shortage of them. This debate stems from the fact that once a nurse is trained, it is very difficult and costly (in terms of opportunity costs) to retrain one in another area for a higher income. Because nursing is so specialized to health care, and especially to hospitals, it has been argued that hospitals exert monopsony (single buyer) power over nurses and therefore underpay them. Two theoretical schools of thought have arisen concerning this issue. First, Blank and Stigler (1957) claimed that a shortage exists when the number of workers increases less rapidly than the number demanded at the salaries offered. Arrow and Capron (1959), however, argued that a shortage arises when demand exceeds supply at the market wage. By virtue of their monopsony power, hospitals can offer wages below the value marginal product of the nurse. In other words, they can afford to pay nurses less than the value of what they are actually producing for the hospital. As long as the overall cost for the nurses to move is positive (and no other employment options exist for them), this gap will persist.

Another reason for the persistence of a nursing shortage may be that the not-for-profit hospitals in particular attempt to maximize public perceptions of high-quality care. One way to achieve this objective is to hire more registered nurses (as opposed to licensed practical nurses). Hence, the nursing shortage may be seen as a consequence of hospital administrations' attempts to maximize quality, which in turn create an artificially high demand for registered nurses. If this is the case, hospitals may respond by substituting licensed practical nurses for registered nurses, which some US hospitals are already doing to contain costs. A counterargument concerning the shortage of nurses is that with the growth of managed care systems and temporary employment services for nurses, the shortages may not be as pronounced as researchers in the past have argued.

🪶 SOCIETY'S INVOLVEMENT IN HEALTH CARE MARKETS AND REGULATION

Economists have argued that perpetuating the current health care system threatens US citizens' future standard of living in three ways:

1. The wasteful and inefficiently organized health system drains resources from other uses (high opportunity costs).
2. The rising cost of government health care programs adds to the federal deficit and reduces national savings.
3. Health care insecurity locks people into existing jobs or welfare rather than allowing them to move into productive employment (Rivlin et al., 1994).

These three factors thus characterize a health care system whose inefficiencies affect other sectors of the economy as well. It is because of this "spillover" that health care costs have become such a controversial issue of public policy.

One fundamental problem facing all health care systems is how to be more cost-effective. An all-encompassing system necessarily has to ensure that the key information required for each decision is available when needed, specifically to those making that decision. The primary objective of health care reform, therefore, has been (and still is) cost containment.

The original purpose of cost containment measures was to constrain the growth of health care spending by either regulating or controlling the prices (or payments) set by health care providers. And studies have found that the most effective cost containment approaches have tended to entail the broadest scope (Gold et al., 1993):

- all-payer versus individual-payer systems
- aggregate payment controls versus per service controls
- total payment limits

The more aggregated approaches restrict the providers' ability to offset their cost pressures by either raising (i.e., transferring) their prices to other payers or increasing the volume of care provided (Williams et al., 1993). A review of major cost-cutting legislation is provided in Table 6.2.

Cost containment would be easier if competing objectives did not exist within the health care system. In principle, the objectives of any health care system will be derived from the ideology of the society it serves. For example, one of the objectives competing with cost containment is access. An egalitarian society would view this as a right, not a privilege, whereas a more individualistic society might see health care as a reward that society offers to its members who manifest both a strong willingness and ability to pay (Williams, 1993). No society, however, exclusively embraces either

Table 6.2 Review of Major Cost Containment Legislation

Legislation	Purpose
Economic Stabilization Program (1971):1	Constrain health care expendiuture growth by controlling prices in health care.
Hospital Containment Act of 1977	Control the growth of hospital costs on an all-payer basis nationwide.
Medicare Hospital Prospective Payment System (1983)	Contain hospital costs by paying basis (based on diagnostic related groups) rather than on a retrospective cost-based scheme.
Resource-Based Relative Value Schedule	Reimburse physicians based on resources used—including cognitive skills—and aim toward reducing procedural reimbursement bias.

of these views in lieu of the other; rather, each interacts with the other so that the patients involved may be treated in both systems during a given episode of illness. The view that currently prevails is thus not the total denial of health care as a right, but rather the attitude that only certain aspects of health care (e.g., emergency care) will be provided to all members of society.

Aside from the above viewpoints, it is also generally assumed that the purpose of health care is to improve health. In this respect, the main criterion seems to be a concern about the overall distribution of the benefits of health care and of health care itself (Williams, 1993). The only solution to this conflict is to encourage the sharing of responsibilities between managers and physicians (as in managed care). Here, incentive structures also need to be reconciled—specifically, the incentives that face participants within the health care system.

In a perverse system, however, the inefficient receive monetary rewards, whereas the efficient obtain budget reductions. Another dilemma facing the health care system is how to educate the general public into believing that it is in their own best interest to engage in cost-effective care. Since cost-effectiveness implies the achievement of a goal (or objective), such as improved health at the lowest cost, it is then entirely consistent with the quality of care provided, which also implies reaching a similar objective.

When applying the conventional distinction between positive and normative economics, a society should ask what *will* happen (positive) as well as what *should* happen (normative). Furthermore, such a society should not confuse financial with economic decision making. In this context economics concerns not only monetary expenditures but also precisely what different people value irrespective of these expenditures. Since health care systems in the United States have rejected willingness and ability to pay as the sole criterion for determining final access to them, it appears inappropriate to examine either revenue flows (or other financial criteria) to place a value on what such a system actually achieves (Williams, 1993). As an alternative to applying financial measures for assessing system operations, we may use the social welfare function, incorporating values from a variety of sources. This function also pursues equity objectives that depart from the Pareto rule (that no judgments can be made about situations if some people are made better off and others worse off), rather taking the view that society as a whole is made better off by combining values from all aspects of society.

Ultimately, the most obvious reason for concern about the type of financial approach employed may be lack of access. And if lack of access is defined as unequal use, it may then be used as a proxy for inappropriately low use. What constitutes either low or inappropriate use cannot be determined on the basis of clinical judgment alone; instead it depends on the value that taxpayers attach to additional use by people who are classified as below-average users (Pauly, 1992). As a result, the high cost of medical services within the United States may explain why Americans generally opt to transfer less to the poor and, according to Pauly, "why our safety net is more porous than those in other countries" (1992). In contrast, when medical costs rise relative to income, those who would not be viewed as poor enough to require subsidized health care may now be regarded as deserving.

The social aspect of the health care market also reveals inducements for government involvement. As stated earlier, the health care market is characterized by market failures. Because of the widespread national effects of these failures, the government has deemed it necessary to respond. For example, the provision of health care services may in some cases lead to externalities, that is, events that occur when one person's actions impose costs (or benefits) on another person not involved in the transaction. In like fashion, the government enters into markets where externalities occur to remedy the situation. Government remedies include (but are not limited to) regulations, taxation, and subsidies. Moreover, a related issue is whether or not property rights are fully recognized. If these rights are fully defined, they can be transferred to the point that externalities cannot exist. Logically, therefore, externalities exist if property rights fail to define ownership.

An example of such a failure to define ownership may be seen in the nonsmoking regulations aboard US airlines. Because nonsmokers suffer from secondhand smoke (either physically or in some other manner), the government has now imposed regulations prohibiting smoking due to the externalities involved. In this case a nonsmoker specifically buys an airline ticket for travel only, and not for the consequences incurred due to smoke encountered in the air.

In addition to dealing with externalities, the government can also encourage positive behavior that leads to societal benefits, such as subsidizing medical education, requiring immunizations, and so on. The public good nature of medical education, (i.e., that all of society benefits from having a trained medical staff) is seen to deserve government subsidies; otherwise, the cost of training individuals to become physicians, nurses, or other medical personnel would be prohibitive. Similarly, since all of society benefits from immunizations, the government therefore constitutes the proper mechanism to ensure adequate production of this service. These are just two examples of public goods found within the health care market.

High health care costs account for another facet of government intervention, especially when hospital costs are so burdensome to society that it can enter further the market and enforce certain changes to curtail further price increases. In this case the government has applied regulations in a further attempt to control more externalities caused by high hospital costs. The government can regulate hospital costs in four areas: price, quantity of services provided, entry into the market, and quality.

First, rate regulation has been shown to control costs because it limits both payment and budget increases. As described above, the more comprehensive the cost control measure, the more likely it is that costs will be reduced rather than being shifted to the unregulated sector. Furthermore, the excessive use of specific services may be controlled by limiting reimbursements.

A more direct way for regulations to control the quantity of services a hospital may provide is through the certificate-of-need (CON) program. Essentially, CON was formed with the intention that local health agencies would approve the capital expansions that hospitals desired to undertake. The point of targeting this aspect of hospital production was that technological advances (and the expensive capital consumed by them) were closely linked to high health care expenditures. The CON program had certain shortcomings, however: defining need was problematic, the process was highly self-regulatory, and decisions were being made primarily on the basis of popular politics.

The government also concerns itself with ensuring that all health care providers and organizations meet certain standards. Consequently, the government has imposed a variety of licensure requirements as barriers to entry. At first this policy may seem antithetical to the typical government role of promoting competition and reducing entry barriers caused by the asymmetrical information between providers and patients. However, the costs of allowing any individual to claim the ability to treat disease and illness would be prohibitively high in terms of possible injury and mortality. Therefore, the government imposes a system of "good" licensure that ensures quality of care while reducing informational and search costs for both patients and potential employers of health care personnel.

Further, both the government and medical boards establish certification requirements to ensure that medical personnel have certain qualifications, including sufficient knowledge of medicine, the possession of information about poor health outcomes, and the ability to identify poor-quality physicians to remove them from practice. This last requirement has been criticized, especially provoking accusations that physicians are inadequate at policing themselves, but new information sources are now available to consumers desiring to search a physician's past record. Here, the cost implication is that increased availability of information to consumers better enables them to make decisions about providers. Consequently, those providers wishing to both maintain and expand their patient base now have added incentives to maintain high-quality medical practices.

Barriers to entry, however, are a function of supply, income and rate of return. For example, as rates of return increase for a given specialty, the number of applicants desiring to enter will also increase. Hence, the most economically rewarding specialties may currently be attracting the "best and the brightest" providers. The government, however, may counteract this trend through the RBRVS, thereby rewarding the primary care specialties essential for the development of managed care systems (and raising both their rate and return). This example represents another way in which government can become involved in directing both the quantity and quality of medical personnel toward larger government objectives.

In addition to these objectives, concerns about health care spending have prompted an extensive study of health care economics as a separate field in itself. At this time, the US health care market is complicated by a health insurance system that leads to (1) increased consumer demand for health services; (2) higher prices due to this increased demand; (3) supplier-induced demand by providers; and (4) reduced access for the approximately 33 to 37 million uninsured, who will have to be cared for if the need arises (either through direct taxation to support public hospitals or through increased premiums for the insured, who cross-subsidize charity care).

Moreover, some concern has also been expressed that rising health care costs have affected US companies' competitive advantages and have in some cases even crowded out government spending in other areas.

In an efficient market, the value of the marginal goods or services received by consumers equals the marginal cost of producing those goods or services (in which case these resources are put to their best use). Unfortunately, the excessive insurance coverage encountered in the health care market causes patients to consume goods to the point where their benefit is zero but the services and goods still retain a positive resource cost. This imbalance then leads to an inefficient overall market.

Moreover, insurance companies further compound market inefficiencies by paying for certain goods and services but not covering less costly, alternative care. For example, under Medicaid, historically emergency room visits are covered, whereas primary care visits are not; it is therefore cheaper for the patient to receive care in an emergency room rather than in the primary care provider's office, which in many cases would be more appropriate—and far less costly overall.

Another defect in the market for health care services is uncertainty about the efficacy of treatment. This uncertainty carries important implications in the allocation of resources (Adair, 1993). These implications are related to practice-pattern variations, where certain traditions (e.g., surgical intervention rather than medical intervention) may affect the standard treatment modality. Even though this variation may be a standard, it does not necessarily result in either the best or most efficient treatment.

The health care industry has been built in large measure on the assumption that when health care is needed, society will pay for it in some fashion, irrespective of the costs involved. This era of unchecked spending has now come to a close, and more conscientious efforts are being made to control costs while continuing to provide necessary medical care. Changes in the delivery of medical care (such as financing intergroup organizations) are now emerging alongside movements toward eliminating the historical format of fees charged for service. In light of these movements, the United States can take stock using the experiences of other countries—specifically, those countries that have achieved greater success in containing medical costs while still delivering high-quality care. These countries have succeeded by emphasizing cooperation with providers (Reinhardt, 1993, as cited in Eckholm, 1993). Such increased cooperation can take place only if both the inherent and current incentive structures within the United States are resolved.

❧ SUMMARY

To summarize, the reasons for the rapid growth in the quantity of health care services in the United States may be explained as follows. First, widespread use of health insurance payments for health care services reduces the out-of-pocket price the consumer faces. This in turn leads to moral hazard, as a result of which the consumer purchases excessive health care services. Second, asymmetric information, a situation in which the physician has more information than the patient, leads the physician to demand increased services on the patient's behalf. Third, the development and use of new medical technologies have increased both the quantity and the cost of health care services.

❧ REFERENCES

Aaron, H. "Equity in the Finance and Delivery of Health Care." *Journal of Health Economics* 11 (1992): 467–471.

Adair, L. "The Role of the Health Care Sector in the U.S. Economy," *EBRI Issue Brief 142*, Washington, DC, EBRI (1993).

Alexander, J., M. Halpern, and S. Lee. "The Short-Term Effects of Merger on Hospital Operations." *Health Services Research* 30 (1996): 827–847.

Arrow, K. and W. Capron. "Dynamic Shortage and Price Rises: The Engineer-Scientist Case." *Quarterly Journal of Economics* 73 (1959): 293–307.

Ashby, J. and C. Lisk. "Why Do Hospital Costs Continue to Increase?" *Health Affairs* Summer (1992): 134–147.

Bays, C. W. "Why Most Private Hospitals are Non Profit." *Journal of Policy Analysis and Management* 2 (1983): 366–385.

Blank, D. and G. Stigler. "The Demand and Supply of Scientific Personnel." New York: National Bureau of Economic Research, 1957.

Detsky, A. "Regional Variation in Medical Care." *New England Journal of Medicine* 333 (1995): 589–590.

Eckholm. E. *Solving America's Health Care Crisis.* New York: Random House (1993).

Feldman, R. and B. Dowd. "What Does the Demand Curve for Medical Care Measure." *Journal of Health Economics* 12 (1992): 193–200.

Feldstein, P. *Health Policy Issues.* Ann Arbor, MI: Health Administration Press (1994).

Folland, S., A. Goodman and M. Stano. *The Economics of Health and Health Care.* New York: Macmillan Publishing Co. 1993.

Frech, H. E. "The Property Rights Theory of the Firm." *Journal of Political Economy* 84 (1976): 143–152.

Gold, M., K. Chu, S. Felt, M. Harrington and T. Lake. "Effects of Selected Cost-Containment Efforts: 1971–1993." *Health Care Financing Review* 14 (1993) 183–225.

Hansmann, H. "The Role of the Non-Profit Enterprise." *Yale Law Review* 89 (1980): 835–901.

Harris, J. "The Internal Organizations of Hospitals: Some Economic Implications," *Bell Journal of Economics* 8 (1977): 467–482.

Institute of Medicine, *Employment and Health Benefits.* Washington, DC: National Academy Press (1993).

Jensen, M. and W. Meckling. "Theory of the Firm: Managerial Behavior, Agency Costs, and Ownership Structure." *Journal of Financial Economics* 12 (1976): 125–135.

Kassirer, J. "Mergers and Acquisitions—Who Benefits? Who Loses?" *The New England Journal of Medicine* 334 (1996): 722–723.

Lee, M. L. "A Conspicuous Production Theory of Hospital Behavior." *Southern Economic Journal* 38 (1971): 48–58.

Medicare and Medicaid Guide, Washington, DC: Commerce Clearing House (1995).

Mooney, G. and M. Ryan. "Agency in Health Care: Getting Beyond First Principles." *Journal of Health Economics* 12 (1993): 125–135.

Newhouse, J. "Toward a Theory of Non-Profit Institutions: An Economic Model of a Hospital." *American Economic Review* 60 (1970): 64–74.

Pauly, M. "Fairness and Feasibility in National Health Care Systems." *Health Economics* 1 (1992): 93–103.

Pauly, M. *Doctors and Their Workshops.* Chicago: University of Chicago Press (1980).

Pauly, M. and M. Redisch. "The Not-for-Profit Hospital as a Physician Cooperative." *American Economic Review* 63 (1973): 87–99.

Phelps, C. *Health Economics.* New York: HarperCollins (1992).

Rasell, E. "Cost Sharing in Health Insurance—A Reexamination," *The New England Journal of Medicine* 332 (1995): 164–168.

Rivlin, A., D. Cutler, and L. Nichols. "Financing, Estimation, and Economic Effects." *Health Affairs* Spring I (1994): 31–49.

Robinson, J. "Payment Mechanisms, Non–Price Incentives, and Organizational Innovation in Health Care," *Inquiry* 30 (1993): 328–333.

Weisbrod, B. *The Nonprofit Economy,* Cambridge, MA: Harvard University Press (1988).

Williams, O. "Corporate Finance and Corporate Governance," *The Journal of Finance* 43 (1988): 567–591.

❧ Glossary of Economic Terms

Asymmetric information   In an economic exchange of goods or services, a situation in which one individual has more information than the other person.

Capitated payment   A payment system that pays a monthly amount per member enrolled in a managed care system irrespective of whether the health care provider treats the enrolled member or not.

Competitive pricing   Prices set at the marginal cost of producing the last unit of a good or service.

Copayment   The proportional amount of the bill for which a patient is responsible, with the insurance paying the balance.

Costs   Resources that are used in the production of goods and services as well as the expenditures that are spent in order to purchase goods and services. The various types of costs include the following:

1. Fixed costs, which are the costs incurred regardless of the amount produced (buildings, contracts, etc.).
2. Average fixed costs, which are the fixed costs divided by output produced.
3. Variable costs, which are the costs associated with the production of each unit of goods and services.
4. Average variable costs, which are variable costs divided by the total number of goods and services produced.
5. Marginal costs, which are the costs of the last unit of goods and services produced.
6. Total costs, which equal fixed costs plus variable costs.
7. Average total costs, which are total costs divided by the total number of output produced.

Deductible   The amount an individual must pay before his or her health insurance becomes responsible for reimbursing the health care provider.

Demand   The representation of consumers' purchase of goods and services. Changes in the quantity demanded are due to changes in prices; changes in demand are due to changes in income, tastes or preferences, and the price of substitute goods.

Efficiency   The allocation of resources to their best use, defined as using resources to the point where their marginal cost equals marginal benefits (or revenues). This relationship implies that the resources required to produce the last unit of a good equal the benefits (or revenues) derived from consuming the last unit of a good.

Elasticity   The responsiveness of the quantity demanded of a good and service to changes in the price of the good and service.

Equilibrium   A condition in which the demand for goods and services equals the supply for goods and services.

Externalities   Effects that arise outside the direct buying and selling of goods and services. For example, pollution is a negative externality in that individuals suffer from the effects of pollution without having purchased the good that produced the pollution.

Indemnity   Payment of insurance benefits.

Marginal benefits   The benefit derived by the last unit of goods and services consumed.

Monopoly   A single seller of goods and services.

Monoposony   A single buyer of goods and services.

Moral hazard   The change in behavior of an individual due to the presence of insurance, for example, consuming more health care services than would have been used if the patient had to pay the full price.

Opportunity costs   The value of the alternative use of resources.

Out-of-pocket prices   The price paid by the individual—either the full price of the health care goods and services or the copayment and deductible for which the individual is responsible.

Preferences   The value and desire that individuals have for goods and services.

Productivity   The use of inputs (such as labor and capital) in order to produce outputs.

Supply   The amount of goods and services produced by an industry.

Welfare loss   Losses in the economy that are due to the inefficient use of resources.

Health Information Systems

7

Charles J. Austin, Medical University of South Carolina
Karen A. Wager, Medical University of South Carolina

T he delivery of health services is an information intensive process. High-quality patient care requires careful documentation of each patient's medical history and present health and wellness status—including psychological and social well-being, current medical conditions, and treatment plans. Administrative and financial information is essential for efficient operational support of the patient care process. Managers need information for formulating strategy and carrying out programs identified in the health care organization's business plan. A strong argument can be made that the health services industry is one of the most information-intensive sectors of the economy.

Information is an important resource that must be planned and managed if it is to be used effectively in supporting organizational goals and objectives. This chapter covers the following topics:

1. The evolution of health information systems,
2. Applications of information technology to patient care and management of health services,
3. Principles of planning, design, implementation, and operation of systems,

4. Recommended guidelines for management oversight of information systems in health care organizations,
5. Future trends in the development of information technology.

〰 HISTORICAL EVOLUTION

The first health information systems date to the early 1960s, when a small number of hospitals began to automate selected administrative operations, usually beginning with payroll and patient accounting functions. These systems were developed by analysts and computer programmers hired by the hospital and were run on large and expensive central mainframe computers (see Figure 7.1). Very little attention was given to automation of clinical information. A few systems were developed for electronic storage of inpatient medical records abstracts for use following discharge. These early hospital information systems were batch-processing systems with no on-line user access to data in the computer files.

Advances in technology during the 1970s expanded the use of information systems in hospitals and marked the beginning of limited applications in physicians' practices. Computers became smaller and less expensive, with more processing power. Some vendors began to develop "applications software packages," generalized computer programs that could be used by any hospital, clinic, or other health services organization that purchased the system. Most of the early software packages supported administrative operations—patient accounting, general accounting, materials management, scheduling, and practice management. Some clinical packages were developed for hospital clinical laboratories, radiology departments, and pharmacies. Users gained direct access to computer files through on-line terminals connected to the systems.

A revolution in computing occurred in the mid-1980s with the development of powerful and inexpensive personal computers (PCs), desktop devices with computing power and storage capacity that equaled or exceeded the large mainframe systems of the 1960s and 1970s (see Figure 7.2). A second major advance was the development of electronic data networks that linked PCs and larger systems together to share information on a decentralized basis. An increasing number of vendors entered the health care software business, and a much larger array of products became available for both administrative and clinical functions.

The 1990s have been marked by dramatic changes in the health care environment, particularly the rapid expansion of managed care and the development of integrated delivery systems. An integrated delivery system (IDS) is a network of hospitals, physicians, and other health care organizations that come together to provide all needed

Figure 7.1   Mainframe Computer (1960s)

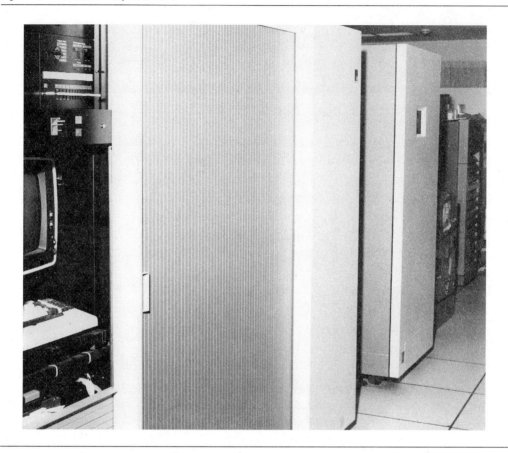

services to a defined patient population. In some cases the IDS provides comprehensive services for a fixed annual fee for each person enrolled in the health plan offered by the system (capitated payment). Integrated networks must be able to share clinical and financial information among the members of the network and with those who purchase health services from the delivery system. As a result, increased priority has been given to the development of computerized patient records that can be shared electronically across the network. A second priority is the development of strategic decision support systems for planning, management, and assessment of the outcomes of care provided by the network.

Health care managers must assume a leadership role in developing and implementing information systems that support patient care, provide information on performance

Figure 7.2   Personal Computer (1980s)

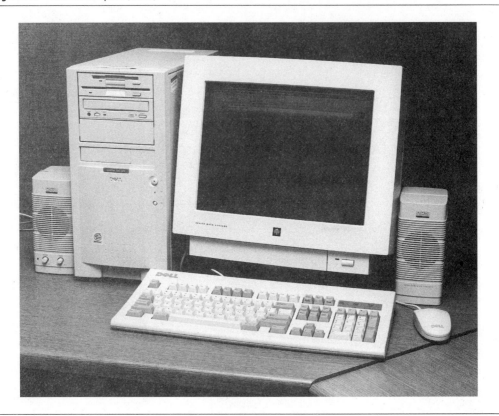

and outcomes, and control health care costs in an integrated environment. Much of the data needed to support these goals is currently captured in health care organizations. However, the data are stored in disparate information systems that often do not communicate with each other. And in spite of more than 30 years of research and development in implementing computer applications in health care organizations, most patient records today are paper records.

The Computer-Based Patient Record (CPR)

In recent years the Institute of Medicine (IOM) of the National Academy of Sciences has brought national attention to the problems associated with managing information using paper records and the need for widespread implementation of the computer-based patient record (CPR). The CPR, as defined by the IOM, is much more than an automated version of current patient records. Rather, the CPR is "an electronic patient record that resides in a system specifically designed to support users through availability of complete and accurate data, practitioner reminders and alerts, clinical decision support systems, links to bodies of medical knowledge, and other aids" (Institute of Medicine, 1991, p. 2). The 12 key attributes of the CPR, as defined in the IOM study, are shown in Figure 7.3. Experts agree that the technology needed to support the CPR is available today; the challenge facing health care managers is to address the organizational, behavioral, and financial issues relating to its widespread implementation.

Although it is an ambitious goal, many health care organizations are moving forward with plans to develop and implement CPR systems within the next decade. Responding to a recent survey in health care computing, 26 percent of leaders indicated that their organizations have already made substantial investments in the equipment and software needed to implement a CPR (HIMSS/HP Leadership Survey, 1995). Another 35 percent either have plans for developing a CPR or have already started a CPR project. A recent study conducted by Coopers and Lybrand and Zinn Enterprises revealed that 60 percent of the 510 health care executives responding believe that the CPR is one of the top technologies to be implemented in the next three years (Morrissey, 1995, p. 66). Leaders of health care organizations that have made significant strides in the development of the CPR caution others not to make the CPR the goal. Rather, the CPR should use technology appropriately to improve the efficiency and effectiveness of the care delivery process (Harrell, 1994, p. 53).

Figure 7.3   The 12 Key Attributes of the Computer-Based Patient Record (CPR)

1. It contains a problem list that clearly delineates the patient's clinical problems and current status of each.
2. It encourages and supports the systematic measurement and recording of the patient's health status and functional levels.
3. It documents the clinical reasoning and rationale for all diagnoses or conclusions.
4. It links patient's clinical records from various settings and time periods to provide a longitudinal record of events that may have influenced his or her health.
5. It addresses patient data confidentiality comprehensively by ensuring that the CPR is accessible only to authorized individuals.
6. It provides simultaneous and remote access to all authorized individuals involved in direct patient care.
7. It allows selective retrieval and formatting of information by users.
8. It provides links to both local and remote knowledge, literature, bibliographic, or administrative databases and systems to assist practitioners in decision making.
9. It facilitates clinical problem solving by providing clinicians with decision analysis tools, clinical reminders, prognostic risk assessment, and other clinical aids.
10. It supports direct data entry by practitioners and stores information using a defined vocabulary.
11. It helps individual practitioners and health care provider institutions to manage and evaluate the quality and costs of care.
12. It provides flexibility to support not only today's basic information needs but also the evolving needs of each clinical specialty and subspecialty.

Source: The Institute of Medicine (1991). *The Computer-Based Patient Record: An Essential Technology for Health Care.*

It may take several years before health care organizations realize the full potential of CPRs. To prepare for their implementation, they should first automate the clinical areas from which most information about patients is generated. They should also integrate information from the various systems into a data communication network so that all relevant patient information is available in a central repository. As a starting point, it is important to understand the computer applications used in health care today.

APPLICATIONS OF INFORMATION TECHNOLOGY
TO PATIENT CARE AND MANAGEMENT OF HEALTH SERVICES

Most computer applications used in health services delivery today fall into three general categories: (1) clinical information systems, (2) administrative and financial systems, and (3) strategic decision support systems (see Figure 7.4). To realize the full

Figure 7.4   Health Care Delivery: An Information-Intensive Process

Information Systems in Health Care	Integrated Delivery Systems

• Clinical Information Systems
  Computer-Based Patient Record (CPR)
  Ancillary Information Systems
     Laboratory
     Pharmacy
     Radiology
  Nursing Information Systems
  Clinical Decision Support Systems
	• Managed Care Systems
	
	• Community Health Information Networks (CHINS)

• Administrative and Financial
  Electronic Claims Processing
  Patient Accounting Systems
  Human Resources
  Materials Management
  Office Automation
	• Electronic Data Interchange (EDI)

• Strategic Decision Support
  Planning and Marketing
  Financial Forecasting
  Resource Allocation
  Performance Measurement
  Outcomes Assessment	

potential of these three categories of information systems, it is essential that the systems be integrated. For example, if a health care provider is to monitor effectively the quality of patient care and control health care costs, the provider must have access both to clinical *and* financial information. The health care industry can no longer afford to support clinical information systems that do not communicate with financial systems. Consequently, it is important to ensure systems integration when designing and implementing clinical, financial, and administrative information systems.

Clinical Information Systems

A *clinical information system* is defined as a system that provides for the organized processing, storage, and retrieval of information to support patient care (Austin, 1992, p. 319). Clinical information systems may include a broad range of functions such as order entry, results reporting, computer-assisted medical instrumentation, and clinical decision support systems. The major goal of a clinical information system is to support patient care by providing the health care practitioner with access to timely, complete, and relevant clinical information. The health care provider uses the clinical information to diagnose, treat, and manage the patient's care effectively. The CPR, as described previously, can be viewed as the "ultimate" clinical information system. However, many types of clinical information systems—including laboratory, pharmacy, radiology, nursing, and clinical decision support systems—are in use today. Many of these systems are entirely or largely text oriented, but advances in diagnostic imaging technology have dramatically increased the amount of nontextual data generated in clinical medicine (Lowe, Buchanan, Cooper, et al., 1995, p. 58).

Laboratory Information Systems.   A *laboratory information system* is a computer-based system that supports laboratory functions for collecting, verifying, and reporting test results. These systems generally support both information processing and laboratory management. Laboratory information systems now use computer technology not only to process the specimens but also to

- analyze the primary data
- store and distribute test results
- monitor testing quality
- document laboratory procedures
- control inventory
- monitor workflow
- assess laboratory productivity

Computer-based laboratory information systems help reduce health care costs while maintaining the quality of services by minimizing the number of tests performed, decreasing the turnaround time between the ordering of a test and the reporting of results, and assisting providers in both the ordering and interpretation of laboratory tests (Smith and Svirbely, 1990, p. 274).

Pharmacy Information Systems. Pharmacy information systems are among the most widely used clinical information systems today. Most *pharmacy systems* simplify and streamline medication dispensing and inventory control, automatically check all drug orders and dosages against the patient profiles to ensure proper dosage, and prevent contraindications (Minard, 1991, p. 15). Such systems generally increase the accuracy and efficiency of distributing drugs and monitoring drug usage. Common functions of pharmacy information systems include

- on-line order entry
- medication administration records
- drug compatibility checks
- automatic refill dispensing reports
- allergy screening
- automatic intravenous scheduling

It is important to integrate pharmacy information with other clinical information systems. For example, a physician should have access to blood and microbiological profiles when ordering medications for a patient. The physician should also be able to monitor changes in laboratory values and drug effectiveness over time. Systems should support the integration of information from various clinical systems and allow the health care provider to view the data graphically.

Radiology Information Systems. The rapid growth of diagnostic imaging technologies over the past two decades has had a profound impact on the development of radiology information systems. *Radiology information systems* have been developed to handle a broad spectrum of functions (Greenes and Brinkley, 1990, p. 325), including

- image generation
- image analysis
- image management
- information management

Picture archiving and communication systems (PACs) were also developed to support the management of digital imaging data. These systems acquire, store, retrieve, and display digital images, replacing the need to store radiological images on film. Traditional PACs are expensive, however, and often not well integrated into other clinical information systems. Therefore, technological advances in image compression and digital video are becoming more widely used, allowing users to view images using real-time, on-screen, color video sequencing (Lowe, Buchanan, Cooper, et al., 1995, p. 58). Systems for classifying, retrieving, and integrating clinical images, however, are still in the early stages of development. As these systems mature, radiological and other clinical images will be stored digitally in CPRs and will be made available to multiple users simultaneously.

Nursing Information Systems. A *nursing information system* is a computer-based system that automates the nursing process from assessment to evaluation, including patient care documentation. It also includes the mechanism for managing the data needed for delivery of patient care—including patient classification, staffing, scheduling, and costs (Hughes and Andrew, 1995, p. 38). Like the ancillary systems discussed earlier in this section, nursing information systems are an integral part of a health care organization's overall information system. Some of the common features of nursing information systems include the following

- patient care decision support (order entry, care planning, assessment/care documentation, flowsheet charting, medication administration recording, patient acuity, and patient education)
- management applications (staffing/scheduling, case scheduling, productivity monitoring, and quality management)
- nursing education and research

A recent article in *Healthcare Informatics* lists over 70 vendors currently offering nursing information systems (Hughes and Andrew, 1995).

Clinical Decision Support Systems. A *clinical decision support system* generally refers to any computer application designed to help health practitioners make clinical decisions (Shortliffe, 1990, p. 469). In a sense, the clinical information systems described above (laboratory, pharmacy, radiology and nursing) are examples of clinical decision support systems. That is, they capture clinical data and give users decision support capabilities. Advanced clinical decision support systems include knowledge-based features that interpret and analyze data. Such systems either take "learned" knowledge and create new knowledge, or they extract knowledge created by human experts and replicate it in a computer system. For example, pharmacy applications include clinical decision support systems that assist in calculating intravenous additive dosages, checking for drug-to-drug conflicts, and recommending substitute drugs based on a patient's response history. Such systems are often also referred to as expert or artificial intelligence systems.

Clinical decision support systems can have a significant impact on improving patient care and managing health care costs. A recent study by Johnston et al. indicates that clinical decision support systems can improve physician performance and improve patient outcomes (Johnston, Langton, Haynes, et al., 1994, p. 135). Other experts agree that clinical decision support systems can contribute both to improving the quality of care and to enhancing the efficiency of care delivery (Haug, Gardner, Tate, et al., p. 1994).

The Health Evaluation through Logical Processing (HELP) system at the University of Utah and the LDS Hospital in Salt Lake City is an excellent example of a clinical information system that supports health practitioners in making clinical decisions. Used to integrate data for clinician review and provide expert advice, the HELP system interfaces with a number of other computer applications—among them a laboratory system, a billing system, an electrocardiography system, a medical record system, and a collection of ancillary department systems. The software that forms the foundation of the HELP system provides tools to support three basic functions: data acquisition, data interpretation, and data review. The HELP system has the following key capabilities:

- It can issue an *alert* to the user, prompting the health care provider to intervene in caring for the patient.
- It can *critique* new orders, either by pointing out disparities between the order and an internal standard of care or by proposing an alternative therapeutic approach.
- It can *suggest* new orders and procedures in response to patient data justifying their need.
- It can conduct *retrospective* quality assurance studies by assessing the average or typical quality of medical decisions and therapeutic interventions made by health care providers (Haug, Gardner, Tate, et al., 1994, p. 398).

Although developers of clinical expert systems often fear that clinicians will not adapt to or appreciate the recommendations of clinical decision support systems, a recent study indicates that many physicians and nurses find such systems useful in managing patient care (Gardner and Hundsgaarde, 1994, p. 428). The study, which evaluated user acceptance of the HELP system, shows that physicians and nurses are extremely satisfied with the accessibility to patient data and clinical alerts (Gardner and Hundsgaarde, 1994, p. 428). Furthermore, respondents did not believe that clinical decision support systems could either increase their liability or reduce their own decision-making power.

Administrative Information Systems

Administrative information systems function primarily at the departmental level in health care organizations. They support administrative operations such as (1) accounting and financial management, (2) scheduling, (3) human resources management, (4) materials management, and (5) office automation. In most cases administrative computer applications in health care are similar to those used in other industries (payroll, general ledger accounting, purchasing, accounts payable, etc.). Patient accounting systems are an exception to this rule because of the industry-specific requirements of private and public health insurance.

Accounting and Financial Management Systems.   Financial information systems support resource allocation, revenue generation, payment for goods and services, and monitoring of the costs of operation for health care organizations. Major applications include the following:

- patient accounting, billing and collections, and processing of accounts receivable
- payroll preparation and accounting
- budgeting and expense reporting
- cost accounting, including direct costs and allocation of overhead
- accounts payable
- financial reporting

Patient accounting systems often employ electronic data interchange (EDI) with major health insurers—Medicare, Medicaid, Blue Cross/Blue Shield, private insurance companies—for billing and claims processing. As discussed below, the expansion of managed care has required major changes to financial information systems, which can no longer be based primarily on fee-for-service payment.

Scheduling Systems.   Information systems are used to support various types of service scheduling in health care organizations:

- appointment scheduling of patients for outpatient clinics
- advanced bed booking and preadmission processing for hospital inpatients
- surgical scheduling in the operating room
- scheduling of patients for services in the clinical laboratory or radiology department

Effective service scheduling provides the dual benefits of improved patient satisfaction and efficient utilization of facilities (Austin, 1992, p. 263).

Human Resources Information Systems.   Employees are the most important resource of the health care organization. A human resources information system (HRIS) is used to support human resources management in a number of areas:

- employee record keeping (linked to payroll system)
- manpower planning
- recruitment of physicians and other professional personnel
- position control and labor cost allocation
- monitoring of employee satisfaction
- productivity analysis

The HRIS establishes an inventory of people, job skills, and positions that is used to "assist managers in establishing objectives and in evaluating the performance of the organization's human resources programs" (Austin, Johnson, and Palestrant, 1994, p. 165).

Materials Management Systems.   Health care organizations use large quantities of supplies and material in providing services to patients. These include drugs and pharmaceuticals, medical supplies, emergency blood supplies, food, office supplies, and parts for equipment repair and maintenance. Information systems are used for

- ordering
- inventory control
- allocation of the cost of materials in the delivery of patient care

Many of the larger suppliers of drugs and medical supplies provide automated order systems in which the health care organization places orders through electronic data interchange with the vendors.

Office Automation.   Computer systems are used extensively to support office operations in health services organizations, just as they are used in most other industries today. Office automation applications include

- word processing
- electronic mail
- maintenance of calendars and meeting schedules
- project management
- management reporting

These systems improve efficiency and reduce the costs of office operations.

❧ STRATEGIC DECISION SUPPORT SYSTEMS

Strategic decision support systems are computer-based systems that provide interactive information support to health care managers in making critical strategic decisions (Jacobs and Pelfrey, 1995, p. 48). In today's highly competitive environment, these systems must provide health care managers with information useful in evaluating key performance indicators and trends, planning strategically, and marketing services. Similarly, strategic decision support systems are needed to measure organizational performance and compare the performance of a given health care organization with other, similar organizations (DesHarnais, Marshall, and Dulski, 1994, p. 635). Although health care executives are beginning to realize the power of information in gaining a strategic advantage, most are not yet using information systems effectively in strategic planning, strategy development, and implementation (Austin, Trimm, and Sobczak, 1995, p. 26).

Strategic decision support systems, also referred to as executive information systems, have several important characteristics. First, they are used to support health care managers, not to replace them. Strategic decision support systems are not decision-making systems. According to Mallach, there must be some human view of the system's recommendation or it is not a decision support system (Mallach, 1994, p. 7). Second, decision support systems are designed to be used for semistructured or unstructured decisions, making them useful tools for strategic planning and marketing activities. Health care organizations can also use these systems to gain a competitive advantage. For example, the technology can be used in a competitive, product-based, externally (market) oriented way. This approach requires management to think conceptually about strategic information systems as *changing* the way in which a service is provided, rather than merely *supporting* current operations (Moriarty, 1992, p. 85). Finally, strategic decision support systems often integrate information from existing clinical, administrative, and financial systems to assist health care executives in evaluating an organization's ability to provide quality care at the most affordable price. The ability to integrate information from various systems is also important to health care executives when negotiating contracts with providers, managed care organizations, and other purchasers.

Managed Care Information Systems

As previously discussed, health care is changing rapidly due to the expansion of managed care and the development of integrated delivery systems. Concerns about rapidly escalating health care costs have led major purchasers of health services—large employers, health insurance companies, and government agencies—to pursue managed care plans vigorously. Wozmak (1995) offers the following functional definition of managed care: "Managed care is a system of providing and paying for medical care that includes a panel of providers who agree to deliver services at an agreed upon fee. Financial incentives are included for patients to use the identified providers that make up the panel . . . Additionally, there is an outside agent . . . that reviews the utilization to assure efficacious use of resources and positive outcomes" (Wozmak, 1995, p. 12).

Three of the more common forms of managed care plans are health maintenance organizations (HMOs), preferred provider organizations (PPOs), and exclusive provider arrangements (EPAs).

HMOs provide coverage of specified health services to their plan members for a fixed, prepaid premium. PPOs are insurance programs in which plan members receive better benefits when they use services offered by preferred providers. Patients can use nonparticipating providers, but at a higher cost. Exclusive provider arrangements (EPAs) are plans in which large employers self-insure by contracting directly with selected providers in their local medical marketplace. Strong financial incentives are employed to limit or exclude services by providers who are not part of the company EPA plan.

Membership in managed care plans has increased rapidly. In 1994 57 million individuals were covered by HMOs, 20 percent more than in 1991 (Marion Merrell Dow, Inc., 1994). Managed care has changed information system priorities for health services organizations. Respondents to a 1995 national survey of trends in health care computing listed "movement to managed care" as the most frequent response to the question, "what issues are driving the increased computerization of health care?" (HIMSS/Hewlett Packard Leadership Survey, 1995, p. 11).

Managers of health care organizations need good demographic information on the medical market, as well as accurate financial forecasts for negotiations with managed care plans. "[A] decision support system might provide information on demographic characteristics of the contract population, historical data on utilization of services, and financial analyses of the impact of alternative pricing arrangements (capitation, discounted fees, etc.) Simulation techniques can be particularly useful in measuring the potential effects of alternative contracting arrangements" (Austin and Sobczak, 1993, p. 34). At the operational level, contract management software is used to track financial results and manage an increasing number of different types of contract arrangements with managed care organizations.

To compete in the medical marketplace, health care managers must be able to monitor and evaluate the *outcomes* of patient care their organizations provide. Managed care plans and self-insured employer groups are using information about outcomes to seek the least expensive services from providers in their communities that result in at least equal patient satisfaction and medical effectiveness. For example, the Cleveland Health Quality Choice Coalition, a voluntary cooperative of employers and

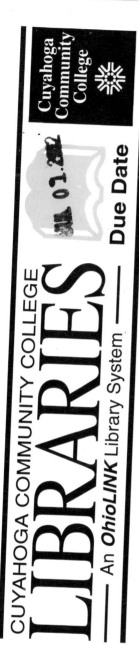

izations in the Cleveland, Ohio, metropolitan area, evaluates the per- ospitals according to the following outcomes: (1) patient satisfaction; ortality; (3) length of hospital stay for different procedures; (4) hospi- plications; and (5) severity-adjusted outcomes for medical, surgical, atients (Rosenthal and Harper, 1994).

successfully in this environment, health care managers must be able mation from their clinical and financial information systems in order utcomes (cost and quality) of the services their organizations provide. et Medical Center in Minneapolis, Minnesota, has developed an ation system to support patient care and strategic management in its 18 facilities. Data from the information system are used to generate a num- nce reports. The scheduling system produces measures of patient satis- patient waiting time on the telephone and the average time interval r an appointment and available openings in the clinic. The system moni- number of patient encounters, patient-staff ratios, and other key indica- quality. After it generates outcome reports on the cost-effectiveness of ment modalities, data from these assessments are used to generate prac- for the clinics. Medical directors receive population-based data to moni- s, illness patterns, prevention and wellness practices, and service usage orting system enables management to assess individual clinics' perfor- ram planning and budgeting purposes (Kralewski et al., 1994, pp. 22–23).

ealth Information Networks

health information network (CHIN) is defined as "an electronic highway mless connectivity to all the components of a health care delivery sys- ns, hospitals, ambulatory care centers, payers, employers, pharmacies, rs, and regulatory agencies" (Weaver, 1993, p. 12) (see Figure 7.5). As livery systems become more widespread and health care organizations boundaries, CHINs are emerging to support them (Hanlon, 1995, p. 9). tended to reduce administrative costs and improve quality of care by pants access to financial, clinical, and administrative information across s. CHINs may also be the first major step to developing a CPR.

Although the potential benefits of CHINs are many, health care managers must appropriately plan for their implementation. To begin with, the health care organization should conduct a formal assessment of its readiness to participate in or develop a CHIN. The purpose of the assessment is to determine whether the organization has the necessary internal capabilities and strategic relationships in place before connecting with payers, purchasers, and other providers to share clinical and financial information.

Figure 7.5   Community Health Information Network (CHIN)

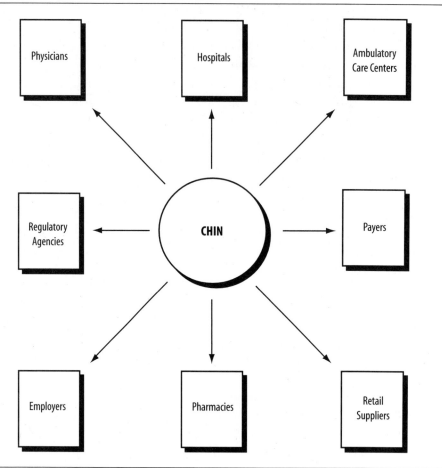

Key representatives from information systems, managed care, executive management, and clinical areas should be involved in this process.

Four primary areas should be addressed in the readiness assessment: (1) business planning, (2) internal environment, (3) information technology, and (4) market readiness (Petry and Chandler, 1995, p. 16). The first three areas measure an organization's internal preparedness; the fourth determines the community's readiness to develop a CHIN. Management should assume a leadership role both in conducting the readiness assessment and in addressing other key issues related to participating in or developing a CHIN. Such issues include defining information systems requirements, establishing data and language standards, planning for systems integration, determining type of ownership, financing the CHIN, and securing confidential patient information.

Advances in *electronic data interchange* (EDI) make CHINs feasible from a technological perspective. EDI provides for the exchange of computer-processable data in a standard format between organizational entities (Moynihan, 1993, p. 1). Although EDI applications were first introduced primarily to process claims and purchase orders electronically, new applications for EDI technology are being developed to transfer both financial and clinical information between health care providers, payers, and purchasers. Future advances in EDI technology will have a profound impact on linking CHINs across the nation.

The Wisconsin Health Information Network (WHIN) was one of the first functional CHINs in the country. It is jointly owned by Ameritech Corporation and Aurora Health Care, a Milwaukee-based integrated provider system. The network, which has been in operation since 1993, now serves over 11 hospitals and more than 1,100 providers in the greater Milwaukee area, including home health and nursing agencies and ambulance services (Bazzoli, 1994, p. 46). Several payers are also participating in the network. The network supports exchange of both clinical and financial information. The clinical information available includes transcribed medical reports, medication reports, post-discharge abstracts and laboratory results. Users can also check on the status of claims from several key payers. In addition, the system offers access to hospital census data and referral information, links to the Internet, and e-mail to users (Bazzoli, 1994, p. 46). Benefits include a lower administrative overhead and a greater focus on patient care.

PLANNING, DESIGN, IMPLEMENTATION, ❧ AND OPERATION OF HEALTH INFORMATION SYSTEMS

Information systems must be carefully planned and managed if they are to support the strategic goals of the health care organization. The first step is development of a strategic information plan.

Strategic information systems planning is the process of identifying and assigning priorities to a portfolio of computer applications that will assist the health care organization in formulating strategy and executing its business plans. Information systems plans must be aligned with the strategic goals and objectives of the organization. The plan should address a number of critical questions for example:

1. How can information systems technology be used to generate new health services in response to market demands?
2. How can information systems technology be used to distinguish services provided by the organization from those of other organizations?
3. Which computer applications and supporting technology infrastructure are needed to make the new strategy work? (Tan, 1995, p. 306)

As health care organizations become more sophisticated in information planning and management, they are increasingly likely to use information to make strategic decisions about positioning their organizations within the environments in which they operate (Austin, Trimm and Sobczak, 1995, p. 27). Although strategic information systems planning has improved in recent years, 19 percent of the respondents to a 1995 national survey of trends in health care computing listed "lack of strategic IS [information system] plan" as their most frustrating information systems problem (HIMSS/Hewlett Packard, 1995). The information systems plan provides the blueprint to ensure that this strategic alignment occurs.

Figure 7.6 lists the major elements for a strategic health information systems plan. The plan should begin with a concise statement of critical *organizational goals and objectives* for the planning period (usually two to five years). As mentioned above, it is

Figure 7.6   Elements of the Information Systems Strategic Plan

1. Statement of corporate/institutional goals and objectives
2. Statement of information systems goals and objectives
   a. Management information needs
   b. Critical success factors
   c. Information priorities
3. Priorities for the applications portfolio
   a. Clinical
   b. Administrative
   c. Decision support
4. Specification of overall system architecture and infrastructure
   a. Level of distribution (centralized to decentralized)
   b. Network architecture
   c. Data location (central data warehouse to total data distribution)
   d. Data security and control requirements
5. Software development plan
   a. Commercial packages
   b. In-house development
   c. Tailor-made applications through contracting
   d. Combination of the above
6. Information systems management plan
   a. Central information systems staff
   b. Outsourcing
   c. Limited central staffing in support of department-level information systems staff
   d. Combinations of the above
7. Statement of resource requirements
   a. Capital budget (hardware, software, network communications, equipment)
   b. Operating budget (staff, supplies, consultants, training, etc.)

essential that *information systems goals and objectives* be aligned with these organizational priorities. For example, if an urban medical center has decided to give priority to expanding ambulatory care services in the community but information system priorities continue to focus on inpatient services, the organization has a serious goal displacement problem.

In his classic *Harvard Business Review* article, Rockart (1979) suggest using the critical success factors approach to define information systems goals and objectives as part of the planning process. Top executives often have difficulty describing their management information needs. However, specifying those key areas where things must go right in order for the organization to flourish helps information systems planners to determine information requirements and establish priorities for system development.

Priorities for the applications portfolio should flow from strategic information systems goals and objectives. Health services organizations will not be able to acquire all the systems they need in any given year. A very important element of the information systems plan is what clinical, administrative, and decision support applications are to be developed. They should be listed in order of importance, with tentative implementation schedules, and the priorities should be reviewed and updated at least once a year.

The first three elements of the information systems plan deal with functional information requirements independent of the technology to be employed. The next two elements specify the technical approach to be followed in system design and implementation.

The plan must specify an *overall system architecture and infrastructure* that includes the following elements:

1. The degree to which computing will be centralized or distributed throughout the organization.
2. The network architecture that specifies how computers and client server workstations will be linked together through communications lines and network servers.
3. The manner in which data will be stored and distributed throughout the organization, including procedures for database security and control.
4. The process by which individual applications will be integrated so that they can exchange information. Options range from a completely open systems approach with interfaces linking software from different vendors to a single vendor approach in which applications are already integrated.

The information systems plan also specifies procedures for *software development*. Most health care organizations now use commercial software packages available from a large number of commercial vendors (see, for example, *Hospital Software Sourcebook*, 1993). Some larger organizations may develop selected applications through in-house programming or use of contractors for tailor-made applications. Combinations of these approaches are possible as well.

The information systems plan should also specify the *information systems management structure* for the organization. Most hospitals and other health service organizations still employ an in-house staff for system management. Decisions must be made concerning the extent to which technical staff will be centralized in an information systems department or distributed among the major user departments of the organization. An increasing number of organizations are outsourcing all or part of their information processing to contractors who provide on-site system development and management services (Gardner, 1991).

The final element of the information systems plan specifies the *resources required* to carry it out. A capital budget should include five- to ten-year projections for the cost of computer hardware, network and telecommunications equipment, and software. The operating budget includes costs for staff, supplies and materials, consultants, training programs, and other recurring expenses. Both budgets should be updated annually.

The entire information systems planning process should be directed by a steering committee with broad representation from major system users throughout the organization (see Figure 7.7). The committee should be chaired by the chief information officer, if such a position has been established. Members should be drawn from corporate administration, medical staff, nursing service, medical records, human resources, and major service departments of the organization.

Working within the framework of the information systems plan, individual computer applications are developed and installed. Project teams should be formed to oversee the process. The teams should include representatives from all user departments as

Figure 7.7   Information Systems Steering Committee

- Chief information officer (CIO)
- Central administration
- Medical staff
- Nursing service
- Medical records
- Human resources
- Major service departments
- Consultant (if needed)

well as information systems staff. Project organization and management includes the following steps:

1. *Systems analysis.* Review of current information practices and determination of new or modified functional requirements for the application.
2. *System specification.* Statement of system requirements that can be incorporated into requests for proposals or requests for information from software vendors or contractors who will bid on the application.
3. *Proposal evaluation.* Review of vendor proposals or standard software packages being considered for the application.
4. *Implementation.* Equipment and software installation, user training, file conversion, and system testing.
5. *Operation and maintenance.* Preventive maintenance for equipment, software maintenance (including periodic upgrades from the vendor), and continued training for new staff members.

Figure 7.8 lists key criteria for evaluating packaged software and vendor proposals. In addition to being certain that the software satisfies the functional requirements determined through systems analysis, the new system must be able to be integrated with other current or projected computer applications. Many health care organizations require software products to meet developing industry standards for data compatibility and interfacing such as Health Level-7, which is being developed under the

---

Figure 7.8   Proposal/Software Evaluation Criteria

---

1. Congruence with organizational requirements
2. Ability to interface/integrate with other applications (e.g., compatibility with Health Level-7 data standards)
3. Financial stability of vendor
4. Level of satisfaction of other users
5. Support available
   a. Training
   b. Documentation
   c. Maintenance
6. Costs
   a. Software lease or purchase
   b. Additional hardware (if any)
   c. Implementation
   d. Operational maintenance and upgrades

NOTE: Use *independent* consultant for assistance with technical evaluation if needed.

---

auspices of the National Standards Institute (Dunbar, 1991). The project team should also investigate the financial stability of the vendor under consideration and check with other users of the product to determine their level of satisfaction. Vendor support services (maintenance and training) are an important component of software implementation. In addition to the initial cost for the software purchase or lease, a complete evaluation must consider the costs of implementation and maintenance, including periodic upgrades. Smaller health care organizations may need to use a consultant to assist in technical evaluation of proposals. It is important, however, that such a consultant be independent and not connected with any specific product or vendor.

Hardware and software purchases can be expensive. In contracting for these services, the health care organization should employ qualified legal counsel to assist in the negotiations and draft the contract. Standard vendor contracts should always be avoided.

As described above, information is an essential resource that must be carefully managed. Given the increased importance of information in strategic decision making and the complexity of modern technology, many health care organizations have established the position of chief information officer (CIO). The CIO usually reports directly to the chief executive officer and is a member of the executive team of the organization. The CIO serves two important functions: (1) assisting the executive team in using information effectively for strategic planning and management; and (2) managing and coordinating information systems and network communications (Austin, 1992, p. 197). The person chosen for this position must possess both strong management and technical skills. In addition to understanding information technology, the CIO should have leadership ability, strong communication skills, vision and imagination, business and financial management skills, and knowledge of health services delivery.

Guidelines For Managing
❦ Information Systems in Health Care Organizations

The reader should take away eight important principles from reading this chapter.

1. **Managers of health care organizations should treat information as an essential organizational resource.** Information is essential to the provision of high-quality, cost-effective health care. Managers must plan and manage the use of this resource just as they manage the human and financial resources of the organization.

2. **Information systems should support strategic planning and management in addition to supporting operations.** In the past, health information systems

have focused primarily on the day-to-day operation of health care facilities. Health care has become highly competitive. Health care executives must learn to use information systems to support decisions about strategy and the positioning of their organizations in the markets where they compete.

3. **Strategic information systems planning is essential.** Given the wide array of information needs and the complexity of modern information technology, such planning is essential to establish priorities among applications, ensure integration among systems, and evaluate alternative approaches to systems development and implementation.

4. **Information systems integration is essential.** Most computer applications cannot stand alone in health care organizations. Individual systems must be able to "talk to one another" electronically. Clinical and financial information must be combined for outcomes assessment of the costs and quality of patient care. Systems integration requires careful planning and adherence to standards for data definition and transmission.

5. **Decisions about information systems should be driven by users rather than by technology.** Those who will use information for strategic and operational support should specify the characteristics of information systems in health care organizations. Technical specialists should provide information on the most suitable hardware and software to meet these user specifications. It is not necessary (or always desirable) to employ the newest technology available.

6. **CPRs will take on increasing importance in the era of managed care and integrated delivery systems.** Health care providers are forming strategic alliances and developing integrated structures for the delivery of service. Those who purchase services must share information on patient satisfaction and clinical outcomes. CHINs are being developed to share information electronically throughout the delivery system. Managers must give priority to computerization of patient records to participate in these activities.

7. **Computer hardware and software must be carefully evaluated before purchases are made.** Health care organizations rely primarily on commercial software for implementing information systems. With a wide variety of products and services available in a volatile marketplace, careful evaluation and vendor selection should precede major purchases.

8. **The CIO plays a critical role in the effective planning and use of information systems in health care organizations.** The CIO performs the critical role of assisting the executive team in effective use of information for strategic planning and management, in addition to managing and coordinating information systems within the organization. Most health care organizations need a well-qualified executive to serve in this position.

&. FUTURE TRENDS

Health services delivery in the 21st century will be radically different from that of today. Integrated delivery systems will become the dominant model, and CHINs will emerge to support them. The expanded use of EDI applications will make it technologically feasible to exchange clinical and financial information across regional and national networks. Advances in voice recognition, imaging systems, and telemedicine will allow health care providers to care for patients anywhere in the world using multimedia technology. Clinical decision support systems will become more widely used in diagnosing, treating, managing, and evaluating patient care. The CPR, as defined by the IOM, will become the standard among health care organizations, and its widespread use will help to control health care costs and conduct outcomes research studies.

In the future, health care executives will rely on sophisticated decision support tools. They will have immediate access to timely, accurate, and complete information in deciding how services will be offered and what resources will be allocated. Information systems planning will become an integral part of the health care organization's overall strategic plan. Health care organizations will address in their strategic plans the organizational, behavioral, and financial issues relating to the implementation of information technology. Clearly, a health care organization's success in this new environment will depend upon its ability to manage information effectively.

&. REFERENCES

Austin, Charles J. 1992: *Information Systems for Health Services Administration.* (4th ed.) Ann Arbor, MI: AUPHA Press/Health Administration Press.

Austin, C., Johnson, J., Palestrant, G. 1994: Information Systems for Human Resource Management in *Strategic Management of Human Resources.* (2nd ed.). Myron D. Fottler, S. Robert Hernandez, Charles L. Joiner (eds.). Albany, NY: Delmar Publishers.

Austin, C. and Sobczak, P. 1993: Information technology and managed care. *Hospital Topics,* 71(3), 33–37.

Austin, C., Trimm, J., and Sobczak, P. 1995: Information systems and strategic management. *Health Care Management Review,* 20(3), 26–33.

Bazzoli, F. (ed.) 1994: Health information networks, where are we headed? *Health Data Management,* 2(9), 39–47.

DesHarnais, S., Marshall, B., and Dulski, J. 1994: Information management in the age of managed competition. *Journal on Quality Improvement*, 20(11), 631–638.

Dick, Richard S. and Steen, Elaine B. (eds.) 1991: *The Computer-Based Patient Record: An Essential Technology for Health Care.* Institute of Medicine. Washington, DC: National Academy Press.

Dunbar, C. 1991: In pursuit of a single health care computing standard. *Computers in Healthcare*, November, 19–24.

Gardner, E. 1991: Going on line with outsiders. *Modern Healthcare,.* July 15, 35–47.

Gardner, R. and Lundsgaarde, H. 1994: Evaluation of user acceptance of a clinical expert system. *Journal of the American Medical Informatics Association*, 1(6), 428–438.

Greenes, Robert A. and Brinkley, James F. 1990: Radiology Systems in *Medical Informatics: Computer Applications in Health Care.* Reading, MA: Addison–Wesley Publishing Company.

Hanlon, P. 1995: Charting the evolution of community health information networks. *The Journal of the Healthcare Information and Management Systems Society*, 9(2), 10–14.

Harrell, A. 1994: Building a patient record system. *Health Progress*, 51–54.

Haug, P., Gardner, R., Tate, K., et al. 1994: Decision support in medicine: examples from the HELP system. *Computers and Biomedical Research*, 27, 396–418.

Healthcare Information and Management Systems Society and Hewlett–Packard Company 1995: *Sixth Annual HIMSS/Hewlett–Packard Leadership Survey: Trends in health care computing.* Chicago, IL: Healthcare Information and Management Systems Society.

Hughes, S. and Andrew, W. 1995: Automating nursing: from assessment to evaluation. *Healthcare Informatics*, 12 (4), 36–50.

Jacobs, S. and Pelfrey, S. 1995: Decision support systems: Using computers to help manage. *Journal of the American Nursing Association*, 25(2), 46–51.

Johnston, M., Langton, K., Haynes, R., et al. 1994: Effects of computer–based clinical decision support systems on clinician performance and patient outcomes. *Annals of Internal Medicine*, 120(2), 135–142.

Kralewski, J. et al. 1994: The development of integrated service networks (ISNs). *A Report for the Minnesota Care Legislative Oversight Committee.* University of Minnesota School of Public Health, February 21.

Lowe, H., Buchanan, B., Cooper, G., et al. 1995: Building a medical multimedia database system to integrate clinical information: An application of high performance computing and communications technology. *Bulletin of the Medical Library Association*, 83 (1), 57–64.

Mallach, Efrem G. 1994: *Understanding Decision Support Systems and Expert Systems.* Burr Ridge, IL: Irwin Publisher.

Marion Merrell Dow, Inc. 1994: *Managed Care Digest.* Medical Group Practice Edition, Volume 1.

McKenzie, J. (ed.) 1993: *Hospital Software Sourcebook.* Rockville, MD: Aspen Publications, Inc.

Minard, Bernie. 1991: *Health Care Computer Systems for the 1990s: Critical Executive Decisions.* Ann Arbor, MI: American College of Healthcare Executives.

Moriarty, D. 1992: Strategic information systems planning for health service providers. *Health Care Management Review* 17(1), 85–90.

Morrissey, J. 1995: Information systems refocus on priorities. *Modern Health care,* 25(7), 65–6, 70, 72.

Moynihan, James J. 1993: EDI: *A Guide for the Healthcare Professional.* Chicago: Probus Publishing Company.

Petry, J. and Chandler, M. 1995: Assessing your CHIN readiness. *The Journal of the Healthcare Information and Management Systems Society,* 9(2), 15–20.

Rockart, J. 1979: Chief executives define their own data needs. *Harvard Business Review,* 57(2), 81–84.

Rosenthal, G. and Harper, D. 1994: Cleveland health quality choice: A model for collaborative community–based outcomes assessment. *Journal on Quality Improvement,* 20(8), 425–442.

Shortliffe, Edward H. 1990: Clinical Decision Support Systems in *Medical Informatics: Computer Applications in Health Care.* Reading, MA: Addison–Wesley Publishing Company.

Smith, Jack W. and Svirbely, John R. 1990: Laboratory Information Systems in *Medical Informatics: Computer Applications in Health Care.* Shortliffe, E. and Perreault, L. (eds.). Reading, MA: Addison–Wesley Publishing Company.

Tan, Joseph K. 1995: *Health Management Information Systems.* Rockville, MD: Aspen Publications, Inc.

Weaver, C. 1993: CHINs: Infrastructure for the future. *Trustee*, December, 12–13.

Wozmak, Mark S. 1995: Managed care: A primer. *American Academy of Medical Administrators Executives*, January/February, 12–14.

Health Care Marketing

Bruce Wrenn
Indiana University South Bend

8

H ealth care organizations are among the last of the service organizations to adopt modern marketing practices into their management systems. Prior to the late 1970s, marketing as we now know it had no significant presence in any health care provider. Those marketing functions that were performed at all were conducted under the auspices of departments with titles like "development" and "public relations" by people who had no formal training or prior experience in marketing outside the health care industry. This lack of interest in the field of marketing was soon to be replaced with a hunger for marketing talent born of the desperate times facing health care providers in the late 1970s and early 1980s.

Marketing is certainly not the only functional department that has undergone sea changes in its role in health care management; but it has been among the most controversial, as administrators have struggled with assessing its value to the organization and in defining its role. This chapter on health care marketing attempts to define the appropriate role for marketing within health care systems by first examining the history of health care marketing, then reviewing the research that seeks to determine the value of marketing to health care organizations, and finally identifying the role of marketing in serving such organizations well, both now and in the future.

ᔰ A History of Health Care Marketing

The Evolution of Competition in the Health Care Industry

Any history of health care marketing must include an exposition on the rise of competition in the market for health services. The evolution of competition in the health care market has been chronicled by numerous authors (Arnold, 1991; Eastaugh, 1992; Feldstein, 1986, 1994; Hillestad and Berkowitz, 1991; Joyce and Cronin, 1985; Malhotra, 1986; Schulz and Johnson, 1983; Vraciu, 1985). From 1935 to 1965 health care costs as a percentage of GNP increased only from 4.1 percent to 5.9 percent. Then in 1966 the government introduced Medicare and Medicaid, basing reimbursement to hospitals according to their costs. Fee-for-service payments by private insurers also generously reimbursed hospitals. Neither the third-party payers (government and insurers) nor patients were overly concerned with the costs of medical care. Consequently, hospitals had little incentive to become efficient, and what competition existed consisted of hospitals trying to offer every possible service and convenience to physicians so that the physicians would not need to refer the patient to another hospital. Certificate-of-need (CON) regulations, which were intended to control growing capital expenditures, were ineffective in limiting hospital investment, since large community hospitals ended up controlling the CON approval process (Feldstein, 1994). HMOs such as Kaiser found it difficult to get a foothold in a market, since they could not get CON approval to build a new facility. Meanwhile, health care expenditures had increased as a percentage of GNP from 5.8 percent in 1966 to over 9 percent by the late 1970s.

While some legislation before the 1970s had the effect of protecting hospitals from the economics of marketplace competition (e.g., Hill Burton legislation, 1945; Medicare and Medicaid legislation, 1965), several other acts laid the groundwork for later competition (Health Professions Educational Assistance Act, 1963; HMO Act, 1973; changes in CON legislation to ensure that those laws would not restrict competition, 1979–80; TEFRA, 1982; DRG legislation, 1983). The change to a more competitive environment in the early 1980s cannot be traced to a specific piece of legislation or single environmental event but was rather the result of two major forces converging on the health care market simultaneously: a desire by third-party payers to reduce increasing health care expenditures and excess capacity among health care providers, particularly physicians and hospitals (Feldstein, 1986).

Diagnosis-related group (DRG) legislation, begun in 1983 and phased in over the next five years, forced hospitals to become more efficient and had the effect of reducing inpatient occupancy rates. Physicians' treatment decisions were more carefully scrutinized in an attempt to reduce costly medical tests and long hospital stays. Other environmental events also contributed to the move toward greater competition. The recession of 1981 and increased foreign competition caused businesses to seek ways of reducing costs to remain competitive, and high medical insurance expenses for employees became an obvious target for cutbacks. To control the rise in their premiums to businesses, insurers instituted programs designed to reduce their payments for medical expenses: preauthorized admissions, mandatory second opinions, lower-cost substitutes for inpatient care, and the development of HMOs and PPOs sponsored by the insurance companies (cf. Johnson and Johnson, 1986, p. 369) with their emphasis on keeping patients out of hospitals and controlling the length of stay for those admitted. Similarly, the federal government's institution of DRG requirements to cut its Medicare expenses, along with court decisions holding that the health care profession was subject to antitrust laws, further promoted market competition. Contributing to hospitals' excess capacity were the increasing competition from large physician group practice clinics and outpatient diagnostic and surgery centers, and the more cost-conscious practice of medicine by physicians, who were being forced to try to shorten patients' stays in hospitals as a result of pressure from insurance companies to reduce the cost of patient care. Social trends emphasizing diet, exercise, and wellness also contributed to a decline in hospital inpatient census. Such environmental shifts have been described not just as rapid change but as a period of destabilization for the health care industry (Ginzberg, 1986).

One of the products of this destabilization of the hospital environment has been a dramatic increase in competition among hospitals for such strategic resources as physician loyalty and consumers (patients) (Coddington and Moore, 1987). Numerous sources have noted the increased level of competition among hospitals as a result of the changes in the environment (Autry and Thomas, 1986; Battistella, 1985; Calder, 1983; Christianson and McClure, 1979; Cooper, 1983; Friedman, 1980; Haines, 1983; Salkever, 1980). One author (Arnold, 1991) suggested that the major environmental forces leading to a rise in competition include excess capacity, inflation and rising health care costs, rapidly advancing technology and increasing specialization, the consumer movement, deregulation of the health care industry, changes in reimbursement systems and declines in occupancy rates, and corporate restructuring and diversification. Such increased competition among health care providers for strategic resources has resulted in a greater interest in marketing.

Rise in Interest in Hospital Marketing

A 1979 bibliography of health care marketing (Robinson and Cooper 1980) listed 166 marketing-related articles for the 25 years prior to 1979, whereas a subsequent bibliography covering only 1979 to 1983 listed 617 marketing-related citations (Cooper, Jones, and Wong, 1984). The year 1977 has been identified as a "landmark" for hospital marketing (Cooper and Kehoe, 1978), when a dramatic increase in articles about hospital marketing began to appear. Articles with titles like "Marketing—An Emerging Management Challenge" (Lachner, 1977); "What Is Marketing" (Wexler, 1977); "Concepts and Strategies for Health Marketers" (Lovelock, 1977); and "Introducing Marketing as a Planning and Management Tool" (Tucker, 1977) are indicative of the nascent quality of hospital marketing in 1977. A 1979 article (Robinson and Whittington, 1979) suggested a number of reasons for the increased interest in health care marketing during the late 1970s (see Table 8.1). Other authors have attributed some of this increased interest to research findings indicating that patients were exercising more discretion in their choice of physicians (Wolinsky and Steiber, 1982) and hospitals (Boscarino and Steiber, 1994). Marketing was viewed as a means for influencing such choice decisions.

Despite the forces promoting the adoption of a marketing orientation for hospitals, marketing received less than unanimous and enthusiastic support by hospital administrators. The difficulties of implementing a marketing orientation in hospitals were evidenced almost immediately by articles with such titles as "Marketing Health Care: Problems in Implementation" (Clarke, 1978); "Roadblocks to Hospital Marketing" (Robinson and Cooper, 1980–81); "Why Marketing Isn't Working in the Health Care Arena" (O'Connor, 1982); "Marketplace Language Harms Health Care" (Hague, 1979); and "Has Marketing Been Oversold to Hospital Administrators?" (Lamb and Finn, 1982).

Marketing and marketers were not enthusiastically welcomed into the health care industry during the early 1980s, although their immediate need was widely recognized. (In 1984, for example, hospital CEOs mentioned marketing as their top priority, and in 1985 recruitment of marketers was given high priority (MacStravic, 1990)). The tenuous nature of marketing's foothold in the industry became immediately obvious when in 1986 and 1987 two leading industry periodicals published articles such as "Hospitals Call a Marketing Time-Out" (*Hospitals*, 1986); "Marketing, Take Two" (*Modern Healthcare*, 1987); and "Will Marketing Ever Grow Up?" (*Hospitals*, 1987). This seemingly stunning reversal of hospital marketers' fortunes is perhaps less dramatic when one realizes that many in the health care field retained a certain wariness of marketing. Witness the following statements published as the marketing wave crested during the 1980s: "Hospital marketing has failed to live up to its promise and its future seems questionable" (*Modern Healthcare*, 1983, p. 75); "The belief persists that hospital markets are fundamentally different from other product/service markets and that conventional marketing approaches are therefore irrelevant for hospital managements" (Cavusgil, 1986, p. 71). Clarke and Shyavitz (1987), commenting on why marketers were finding it so difficult to be adopted and fully assimilated into the health care field, noted that many of the people with marketing titles were former public or

Table 8.1   Some Reasons for Rising Levels of Interest in Health Care Marketing in the Late 1970s

Reason	Explanation
1. Rising costs.	With rapid escalation of health care costs has come a search for methods and techniques to slow the rate of increase. Marketing may be useful to health care administrators in effecting cost containment measures.
2. Rising accountability .	Legislation has created mechanisms for evaluating of health care service providers. Providers are now required to give information to support requests for additional services and to defend the allocation of resources. Marketing techniques and concepts are useful in the development of such information.
3. Increasing emphasis by trustees and directors on the health care consumer's needs.	Administrators must demonstrate to governing boards that health care consumers have been consulted and their needs considered in planning and operating the services offered.
4. Increase in proprietary health care services.	The successes of such profit-making health care services as hospital management firms, proprietary hospitals, health maintenance organizations, group practices, and emergency clinics have been widely reported. As a result, many health care organizations believe that they must become more competitive and devote increased attention to their principal markets.
5. Underutilization viewed as a waste.	Marketing provides the administration with concepts and techniques to smooth irregular demand patterns, review consumer needs, identify and reach target markets, and measure customer satisfaction with services offered. Thus, marketing may be useful in increasing levels of utilization without creating a demand for unnecessary services.
6. Duplication of services.	Marketing can help administrators measure total demand, assess the level and quality of services offered by other health care providers, and determine which services should be offered to meet effectively the needs of the markets served by the organization. Thus, marketing can provide information to assist decision makers in their quest to achieve effective utilization of available financial, human, and equipment resources.
7. Rising sense of professionalism by staff.	Increasingly, nurses, pharmacists, respiratory therapists, and other staff members seek recognition for their contributions. Marketing, with its emphasis on exchange relationships with key publics, offers a useful approach for to administrators faced with an increasingly complex set of staff needs and expectations.
8. Changing nature of patient-physician relationship.	Patients have become more active participants in decisions affecting their health care. Choices with respect to where, how, and what health care services are sought are increasingly influenced by consumer awareness and knowledge. Marketing techniques are useful in developing consumer awareness and providing information about alternative services.
9. Rising interest in prevention.	While most consumers still seek health care on an episodic, curative crisis basis, there is a clear trend toward preventive health services, which are amenable to marketing efforts and can substantially reduce the overall costs of health care.
10. Rising consumer dissatisfaction with health care providers.	Expectation levels of health care consumers are rising. Therefore, health care providers must develop a better understanding of consumer expectations and satisfaction levels. Marketing provides the measurement techniques needed to determine patient expectation and satisfaction.
11. Health care as a business.	Many observers believe that health care possesses the elements of a business. That is, competing organizations offer products and services to consumers at prices and locations that differ substantially. Effective public relations and promotional techniques use the same principles, as do business firms.

Source: Robinson and Whittington (1979).

community relation directors or planning directors who merely had a job title change; very few of them had any training as health care marketers; those trained marketers who came from other industries were novices in health care; and marketing programs, despite large increases in marketing budgets, were still severely underfunded relative to other industries facing similar competitive environments. They concluded that while there was "lots of talk" about marketing, very little authentic marketing was taking place.

Continued competition kept marketing budgets increasing throughout the 1980s in spite of questions about the effectiveness of marketing efforts. However, in 1990 hospital marketing budgets began to oscillate significantly from one year to the next (*Marketing News*, 1994), and in a survey of health care executives in the early 1990s, marketing issues ranked last out of a list of nine in terms of future importance to health care administration (Hudak, Brooke, Finstuen, and Riley, 1993). Oscillating marketing budgets and declining importance may be a manifestation of two phenomena: (1) uncertainty as to the value of marketing to health care organizations, and (2) a belief that marketing essentially consists of image enhancement and demand stimulation activities, the need for which varies over time with market conditions and with organizational structures.

₰ Does Marketing Make a Difference to Health Care System Success?

Research attempting to determine whether marketing contributes to the success of health care organizations has focused on testing the hypothesis that marketing-oriented organizations are more successful than those that are not. We examine this hypothesis for health care organizations by first briefly describing the construct "marketing orientation" and its history as a subject for research and then looking at the empirical evidence that tests the hypothesis in health care settings.

Marketing Orientation

Marketing orientation is grounded in the marketing concept. The marketing concept was formally articulated in the writings of McKitterick (1957), Felton (1959), and Keith (1960), although earlier writings by Alderson (1955), Drucker (1954), and Converse and Heugy (1946) stressed the need for marketers to help their firms become customer-centered. In fact, McKitterick mentions reading issues of the *Journal of Marketing* and *Harvard Business Review* of the 1930s and 1940s in which the elements of the marketing concept were being discussed.

The marketing concept is generally acknowledged as consisting of three elements (Cravens, 1987; Cravens, Hills, and Woodruff, 1987; Dalrymple and Parsons, 1990; Houston, 1986; McCarthy and Perrault, 1990):

1. Customer philosophy—attention to identifying and satisfying exchange partners' wants and needs.
2. Goal attainment—the means by which an organization can achieve its goals most efficiently while satisfying customer needs.
3. Integrated marketing organization—integration of effort by all areas of the organization to satisfy corporate goals by satisfying customer needs and wants.

The degree to which an organization has successfully implemented the marketing concept has been referred to as the organization's "marketing orientation" (McCarthy and Perrault, 1990) and serves as our definition of this construct.

The three components of the marketing concept are contained in Kohli and Jaworski's (1990) definition of market orientation: "Market orientation is the organization-wide *generation* of market intelligence pertaining to current and future customer needs [i.e., customer philosophy], *dissemination* of the intelligence across departments [i.e., integrated marketing organization], and organizationwide *responsiveness to it* [i.e., goal attainment]" (p.6). A literature review (Wrenn, 1995) of studies measuring the effect of marketing orientation reported the following general conclusions:

1. Perhaps most significantly for marketing theorists and practitioners is the consistent finding that being marketing oriented does improve organizational performance. This has been shown to be true for large (Jaworski and Kohli, 1993) as well as small firms (Naidu and Narayana, 1991), product producers (Narver and Slater, 1990) as well as service suppliers (Decker, 1985), for-profit (Slater and Narver, 1994), as well as not-for-profit organizations (Qureshi, 1993).
2. Also of interest to proponents of the adoption of a marketing orientation are the recent findings that environmental conditions (market turbulence, competitive intensity, technological turbulence) do little to moderate the positive impact of marketing orientation on firm performance (Jaworski and Kohli, 1993; Slater and Narver, 1994).
3. Adopting a market orientation can have significant internal benefits in addition to the external market performance benefits attributable to its adoption. Siguaw, Brown, and Widing (1994) report that if the firm is perceived as having a high marketing orientation, the sales force practices a greater customer orientation, has reduced role stress, and expresses greater job satisfaction and organizational

commitment. Likewise, Jaworski and Kohli (1993) discovered a significant positive relationship between a firm's marketing orientation and employee commitment to the firm.

4. Marketing orientation has also been found to be positively related to customer satisfaction (McCullough, Heng, and Khem, 1986). However, more studies are needed to determine if this finding holds across industries.

Marketing Orientation in Health Care Organizations

Within a hospital setting, the marketing concept has been defined (Arnold, Capella, and Sumrall, 1987b) as: "...a patient orientation backed by integrated marketing aimed at generating patient satisfaction as the key to satisfying the hospital's goals" (p. 20). Such a definition is consistent with the general definition encompassing customer philosophy, integrated marketing organization, and goal-directed behavior. Although health professionals have long accepted the belief that the health needs of the public should govern the behavior of hospitals and other health care institutions, the predominant practice has been to define needs "in terms of how the health professional felt people should behave rather than the actual utilities sought by the consumer or motivations that influence human behavior" (Cooper, 1985, p. 7). This notion that health professionals are in a better position to define the entire needs of consumers, who have only limited ability to express their health needs, is similar to the belief held by critics of the marketing concept that it relies too much on consumers, who are not able to articulate their needs because they are unaware of what technology can produce (Bennett and Cooper, 1979; Hayes and Abernathy, 1980; Kaldor, 1971; Riesz, 1980; Sachs and Benson, 1978; Weeks and Marks, 1968). Several authors have defended the marketing concept against such criticism (Houston, 1986; Kiel, 1984; McGee and Spiro, 1988; Parasuraman, 1981; Samli, Palda, and Barker, 1987); they argue that the marketing concept does not expect customers themselves to be the sole source of product ideas, or even know their own needs; it simply says that management should be guided by a willingness to recognize and understand customer needs and to adjust the organization's offering in light of such understanding. Such a rebuttal seems equally valid for the health care managers who do not consider the marketing concept to be an appropriate philosophy for their organization. In fact, many people believe that the marketing concept is an appropriate guiding philosophy for health care organizations, and that they could benefit from having a marketing orientation (Arnold, Capella, and Sumrall, 1987a, 1987b; Cavugil, 1986; Clarke and Shyavitz, 1987; Cooper, 1985; Kaplan, 1979; Kotler and Clarke, 1987; Malhotra, 1987; Stensrud and Arrington, 1988).

Experts disagree, however, about the degree to which health care organizations in general have adopted a marketing orientation. Some believe that a true marketing orientation is rare among such organizations (Arnold, Capella, and Sumrall, 1987b; Clarke and Shyavitz, 1987; McDevitt, 1987; Robbins, Kane, and Sullivan, 1988; Stensrud and Arrington, 1988), while others claim that there was evidence of a higher level of marketing orientation in hospitals in the mid- to late 1980s (Bartlett, Schewe, and Allen, 1984; McDevitt and Shields, 1985). The degree to which hospitals and other health care organizations and systems have adopted a true marketing orientation remains a debatable issue in the 1990s as well, with two studies in the same issue of the *Journal of Health Care Marketing* making these seemingly incompatible claims:

> Our findings indicate that the health care industry, despite the competitive hardships during the past several years, has not embraced a marketing philosophy. (Naidu and Narayana, 1991, p. 27)

> A majority of hospitals responding [to the survey] have a strategic marketing planning process that is moderately to highly mature. (Zallocco and Joseph, 1991, p. 9)

The uncertain state of marketing orientation within hospitals is evident even from an examination of the opinions of administrators and marketers within the same hospital on the subject. One study (Wrenn, LaTour, and Calder, 1994) revealed no significant agreement between CEOs/COOs and their marketing officers regarding the marketing activities in their hospital.

While the debate over the extent of their marketing orientation continues, what does appear clear is that health care organizations, like organizations in other industries, do benefit from such an orientation. This conclusion appears very robust since it has been supported by findings from research conducted with a cross-section of hospitals at different times by different researchers using different methodologies (see Table 8.2). We can then safely conclude that the use of marketing practices that reflect a true marketing orientation will help health care service organizations become more successful. Why, then, does controversy continue concerning the use of marketing in health care systems as we near the year 2000?

❧ THE PRESENT AND FUTURE ROLE OF MARKETING IN HEALTH CARE SYSTEMS

Some health care administrators still cling to the perception that marketing is primarily a set of demand stimulation tools that are useful only when the organization needs to appeal directly to consumers: "Some hospitals overreacted to managed cared in 1994, slashing marketing budgets in the belief that the opinions of individual consumers no longer matter . . ." (*Modern Healthcare*, 1995, p. 44). This perception

Table 8.2 Studies of the Effect of Marketing on Hospital Performance

	McKee, Varadarajan and Vassar (1986)	Naidu and Narayana (1991)	Naidu, Kleimenhagen, and Pillari (1992)	McDermott, Franzak, and Little (1993)	Gruca and Nath (1994)	Wrenn, LaTour, and Calder (1994)
Types of Hospitals:						
Not-for-Profit	X	X	X	N/A	X	X
For-Profit	X	X	X			X
Size of Hospitals						
Under 250 beds	X	X	X			X
Over 250 beds	X	X	X	X		X
Object of Measurement-Marketing	Marketing planning orientation	Marketing orientation	Marketing orientation	Marketing orientation	Traditional and innovative marketing activities	Marketing orientation
Object of Measurement-Performance	Occupancy rate	Occupancy rate	Occupancy rate	Operating margins	Return on assets, occupancy rate, market share	Occupancy rate, revenue, total patient days
Notable Findings	"...more comprehensive [marketing] planning is associated with higher hospital occupancy rate."	"...the evidence suggests that marketing orientation helps the health care facility in the long run."	"Empirical evidence tends to indicate that higher return on equity is associated with higher marketing orientation."	"...hospital executives who are 'data drivers' and who emphasize teamwork regarding their marketing decision making will achieve a higher financial performance than those who manage either by instinct or tradition."	"Traditional marketing factors significantly ($p < 0.05$) accounted for differences in return on assets."	"Roughly a 10 percent improvement in marketing orientation is associated with a $25 million increase in total patient revenue and an 8 percentage point improvement in occupancy rate."

of marketing as having dubious value unless it will directly stimulate market desire for a particular "brand" of health care has existed for some time. The following comments by the president of Jewish Hospital in Louisville reflect such a perception:

> . . . the [marketing] department's objective was to build the business and steal market share from competitors. It didn't. . . . We aren't sure that marketing works. In examining our 1987 business plans, I wasn't convinced that we were getting a return on our marketing spending. Rather, our success has come from building quality programs, diversifying, and using a product-line management approach, and working closely with our medical staff (*Hospitals,* 1987, p. 44). [comments made after dismantling the hospital's marketing department]

Many marketing theorists would argue that marketing, when fully exploited, can and should contribute to the building of quality programs, determine which diversification plans are best, design and operate product-line management approaches, and establish closer relationships with medical staff. Such anecdotal comments are emblematic of the belief that marketing and selling are synonymous terms and that marketing consists of a set of tools for arousing consumer interest in a particular health care organization—either to enhance the organization's image or to stimulate demand for its services. Authentic marketing consists of much more than promotion and selling. In commenting on how marketing is perceived in the most successful, market-focused organizations, Kotler noted:

> Marketing is seen as more than a department. Marketers get involved in management decision making long before any product is designed and they continue their work long after the product is sold. Marketers identify customer needs that represent profitable opportunities; they participate in the design of the product and service mix; they heavily influence the pricing of the offerings; they work hard to communicate and promote the company's products, services, and image; they monitor customer satisfaction; and they constantly improve the company's offerings and performance on the basis of market feedback (Kotler, 1994, p. *xxv*).

Table 8.3 illustrates the differences between the perception of marketing as selling versus authentic marketing in health care systems.

Although authentic marketing, as Kotler noted, encompasses numerous activities, two are central to the successful use of marketing in health care organizations as the 21st century approaches: (1) promoting the adoption of a true marketing orientation in the health care system and (2) identifying and exploiting a competitive advantage.

Table 8.3   Perception of Health Care Marketing as Selling versus Authentic Marketing

	Marketing as selling	Authentic marketing
Objective of Health Care Provider	Getting you well—marketing not involved in provision of services	Treating you well—marketing integrally involved in generating satisfied customers
When Marketing Is Used	Only when facing zero sum situation with competitors	Constantly—both internally and externally
Who Does Marketing	Marketing department	Everyone in system
Contribution of Marketing	Generating revenues	Mutually beneficial exchanges—to customer and organization
Major Requirements for Achievement of Marketing Objectives	Communication budget	Adoption of true marketing orientation by everyone in the system

Promotion of a Marketing Orientation

Several writers have commented that one of the most important contributions, if not *the* most important, that marketers can make to health care providers is to foster the adoption of a marketing orientation by the organization:

> Perhaps the most important contribution marketing can make [to hospitals] is to infuse a management philosophy, a marketing orientation throughout the operation (Cavusgil, 1986, p. 72).

> Teaching market orientation . . . throughout the [health care] organization may well be the core task of the marketer today (Parrington and Stone, 1991, p. 48).

> The health care marketing executive's primary challenge is not convincing the marketplace that it should be enamored with a particular health care organization, but convincing the health care organization that it should be enamored with the marketplace. The health care executive's first responsibility is not marketing the organization to the market, but institutionalizing the market concept throughout the health care organization (Rynne, 1995, p. 69).

What exactly does a marketing orientation consist of in a health care setting? Kotler and Clarke (1987, p. 32) specify five components of a health care marketing orientation:

    1. *Customer philosophy.* Does management acknowledge the primacy of the marketplace and of customer needs and wants in shaping the organization's plans and operations?

2. *Adequate marketing information.* Does management receive the kind and quality of information needed to conduct effective marketing?
3. *Strategic orientation.* Does management generate innovative strategies and plans for achieving its long-run objectives?
4. *Operational efficiency.* Are marketing activities selected and handled in a cost-effective manner?
5. *Integrated marketing organization.* Is the organization staffed to carry out marketing analysis, planning, implementation and control?

Wrenn, LaTour, and Calder (1994) identified five tasks for health care marketers that flow from these components of a marketing orientation:

1. Define and train people to understand what it means to adopt a customer philosophy.
2. Obtain, analyze and interpret information concerning what services the health care organization's markets are suggesting the organization should effectively operate.
3. Assist line officers in designing and implementing strategic plans that use such information and obtain competitive advantages for the health care organization.
4. Monitor performance and suggest corrective actions where needed.
5. Ensure that such market-driven thinking is integrated throughout the organization.

Implementation of the last task is of particular importance if the organization is to reap the rewards of a marketing orientation. This claim has empirical support (McDermott, Franzak, and Little, 1993), as well as intuitive appeal. Rynne (1995), for example, demonstrates the importance of organizationwide, market-driven thinking with the authentic story of a woman with cancer who established a close relationship with her oncologist. She depended on him, respected him, and felt appreciated by him, while he admired her spirit and tried to do his best by her. Their relationship was so strong that she continued to see him for treatment after he left one university hospital for another. One day, in severe pain, she called for an appointment, which he readily agreed to. Upon arrival at his office the receptionist told the woman that she didn't have an appointment, causing her acute embarrassment and anxiety. After requesting the receptionist to ask the doctor, she was informed that she did have an appointment. She waited an hour before being shown to the examining room, and then waited another hour. Finally, the doctor arrived and after a brief but fairly satisfying conversation wrote a prescription and explained it to her. As the woman left, she approached the desk and attempted to pay for all services with a single check as she had previously arranged by phone. She was told she couldn't, that lab and x-ray services required separate payment. After much explaining and discussion, she was finally allowed to write the check. The upshot of this experience was that the woman resolved never to return to the hospital. She changed oncologists, returning to the original hospital from which her doctor had moved. Rynne concluded the story this way:

> What is the product or service? The product is actually much more than the interpersonal encounter with the caregiver. It is the *whole experience*—from receptionist through waiting through nurse through physician through transport through billing. That total experience was so negative, so enervating, so different from the entire staff of the oncology service at the original hospital that it wore her down. Rather than endure it, she left her physician to find health care . . . . To break the complicated product health care into its component parts and put it back together again for customer satisfaction is precisely the health care marketing challenge . . . . The health care marketing executive's first obligation is to focus on his or her colleagues in line management, to help them define their roles in terms of marketing, and to give them all the help they need to successfully carry out *their* marketing challenges. Given the range of businesses under a health care organization's umbrella and the range of the departments, functions, and people involved, the health care marketing executive's more than full-time challenge is to—might and main—get all those functions and departments—working through existing structures and systems—to embrace the marketing concept (pp. 80–81).

Rynne went on to suggest four strategies marketers can use to instill a marketing orientation throughout the health care organization:

1. Demonstrate, codify, and then institutionalize market research as the fount of service design and delivery.
2. Imitate how finance has worked a cultural change in health care organizations—make marketing the subject of a management system.
3. Provide opportunities for operating units across the organization to learn marketing by doing it.
4. Fight and win a few key battles over operations issues in the name of the customer.

Identification of a Competitive Advantage

Boyd, Walker, and Larreche (1995) have made the point that it is common today for high-level executives to desire their organization to become more market-driven, and as we have stated here, that means that "in the sense of doing what is necessary to serve and satisfy customers, marketing is every employee's business." However, as they also note:

> . . . even when the day-to-day responsibility for marketing activities is delegated to all employees, someone still has to plan, coordinate, and control those activities for each of the firm's product-market entries. A marketing strategy must be formulated which brings value to the consumer and attains an enduring competitive advantage . . . Such activities are, typically, the responsibility of . . . marketing personnel . . . (Boyd, Walker, and Larreche, 1995, p. *v*).

The important responsibility of marketers to formulate a marketing strategy for the firm that identifies and exploits a competitive advantage in the organization's markets was asserted earlier by Day and Wensley (1983). Day (1990, p. 42), later expressed the importance of successfully finding a competitive advantage this way: "There is no alternative to persuasive evidence of competitive advantage, for this is what produces the profits and revenues." Ansoff (1965), a strategic management planning theorist, is usually credited with originating the idea of competitive advantage, although it is now accorded a central place in the works of many writers on marketing strategy as well; see, for example, Aaker (1995), Day (1990), Schnaars (1991), Sudharshan (1995).

To understand the concept of competitive advantage and why it plays such a central role in marketing strategy, one must understand how marketers view competition. The most successful marketers do not have a desire to "beat the competition"; their desire is to make competitors totally irrelevant to their customers. That is, marketers want to establish such a close, satisfying, long-term relationship with their customers that those customers have no interest in considering alternatives. Ideally, the strength of the relationship makes movement to a competitor so inconvenient, risky, and unnecessary that the customer exercises a "willful suspension of choice" and determines to continue to give the company his or her business. In a sense, what marketers are trying to do is to satisfy the customer so completely that the barriers to exit from the relationship are too high in the customer's minds to justify seeking an alternative means of addressing his or her needs. A marketer who is successful in establishing such a relationship with a customer has made competition irrelevant. Accomplishing this goal requires the identification and exploitation of a significant competitive advantage.

A competitive advantage is "something special that a firm does, or possesses, that gives it an edge against competitors" (Schnaars, 1991). Cohen (1995) states four characteristics that must be present for a competitive advantage to be exploitable:

1. The advantage(s) must be *real*. Just wishing it to be there does not make it so. Saying you have the lowest prices does not make it true.

2. They must be *important to the customer*. Competitive advantages exist only when they ultimately translate into a benefit that the customer seeks and values. Merely being different from competitors along some dimension that you, the company, thinks is important does not mean that you have a true competitive advantage. "When the perception of competitive advantage differs between the marketer and customer, the customer always wins."

3. They must be *specific*. "It is not enough to say, 'We're the best.' The question is, the best what? And why? To the customer nonspecificity translates into mere puffery and is not a competitive advantage."

4. They must be *promotable*. Meaning, you must be able to communicate the advantage to the customer in language which he or she not only understands but which is also highly motivating. The first three characteristics above must be present before this fourth characteristic has relevance, but unless this fourth point is implemented, the value of the first three goes wanting. Also implied in this point is that a marketing budget of sufficient size is in place so that the competitive advantage can be promoted with enough frequency and reach to attract the target market audience.

Applying Porter's (1985) model of competitive advantage to the health care field, Coddington and Moore (1987) identify ten broad strategies for exploiting a competitive advantage.

1. *Differentiation on the basis of quality.* Obviously, quality is of tremendous interest to all parties in today's health care market, so all health care systems would like to differentiate themselves from competitors on this basis. We are not talking here about quality as it might be defined by the Joint Commission on Accreditation of Hospitals but rather about how customers perceive it. Coddington and Moore devote a chapter in their book to discussing what different customer groups such as patients, benefit managers (employers), and health care professionals regard as quality in hospital services and physician services; they then explore the strategic implications of using such quality indicators to gain a competitive advantage. More recently, Bowers, Swan, and Koehler (1994) have identified five attributes of health care delivery that define patients' perception of

quality and satisfaction—empathy, reliability, responsiveness, communication, and caring—and specified the managerial implications for their findings.

2. *Aggressive pursuit of alternative delivery system contracts.*

3. *Diversification.*

4. *Vertical integration.*

5. *Networking.* In 1987 Coddington and Moore distinguished these last four as different strategies. Today, they might be thought of as different components of a single strategy by many health care providers to build an integrated health care delivery system in order to effectively pursue contracts with employee groups, spread their risk by diversification, maximize market coverage, gain control over several related links in the service delivery chain, and provide a continuum of care and financial control within an internal feeder network via vertical integration or strategic alliance. This chapter is not the place to discuss the organizational structures best suited to meet the challenges of an uncertain future in health care. Interested readers are instead referred to some of the more recent attempts to address which organizational structures and mechanisms are best suited to a highly competitive future health care market: cf. Zuckerman, Kaluzny, and Ricketts (1995); Wolford, Brown, and McCool (1993); Brown and McCool (1990); Cave (1995); E. Johnson (1995); R. Johnson (1995); and Weil (1995).

While many predict that integrated health care networks will dominate all markets (*Hospitals and Health Networks,* 1995), others (Coile, 1995; Goldsmith, 1994) suggest that the wisest course is to avoid asset-based integration in favor of "virtual integration," which emphasizes coordination through patient-management agreements, provider incentives, and information systems rather than investment in a large number of facilities. Whatever the future of the health care market, the objective of the formation of any integrational structure is to gain a competitive advantage. Depending on the degree to which the chosen structure fits the market environment's key success factors (Ohmae, 1982), such strategies for configuring the organization may or may not provide the benefits sought by the strategists.

6. *Aggressive marketing.*

7. *Centers of excellence.* These two strategies for competitive advantage may also be thought of as the single strategy of correctly identifying key target markets that offer an opportunity to achieve growth objectives and then successfully using the organization's marketing mix to attract customers in that segment. Hillestad and Berkowitz (1991) illustrate this idea by describing how Abbott Northwestern Hospital achieved a competitive advantage by targeting women; designing WomenCare, a center of excellence for women's

medicine; and aggressively marketing the program to its target market. Of course, the achievement of a competitive advantage through greater marketing skill could result from many activities related to the analysis of market information and the planning, implementation, and control of marketing programs. Books such as *Marketing in Transition: Practical Answers to Pressing Questions* (Rynne, 1995) can be used to develop programs specifically designed to achieve a competitive advantage through the use of marketing.

8. *Physician bonding.* Coddington and Moore suggest that hospitals may gain a competitive advantage by forming some type of formal association with physicians. As with each of these ten competitive advantage strategies, a separate chapter is devoted to a discussion of the types of alliances hospitals and physicians can form to achieve this goal. Cave (1995) describes seven different forms such an alliance can take and maintains that an equity model is the most sustainable and also most cost-effective in delivery of services over the long term.

9. *Being a low-cost provider.* Given the current scrutiny of health care costs, some might argue that being a low-cost provider is a strategy for *survival*, not for gaining a competitive advantage. Because all providers are being squeezed on cost, this cannot become a solitary basis for competitive advantage—and it is probably the most difficult of all the strategies to sustain. However, it can be an effective strategy when combined with one or more of the others, particularly number one (differentiation on the basis of quality), because raising quality is the preferred way to lower total cost. Those interested in learning more about the low-cost strategy for competitive advantage are referred to Porter (1980).

10. *Downsizing.* The objective in reducing the size of health care institutions is to get rid of excess capacity while simultaneously improving quality of operations. Many institutions seek to find the "right size," which provides the greatest economic advantages while enhancing the ability to serve its markets well: "The only purposes of downsizing are to render the [health care institution] more efficient and maximize its competitive community position" (Doherty, O'Donovan, and O'Donovan, 1986). Coddington and Moore cite several case studies that lead them to a number of conclusions about downsizing in the health care industry: Downsizing can be accomplished without the loss of scale economies; it can actually lead to an increase in profitability; if done hastily it can have a deleterious effect on the confidence of physicians and consumers; staff reductions without layoffs are possible; successful downsizing efforts include good communication with employees and physicians; and the medical staff and board of trustees should be involved in downsizing decisions.

In a later book Coddington, Keen, Moore, and Clarke (1990) describe in detail four possible future scenarios for the health care industry during the 1990s and then identify the best marketing strategies for physicians and hospitals seeking to gain a competitive advantage according to each of these respective scenarios. Such contingency planning for different future environments is becoming more commonplace (cf. *Hospitals and Health Networks,* 1995) and reflects the uncertainty surrounding long-term marketing planning in the health care industry.

An excellent example of how to develop different marketing programs for different purchase decision/paradigms is Terrence Rynne's (1995) book, which contains a detailed discussion of the challenges facing health care marketers according to several scenarios and of the differences between marketing conducted for an individual organization and marketing for an integrated health care delivery system. As long as the health care industry remains in such a turbulent condition and in transition to an unknown future state, obtaining a sustainable competitive advantage is problematic. Health care marketers may have to be content with obtaining a short-term advantage and preparing themselves with the skills needed to master future challenges.

The Future of Health Care Marketing

Health care marketers must master many skills to perform well in what promises to remain a turbulent environment. One set of suggestions for preparing for future marketing environments is listed below (Beckham, 1991):

1. Articulate a philosophy of marketing that has a role for everybody in the organization.
2. Spend as much time with the people who make the product as with the people who buy it.
3. Get your hands around the basic tenets of quality improvement and apply them in your work.
4. Get friendly with your computer and with the people who own your organization's transaction data.
5. Bring consumers, physicians, and employers right into the product development process.
6. Look outside your own organization to find some of what you need to create a sustainable competitive advantage.
7. Recognize that some of what you do has real ethical implications.
8. View your organization within the broader context of an industry that, despite its many shortcomings, is still the largest and most vital in the nation.
9. Create new markets; don't just take old markets.
10. Engender a flexibility and quickness that facilitates a fluid responsiveness to markets.
11. Get some help at the top.

Other health care marketing writers have attempted to identify those skills and qualifications that health care marketers will need to manage marketing programs successfully in the future (Winston, 1994a):

1. Education and experience in a wide range of professional services marketing.
2. Specific sophistication in such skills as negotiation, contracting, networking, targeting, sales management, relationship marketing, governance, strategic planning, outcome measurement, computer database analysis, customer service and cost-benefit analysis.
3. Readiness to update skills, knowledge, and awareness of spending issues.
4. Systems orientation, enabling participation in strategic planning, marketing planning, and policy and governance decisions.
5. Ability to relate well to a wide range of professionals, providers, insurers, health care delivery systems, and consumers.
6. Effectiveness in using external resources such as attorneys, consultants, legislators, contractors, and traditional media placement professionals.
7. Willingness to contribute to organizational reengineering and restructuring.
8. Proven and continuing cost-effectiveness and value to the organization.
9. Ability to demonstrate the true value of their products and services to a wide range of target groups.

Interested readers are referred to other lists of marketing skills, tasks, and strategies useful in the future (cf. Schaupp, Ponzurick and Schaupp, 1994; Winston, 1994b; Cooper, 1992; Klein, 1990; Boscarino and Steiber, 1994).

BIBLIOGRAPHY

The following books are recommended reading for health care marketers.

Terrence Rynne, *Health Care Marketing in Transition*, Burr Ridge, IL: R. D. Irwin, 1995.

Philip D. Cooper, ed., *Health Care Marketing*, 3rd ed., Gaithersburg, MD: Aspen Publishers, 1994.

Steven G. Hillestad and Eric Berkowitz, *Health Care Marketing Plans*, 2nd ed., Gaithersburg, MD: Aspen Publishers, 1991.

Paul J. Feldstein, *Health Policy Issues*, Ann Arbor, MI: AUPHA Press/Health Administration Press, 1994.

Steven R. Eastaugh, *Health Economics*, Westport, CT: Auburn House, 1992.

Curtis P. McLaughlin and Arnold D. Kaluzny, eds., *Continuous Quality Improvement in Health Care*, Gaithersburg, MD: Aspen Publishers, 1994.

Wendy Leebov and Gail Scott, *Service Quality Improvement: The Customer Satisfaction Strategy for Health Care*, Chicago: American Hospital Association, 1994.

Steven Stelber and William J. Krowinski, *Measuring and Managing Patient Satisfaction*, Chicago: American Hospital Association, 1990.

Joint Commission on Accreditation of Health Care Organizations, *The Measurement Mandate*, Oakbrook Terrace, IL: JCAHO, 1993.

Emily Friedman, ed. *Choices and Conflict: Explorations in Health Care Ethics*, Chicago: American Hospital Association, 1992.

Stephen Shortell and Arnold Kaluzny, *Health Care Management: Organization Design & Behavior*, 3rd ed., Albany, NY: Delmar Publishers, 1994.

&. REFERENCES

Aaker, David A. (1995), *Strategic Market Management*, 4th ed., New York: John Wiley & Sons.

Alderson, Wroe (1955), "A Marketing View of Business Policy," *Cost and Profit Outlook,* 8 (December), 1.

Ansoff, H. Igor (1965), *Corporate Strategy,* New York: McGraw–Hill.

Arnold, Aline (1991), "The 'Big Bang' Theory of Competition in Health Care," *Business Forum*, 15 (4), 6–9.

Arnold, Danny R., Louis M. Capella, and Delia A. Sumrall (1987a), "Hospital Challenge: Using Change Theory and Processes to Adopt and Implement the Marketing Concept," *Journal of Health Care Marketing*, 7 (June), 15–24.

Arnold, Danny R., Louis M. Capella, and Delia A. Sumrall (1987b), "Organization Culture and the Marketing Concept: Diagnostic Keys for Hospitals," *Journal of Health Care Marketing*, 7 (March), 18–28.

Autrey, Pam and Dennis Thomas (1986), "Competitive Strategy in the Hospital Industry," *Health Care Management Review*, 11 (Winter), 7–14.

Bartlett, Pamela J., Charles D. Schewe, and Chris T. Allen (1984), "Marketing Orientation: How Do Hospital Administrators Compare with Marketing Managers?" *Health Care Management Review*, 9 (Winter), 77–86.

Battistella, Roger M. (1985), "Hospital Receptivity to Market Competition: Image and Reality," *Health Care Management Review,* 10 (Summer), 19–26.

Beckham, J. Daniel (1991), "The New Marketing," *Healthcare Forum Journal,* 34(5), (September/October), 48–52.

Bennett, R. C. and R. G. Cooper (1979), "Beyond the Marketing Concept," *Business Horizons,* 22 (June), 76–83.

Boscarino, Joseph A., and Steven R. Steiber (1994), "The Future of 'Marketing' Health Care Services," in *Health Care Marketing,* Philip D. Cooper, ed., Gaithersburg, MD: Aspen Publishers.

Boscarino, J.A. and S.R. Steiber (1982), "Hospital Shopping and Consumer Choice," *Journal of Health Care Marketing,* 2, 15–23.

Bowers, Michael R., John E. Swan, and William F. Koehler (1994), "What Attributes Determine Quality and Satisfaction with Health Care Delivery?" *Health Care Management Review,* 19(4), 49–55.

Boyd, Harper W., Orville C. Walker, and Jean–Claude Larreche (1995), *Marketing Management,* Chicago: Richard D. Irwin.

Brown, Montague and Barbara P. McCool (1990), "Health Care Systems: Predictions for the Future," *Health Care Management Review,* 15(3), 87–94.

Calder, Bobby J. (1983), "Competition Getting Even Hotter," *Modern Healthcare,* 13 (April), 80–91.

Cave, Douglas (1995), "Vertical Integration Models to Prepare Health Systems for Capitation," *Health Care Management Review,* 20(1), 26–39.

Cavusgil, S. James (1986), "Marketing's Promise for Hospitals," *Business Horizons,* 29 (September–October), 71–76.

Christianson, Jon B. and Walter McClure (1979), "Competition in the Delivery of Medical Care," *The New England Journal of Medicine,* 301, 812–818.

Clarke, Roberta N. (1978), "Marketing Health Care: Problems in Implementation," *Health Care Management Review,* 3 (Winter), 21–27.

Clarke, Roberta N. and Linda Shyavitz (1987), "Health Care Marketing: Lots of Talk, Any Action?" *Health Care Management Review,* 12 (1), 31–36.

Coddington, Dean C. and Keith D. Moore (1987), *Market-Driven Strategies in Health Care,* San Francisco: Jossey–Bass.

Coddington, Dean C., David J. Keen, Keith D. Moore, and Richard L. Clarke (1990), *The Crisis in Health Care*, San Francisco: Jossey–Bass.

Cohen, William A. (1995), *The Marketing Plan*, New York: John Wiley & Sons.

Colie, Russell C. (1995), "Assessing Healthcare Market Trends and Capital Needs: 1996–2000" *Healthcare Financial Management*," (August), 60–65.

Converse, P. D. and H. W. Huegy (1946), *The Elements of Marketing*, New York: Prentice Hall.

Cooper, Philip (1992), "Positive Perspectives, Concerned Perspectives, and Action Suggestions for Long-term Health Care Marketing Success," *Journal of Health Care Marketing*, 12(1), 2–3.

Cooper, Philip D. (1985), "What Is Health Care Marketing?," in *Health Care Marketing: Issues and Trends*, Philip D. Cooper, ed., Rockville, MD: Aspen.

Cooper, Philip D., Karen M. Jones, and John K. Wong (1984), *An Annotated and Extended Bibliography of Health Care Marketing*, Chicago: American Marketing Association.

Cooper, Philip D., and William J. Kehoe (1978), "Health Care Marketing: An Idea Whose Time Has Come," in *Proceedings of the 1978 Educator's Conference*, Subhash C. Jain, ed., Chicago: American Marketing Association, 369–372.

Cooper, Robert B. (1983), "Market Strategies for Hospitals in a Competitive Environment," *Hospital and Health Services Administration*, 28 (May–June), 9–15.

Cravens, David W. (1987), *Strategic Marketing*, Homewood, IL: Irwin.

Cravens, David W., Gerald E. Hills, and Robert B. Woodruff (1987), *Marketing Management*, Homewood, IL: Irwin.

Dalrymple, Douglas J. and Leonard J. Parsons (1990), *Marketing Management*, New York: John Wiley & Sons.

Day, George S. and Robin Wensley (1983), "Marketing Theory With a Strategic Orientation," *Journal of Marketing*, 47 (Fall), 79–89.

Day, George S. (1990), *Market Driven Strategy*, New York: The Free Press.

Decker, Betty L. (1985), "A Description and Analysis in Terms of Kotler's Marketing Orientation of Selected University Marketing Agencies Which Sell Faculty-Developed Non-Profit Materials," Ph.D. dissertation, Michigan State University.

Doherty, V., T. O'Donovan, and P. O'Donovan (1986), "Downsizing Hospital Capacity," *Health Care Strategic Management*, 4(4), 4–7.

Drucker, Peter F. (1954), *The Practice of Management*, New York: Harper & Row.

Eastaugh, Steven R. (1992), *Health Economics*, Westport, CT: Auburn House.

Feldstein, Paul J. (1986), "The Changing Health Care Delivery System," *Trustee*, 39 (February), 15–21.

Feldstein, Paul J. (1994), *Health Policy Issues*, Ann Arbor, MI: AUPHA Press/Health Administration Press.

Felton, Arthur P. (1959), "Making the Marketing Concept Work," *Harvard Business Review*, 37 (July/August), 55–65.

Friedman, Emily (1980), "Does Market Competition Belong in Health Care?" *Hospitals*, 54 (July 1), 47–50.

Ginzberg, E. (1986), "The Destabilization of Health Care," *New England Journal of Medicine*, 315, 757–761.

Goldsmith, Jeff C. (1994), "The Illusive Logic of Integration," *Healthcare Forum Journal*, 37(5), 26–31.

Gruca, Thomas S. and Deepika Nath (1994), "The Impact of Marketing on Hospital Performance," *Journal of Hospital Marketing*, 8(2), 87–112.

Hague, James E. (1979), "Marketplace Language Harms Health Care," *Hospital Progress*, 60 (October), 6ff.

Haines, Arthur C. (1983), "Impressions of Marketplace Competition in the Twin Cities," *Hospital and Health Services Administration*, 28 (May–June), 27–42.

Hayes, Robert A. and William J. Abernathy (1980), "Managing Our Way to Economic Decline," *Harvard Business Review*, 58 (July–August), 67–77.

Hillestad, Steven G. and Eric N. Berkowitz (1991), *Health Care Marketing Plans*, 2nd ed., Gaithersburg, MD: Aspen Publishers.

Hospitals (1986), "Hospitals Call a Marketing Time-Out," 60 (June 5), 50–55.

Hospitals (1987), "Will Marketing Ever Grow Up?" 61 (June 5), 42–47.

Hospitals and Health Networks (1995), "Choose Your Tomorrow," (August 20), 38–40.

Houston, Franklin S. (1986), "The Marketing Concept: What It Is and What It Is Not," *Journal of Marketing*, 50 (April), 81–87.

Hudak, Ronald P., Paul P. Brooke, Kenn Finstuen, and Pat Riley (1993) "Health Care Administration in the Year 2000: Practitioners' Views of Future Issues and Job Requirements," *Hospital and Health Services Administration*, 38(2), 181–195.

Jaworski, Bernard J. and Ajay K. Kohli (1993), "Market Orientation: Antecedents and Consequences," *Journal of Marketing*, 57 (July), 53–70.

Johnson, Everett (1995), "The Public's Future Perspective on Managed Care," *Health Care Management Review*, 20(2), 45–47.

Johnson, Everett A. and Richard L. Johnson (1986), *Hospitals Under Fire*, Rockville, MD: Aspen Publishers.

Johnson, Richard L. (1995), "'Hospital Governance in a Competitive Environment," *Health Care Management Review*, 20(1), 75–83.

Joyce, Mary L., and J. Joseph Cronin (1985), "An Application of Institutional Change Theories in the Health Care Industry: Implications for Planning," *Journal of Health Care Marketing*, 5 (Spring), 9–18.

Kaldor, A. G. (1971), "Imbricative Marketing," *Journal of Marketing*, 35 (April), 19–25.

Kaplan, Michael D. (1979), "What It Is, What It Isn't," *Hospitals*, 53 (September 16), 176ff.

Keith, R. J. (1960), "The Marketing Revolution," *Journal of Marketing*, 24 (January), 35–38.

Kiel, Geoffrey (1984), "Technology and Marketing: The Magic Mix?" *Business Horizons*, 22 (May–June), 7–14.

Klein, Richard C. (1990), "Will the Real Health Care Marketer Please Stand Up?" *Journal of Health Care Marketing*, 10(2), 2–4.

Kohli, Ajay D. and Bernard T. Jaworski (1990), "Market Orientation: The Construct, Research Propositions, and Managerial Implications," *Journal of Marketing*, 54 (April), 1–8.

Kotler, Philip (1994), *Marketing Management*, Englewood Cliffs, N.J.: Prentice Hall.

Kotler, Philip and Roberta N. Clarke (1987), *Marketing for Health Care Organizations*, Englewood Cliffs, N.J.: Prentice Hall.

Lachner, Bernard J. (1977), "Marketing—An Emerging Management Challenge," *Health Care Management Review*, 2 (Fall), 25–30.

Lamb, Charles W. and David W. Finn (1982), "Has Marketing Been Oversold to Hospital Administrators?" *Journal of Health Care Marketing*, 2 (Fall), 43–46.

Lovelock, Christopher H. (1977), "Concepts and Strategies for Health Marketers," *Hospitals and Health Services Administration*, 22 (Fall), 50–62.

MacStravic, Scott (1990), "The End of Health Care Marketing?" *Health Marketing Quarterly,* 7(1/2), 28–37.

Malhotra, Naresh K. (1987), "A Marketing Orientation to Modeling the Hospital-Supplier Interface: a Probabilistic Approach," *Journal of Health Care Marketing,* 7 (June), 6–14.

Malhotra, Naresh K. (1986), "Hospital Marketing in the Changing Health Care Environment," *Journal of Health Care Marketing,* 6 (September), 37–48.

Marketing News (1994), "Health Care Marketers Plot Strategy in Face of Reform," 28 (1), (January 3), 1ff.

McCarthy, Jerome E. and William D. Perreault Jr. (1990), *Basic Marketing—A Managerial Approach,* 10th ed., Homewood, IL: Irwin.

McCullough, James, Lim Ser Heng, and Gan See Khem (1986), "Measuring the Marketing Orientation of Retail Operations of International Banks," *International Journal of Bank Marketing,* 4(3), 9–18.

McDermott, Dennis R., Frank J. Franzak, and Michael W. Little (1993), "Does Marketing Relate to Hospital Profitability?" *Journal of Health Care Marketing,* 13(2), 18–25.

McDevitt, Paul (1987), "Learning by Doing: Strategic Marketing Management in Hospitals," *Health Care Management Review,* 12(1), 23–30.

McDevitt, Paul K. and Lisa A. Shields (1985), "Tactical Hospital Marketing: A Survey of the State of the Art," *Journal of Health Care Marketing,* 5 (1985), 9 –16.

McGee, Lynn W. and Rosann L. Spiro (1988), "The Marketing Concept in Perspective," *Business Horizons,* 31, (May–June), 40–45.

McKee, Daryl P., "Rajan" Varadarajan, and John Vassar (1986), "The Marketing Planning Orientation of Hospitals: An Empirical Inquiry," *Journal of Health Care Marketing,* 6 (1986), 50–60.

McKittrick, J. B. (1957), "What Is the Marketing Management Concept," in *The Frontiers of Marketing Thought and Science,* Frank M. Bass, ed., Chicago: American Marketing Association, 71–81.

Modern Healthcare (1995), "Marketing Will Resurface, But With Fresh Approach," (January 2), 44.

Modern Healthcare (1987), "Marketing, Take Two," 17 (April 10), 46–55.

Modern Healthcare (1983), "Lack of Expertise, Funding Shackles Marketing Moves," (April), 75–78.

Naidu, G. M., Arno Kleimenhagen, and George D. Pillari (1992), "Organization of Marketing in U.S. Hospitals: An Empirical Investigation," *Health Care Management Review,* 17 (4), 29–43.

Naidu, G. M. and Chem L. Narayana (1991), "How Marketing Oriented Are Hospitals in a Declining Market?" *Journal of Health Care Marketing,* 11 (March), 23–30.

Narver, John C. and Stanley F. Slater (1990), "The Effect of a Market Orientation on Business Profitability," *Journal of Marketing,* 54 (October), 20–35.

O'Connor, C.P. (1982), "Why Marketing Isn't Working in the Health Care Arena," *Journal of Health Care Marketing,* 2 (Winter), 31–36.

Ohmae, Kenichi (1982), *The Mind of the Strategist,* New York: McGraw-Hill.

Parasuraman, A. (1981), "Hang On to the Marketing Concept!" *Business Horizons,* 24 (September–October), 38–40.

Parrington, Mark and Betsy C. Stone (1991), "The Marketing Decade: A Desktop View," *Journal of Health Care Marketing,* 11(1), 45–50.

Porter, Michael (1985), *Competitive Advantage: Creating and Sustaining Superior Performance,* New York: The Free Press.

Porter, Michael (1980), *Competitive Strategy,* New York: The Free Press.

Qureshi, Salim (1993), "Market Driven Public Institutions Attract Resources," *Journal of Professional Services Marketing,* 9(2), 83–92.

Riesz, Peter C. (1980), "Revenge of the Marketing Concept," *Business Horizons,* 23 (June), 49–53.

Robbins, Stephen A., Christopher M. Kane, and Daniel J. Sullivan (1988), "The Amherst Study of Hospital Marketing Practices," *Journal of Health Care Marketing,* 8 (March), 86–87.

Robinson, Larry M. and Philip D. Cooper (1980), *Health Care Marketing: An Annotated Bibliography,* Atlanta: U.S. Department of H.E.W., Public Health Service, Centers for Disease Control, Bureau of Health Education.

Robinson, Larry M. and Philip D. Cooper (1980–81), "Roadblocks to Hospital Marketing," *Journal of Health Care Marketing,* 1 (Winter), 18–24.

Robinson, Larry M. and F. Brown Whitington (1979), "Marketing as Viewed by Hospital Administrators," in *Health Care Marketing: Issues and Trends,* Rockville, MD: Aspen, 39–54.

Rynne, Terrence J. (1995), *Healthcare Marketing in Transition*, Burr Ridge, IL: R. D. Irwin.

Sachs, William S., and G. Benson (1978), "Is It Not Time to Discard the Marketing Concept?" *Business Horizons*, 21 (August), 68–74.

Salkever, David S. (1980), "Competition Among Hospitals," *Hospitals and Health Services Administration*, 25 (Spring), 56–70.

Samli, A. Coskun, Kristian Palda, and A. Tansu Barker (1987), "Toward a Mature Marketing Concept," *Sloan Management Review*, 29 (Winter), 45–51.

Schaupp, Dietrich L., Thomas G. Ponzurick, Frederick W. Schaupp (1994), "Survival Tactics for Managing the Hospital Marketing Effort," *Journal of Hospital Marketing*, 8(2), 113–119.

Schnaars, Steven P. (1991), *Marketing Strategy*, New York: The Free Press.

Schulz, Rockwell and Alton C. Johnson (1983), *Management of Hospitals,* 2nd ed., New York: McGraw–Hill.

Slater, Stanley F. and John C. Narver (1994), "Does Competitive Environment Moderate The Market Orientation–Performance Relationship?" *Journal of Marketing,* 58 (January), 46–55.

Siguaw, Judy A., Gene Brown, and Robert E. Widing (1994), "The Influence of the Market Orientation of the Firm on Sales Force Behavior and Attitudes," *Journal of Marketing Research*, 31 (February), 106–116.

Stensrud, Robert and Barbara Arrington (1988), "Marketing–Oriented Organizations: An Integrated Approach," *Health Progress*, 69 (March), 86–95.

Sudharshav, D. (1995), *Marketing Strategy*, Englewood Cliffs, NJ: Prentice Hall.

Tucker, Stephen L. (1977), "Introducing Marketing as a Planning and Management Tool," *Hospital and Health Services Administration*, 22 (Winter), 37–44.

Vraciu, Robert A. (1985), "Hospital Strategies for the Eighties: a Mid-Decade Look," *Health Care Management Review*, 10 (Fall), 9–19.

Weeks, Richard R. and William J. Marks (1968), "The Marketing Concept: Problems and Promises," *Business and Society*, 9 (Autumn), 39–42.

Weil, Thomas (1995), "Close to a Bull's Eye—A Concurring Opinion," *Health Care Management Review,"* 20(2), 35–44.

Wexler, Nat N. (1977), "What Is Marketing?," *Hospitals*, 51 (June 1), 52–53.

Winston, William (1994a), "Health Care Marketing's Role in the Future," *Health Marketing Quarterly*, 12(1), 5–8.

Winston, William (1994b), "Why Most Hospital Marketing Programs Still Fail," *Journal of Hospital Marketing*, 8(2), 5–14.

Wolford, G. Rodney, Montague Brown, and Barbara P. McCool (1993), "Getting to Go in Managed Care," *Health Care Management Review*, 18(1), 7–19.

Wolinsky, F. D. and S. R. Steiber (1982), "Salient Issues in Choosing a New Doctor," *Social Science and Medicine*, 16A, 1–9.

Wrenn, Bruce, Stephen A. LaTour, and Bobby J. Calder (1994), "Differences in Perceptions of Hospital Marketing Orientation Between Administrators and Marketing Officers," *Hospital and Health Services Administration*, 39(3), 341–358.

Wrenn, Bruce (1995), "Marketing Orientation: Past, Present, and Future," in *Developments in Marketing Science*, Roger Gomes, ed., Vol. 18, Coral Gables, FL: Academy of Marketing Science, 56–62.

Zallocco, Ronald L., and W. Benoy Joseph (1991), "Strategic Market Planning in Hospitals: Is It Done? Does It Work?" *Journal of Health Care Marketing*, 11(1), 5–11.

Zuckerman, Howard, Arnold Kaluzny, and Thomas C. Ricketts (1995), "Alliances in Health Care: What We Know, What We Think We Know, and What We Should Know," *Health Care Management Review*, 20(1), 54–64.

Quality Management and Improvement 9

Barbara Arrington, Saint Louis University
Richard S. Kurz, Saint Louis University

As the US health care system restructures under the pressures of managed care market reform and government demands, health care organizations need to provide increasingly high-quality, cost-effective care. There is much in the "cutting edge" organizational performance literature recommending implementation of "total quality management" and/or "continuous quality improvement" in response to this need for quality and cost improvements. Common to these phrases—"total quality management" and "continuous quality improvement"—is the word *quality*. What is quality in health care? How do health care organizations manage and continually improve the quality of the health care they provide? How successful have they been to date in managing and improving quality? This chapter explores these questions.

✑ WHAT IS QUALITY?

Our understanding of what constitutes quality in health care has evolved over this century from a very narrow conception to one that is increasingly broad. "Stated in the most general terms, quality consists in the ability to achieve desirable objectives using legitimate means" (Donabedian, 1988, p. 173).

The Structure-Process-Outcome Paradigm

In 1966 Donabedian explicated an integrated paradigm of health care quality that identified and delineated three categories of interdependent quality determinants: structure, process, and outcome. Structure comprises such elements as strategy, facilities and equipment, money, staff, and other resources, which create the system through which services are provided. Process consists of those characteristics of service delivery, such as appropriateness and safety, that create value (or not) for the recipient of service and are constructed by linked, sometimes sequential steps designed to effect an outcome or set of outcomes (James, 1995). Outcomes are the result of actions taken in the process. None of these independently explains quality. Quality must be understood in terms of the interdependence of structure, process, and outcomes, that is, in terms of the structures and processes that promote the actions leading to better (or worse) outcomes for patients. This structure-process-outcome paradigm has organized and informed Donabedian's subsequent work on the quality of health care (1988, 1993) as well as the work of many others over the last 30 years. Most recently, the definition of quality in health care has been broadened to include meeting internal and external customer needs and expectations. This change has come about through application of the work of Crosby (1984), Deming (1993, 1986), Juran (1989), and others on the principles, practices, and methods of industrial and manufacturing quality to health care organizations.

Quality Management and Improvement Theory

The terms "total quality management" and "continuous quality improvement" are both used to describe the managerial philosophy, knowledge, and skills needed to support the management and improvement of organizational quality. Sometimes these terms are used synonymously; at other times writers or speakers take great pains to differentiate the two. We leave it to our readers to choose their preferred term. For the purposes of this chapter, we will refer simply to managing and improving quality.

An emphasis on quality management and improvement is a logical advancement in management science and practice related to understanding and improving organizational performance (Kurz, 1995). At the beginning of this century, early management theory focused on rational, closed systems models, as represented by the work of Frederick Taylor on scientific management and Max Weber on bureaucracy. Somewhat later theory investigation extended to consider closed, natural systems as in the studies of the human relations school. In the 1950s and 1960s attention turned to rational, open systems models through the work of Herbert Simon on administrative behavior and Paul Lawrence and Jay Lorsch on contingency theory. This expansion of theory continued in the 1970s with a shift to natural, open systems models that emphasized organizational survival over efficient performance as the primary goal of organizational performance. Jeffrey Pfeffer and Gerald Salancik produced excellent scholarship on resource dependence that profoundly affected management thought in regard to the strategic and operational performance of organizations.

Current thinking on quality management and improvement represents a synthesis of the natural systems view. It expands our understanding of organizational operational performance by exploring how organizations do what they do and how they can improve their outcomes. Quality management and improvement thinking focuses on the centrality of processes in enabling employees to perform well by empowering and supporting their endeavors. It recognizes that performance "is not an individual matter, it is an organizational, group, and team effort." (Brodeur, 1995, p. 116) Moreover, quality management and improvement thinking links these questions of operational performance to the more basic strategic performance consideration of why organizations do what they do, completing a circle of ideas that begins with strategic action and continues through process and outcomes improvement based on meeting consumer and community expectations and needs.

Quality Defined

What, then, is quality? Quality is the extent to which patient, organizational, and community health outcomes (Kaluzny et al., 1995) resulting from the interaction of relevant structures and processes meet or exceed the needs and expectations of internal and external customers (see Figure 9.1). At the least, internal and external customers comprise patients and their families, the community, payers, physicians, employers, employees, and regulatory/government agencies.

> By recognizing that health is the true product of the health care enterprise, we understand in a way not otherwise possible the pivotal role of quality. . . . A knowledge of quality is indispensable to rational management. Without it we cannot judge productivity or efficiency or arrive at a reasoned allocation of resources. Without it, recruitment, remuneration, and advancement could become arbitrary, prices idiosyncratic, and competition blind. . . . We also need to understand that the concept of quality itself is in large measure a social construct. It represents our conceptions and valuations of health, our expectations of the client-provider relationship, and our views of the legitimate roles of the

Figure 9.1   Quality Defined

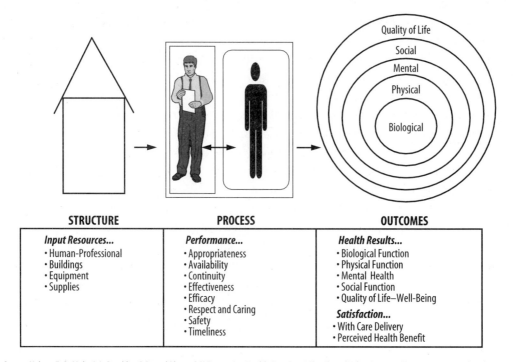

STRUCTURE	PROCESS	OUTCOMES
Input Resources... • Human-Professional • Buildings • Equipment • Supplies	***Performance...*** • Appropriateness • Availability • Continuity • Effectiveness • Efficacy • Respect and Caring • Safety • Timeliness	***Health Results...*** • Biological Function • Physical Function • Mental Health • Social Function • Quality of Life–Well-Being ***Satisfaction...*** • With Care Delivery • Perceived Health Benefit

Source: Nelson, E. C., Mohr, J. J., Batalden, P. B., and Plume, S. K. "Improving Health Care: Part I. The Clinical Value Compass." Presentation, Woodstock, VT. 13 July 1995.

health care enterprise. . . . Within the bound set by our values, traditions, and institutions there is much we can do to advance the quality of care. It is important to understand, however, that quality is something more than an attribute we can choose—or not choose—to work into health care to a greater or lesser degree. It is rather, the moral force that must animate all who devote their lives to health care (Donabedian, 1988, p. 190).

Several management principles underlie this understanding of quality management and improvement:

- Failures in performance result from problems in underlying systems and processes, not in people.
- Quality is best improved when statistically based, problem-solving approaches are employed to diagnose problems and observe progress.

- Organizationwide, cross-departmental and cross-functional teams are a fundamental tool of quality management and improvement.
- The use of structured group processes to improve organizational systems and processes prospectively rather than correcting them after the fact leads to better quality over time.
- Quality is best improved when employees are empowered to identify problems and improvement opportunities, act to resolve problems, and take opportunities.
- Internal and external customers are key drivers of performance expectations and performance evaluation (Shortell et al., 1995a; Deming, 1986).

❧ MANAGEMENT AND CONTINUAL IMPROVEMENT OF QUALITY

History

Clearly, quality is of central concern to health care organizations and must therefore be a primary managerial focus. How do health care organizations manage and continually improve the quality of the health care they provide? The answer to this question has changed radically over the last 50 years.

Traditionally, health care quality was considered the direct responsibility of the provider, most often a physician, and was managed and improved through the application of professional values and scientifically based professional subject and discipline knowledge (Batalden, 1995, 1993; Berwick, 1995, 1989; Flood, 1994).

> Early quality assurance efforts were aimed at ensuring that medical students mastered the basic materials and that established physicians demonstrated their credentials through licensing and certification processes. . . . [T]he work of the physician was so complex and uncertain that it required extraordinary skill and training, and autonomy from other professionals as well as from organizations, to carry it out. . . . [A] process of training and professionalization was needed to instill in the physician the appropriate values, skills, and knowledge to accomplish these tasks rather than relying on organizational oversight to ensure them. Each physician had to act like a mini-organization, to perform and control the quality of his or her work. In this context, most assumed that the organizational contributions [to quality] were limited to providing good "workshop" conditions in terms of safety and sanitation, support staff, and facilities (Flood, 1994).

As physicians' scientific ability to prevent, diagnose, and treat illness and disease has grown dramatically over this century, so too has their capacity to support quality management and improvement (Berwick, 1995, Lengnick-Hall, 1995).

The adequacy of the individual provider's knowledge, skills and credentials continues to be a central component of quality management and improvement. Today, however, more and more of our focus is on understanding how organizations contribute to quality in health care. In the latter half of this century, we have developed an increasingly sophisticated understanding of the way in which organizational structures and processes influence provider behavior, both in terms of the processes they employ and the outcomes their patients experience.

Extension of responsibility for quality beyond the immediate purview of the direct care provider began with the involvement of organized physician entities (e.g., hospital medical staffs, in both their credentialing and quality assurance roles), professional organizations (e.g., the American Medical Association), organizational accrediting bodies (e.g., the Joint Commission on the Accreditation of Healthcare Organizations), and government agencies (e.g., professional review organizations). The primary role of these organizations has been to oversee and regulate quality by reviewing health care delivery and, based on their reviews, to reward good performance, call attention to poor quality behavior, and sanction poor performance. Currently, activities of organizations like the Joint Commission (O'Leary, 1993) and the application of performance criteria such as those of the Malcolm Baldrige National Quality Award (US Chamber of Commerce, 1993) are modifying and expanding to link structure, process, and outcome in the evaluation of quality.

As we approach the new century, those thinking and writing about these issues in general and health care in particular identify four areas of management development essential to the continued growth of quality management and improvement. (Arrington et al., 1995; Batalden, 1995; Deming, 1993; Hamel and Prahalad, 1993):

- Management must develop knowledge specifically supportive of improvement efforts.
- Management must use strategic leadership to leverage organizational quality improvement efforts by cultivating a shared sense of purpose and focus, encouraging improved performance, and promoting organizational learning.
- Management must master methods and tools that accelerate improved performance.
- Management must demonstrate an ever-increasing ability to develop new knowledge and apply it to improving the processes of daily work.

Most of the remainder of this chapter is devoted to exploring these four imperatives and proposing appropriate management efforts.

Knowledge for Improvement

It is increasingly understood that the continuing improvements in quality that health care needs—in terms of both efficiency and effectiveness—are provider and organizational improvements for which professional values and expert knowledge are necessary but not sufficient. Deming (1986) identified a second body of necessary, scientifically based knowledge, which he labeled "profound knowledge" or "knowledge for improvement" (Berwick, 1995). Professional knowledge includes the basic biomedical and clinical subjects and disciplines and the profession's shared moral and social values. Knowledge for improvement is complementary to, but very different from, professional knowledge—and much less familiar. Knowledge for improvement derives from modern managerial ability to understand and improve human systems. Knowledge for improvement combines an understanding of systems, variation, psychology (especially, the psychology of work and of change), and theory of knowledge (Batalden, 1995; Berwick, 1995). Combining professional knowledge with knowledge of improvement helps us to manage and continually improve the quality of health care, both in terms of the nature of the improvements that are made and the speed with which they can be implemented. (Young et al., 1995). The following paragraphs briefly describe the components of knowledge for improvement—the improvement sciences.

Understanding Systems. The first improvement science is the science of understanding systems. Deming (1993), Juran (1989), Senge (1990) and Ferguson et al. (1993) maintain that the essential work of an organization must be understood in relation to its "systemness." In order to improve, we must first understand the structure of the system that supports performance and outcomes as a "whole," that is, as a system—a group of interdependent parts (people, processes, products, services) sharing a common purpose. To understand a system we must first know its aim or purpose. We must then master not only its interdependent parts but also, and most important, the dynamics of their interdependence. A system is a set of interconnected elements that meets the following conditions:

- The behavior of each element has an effect on the behavior of the whole.
- The behavior of the elements and their effects on the whole are interdependent.
- However subgroups of the elements are formed, each has an effect on the behavior of the whole and none has an independent effect (Ackoff, as quoted in Ferguson et al., 1993, p. 1).

Batalden (1995) and others working with him have identified the generic elements of a health care system capable of continual improvement (see Figure 9.2). Such a system can clearly articulate shared answers among its members to the following questions:

- *Why* do we make what we make in our organization?
- *How* do we make what we make?
- How do we *improve* what we make?

Understanding organizational performance from a systematic point of view requires synthesis, that is, understanding the parts of a system in terms of their dynamic interactions (the arrows between the parts) and what is produced through their interactions. In Figure 9.3, Batalden expands on the simpler conception of Figure 9.2 by indicating the foci of attention, the needed information, and the strategic and operational activity that supports a response to each of these three system-related questions.

- *Why do we make what we make in our organization?* The primary concerns in this regard are the demands of the environments in which the organization must act, the underlying social and health care needs the organizational system is

Figure 9.2   A Simple View of a System

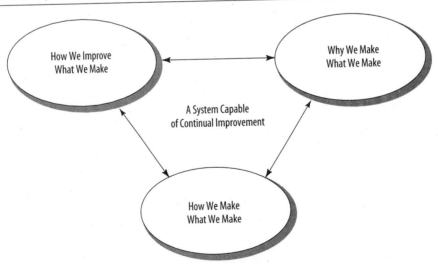

Source: Batalden, P. "Organizing the Production of Health Care as a System." Presentation, Woodstock, VT. 11 July 1995.

Figure 9.3   Understanding a System Capable of Continual Improvement

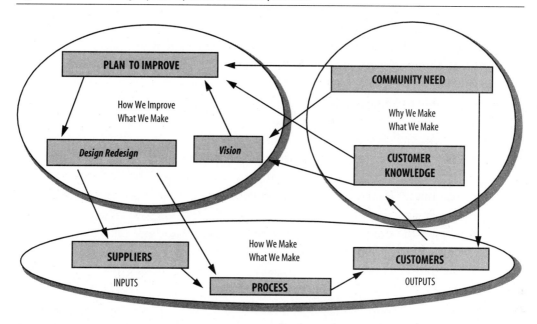

Source: Batalden, P. "Organizing the Production of Health Care as a System." Presentation, Woodstock, VT. 11 July 1995.

constructed to meet, and the preferences of the customers it serves. We must develop *customer knowledge* which allows us to determine *community need*.

- *How* do we make what we make? The methods and approaches used to meet social and health care needs are of concern in relation to this question, that is, the structures and processes that create the organization's services and products and, therefore, its outcomes. Our primary subquestions relate to identifying our *suppliers (inputs),* our *core processes,* and our *customer-driven outputs.*

- How do we *improve* what we make? The foci of this question are the nature and character of organizational performance that the system wants to achieve. What *vision* of the future do we want to create for our organization and the people it serves? What is our *plan to improve*? What are the *design and redesign requirements* of our plan?

Understanding Variation.   Variation is inherently present in people, processes, and products (Deming, 1986). Understanding variation—or lack of variation (stability)—over time is essential to recognizing, interpreting, and using observed differences for the purpose of improvement (Berwick, 1995). Differences in health care outcomes after the use of comparable procedures, therapies, or hospitalizations result from one of two closely related processes: deciding what care to provide and then providing it (Mulley, 1995). Quality management and improvement requires us to describe and understand the nature and sources of variation in organizational outcomes and their related structures and processes. Methods of statistical process control are the primary tools we use to describe and understand variation (Batalden et al., 1984). If we understand variation, we can then do the following:

- Understand and apply basic improvement concepts such as "special cause," "common cause," and "tampering."
- Accurately select and measure important structure, process, and outcome variables in actual work settings.
- Display those measures in the most informative format, especially to reduce tampering and support process improvement cycles.
- Integrate improvement into the daily life of our organization.

Understanding Psychology.   The third improvement science is psychology, specifically as it relates to understanding what affects human behavior and conceiving mechanisms for removing barriers to joy and pride in work. Four areas of psychology are particularly important in this regard: understanding group process, understanding conflict (its sources and its resolution), understanding motivation, and understanding creativity (Batalden, 1995; Berwick, 1995; Haddock et al., 1995).

Group process: Work in systems is accomplished through a series of frequently complex exchanges and interactions between and among people. To understand the interactions among the elements in human systems, we must recognize how groups function effectively. Any organization intent on developing competence in quality management and improvement focuses on increasing its ability to work and be effective in and through teams (Shortell et al., 1995b).

Conflict: Groups function most effectively when they are able to cooperate, that is, when friction and its costs are minimized. For systems to function, processes must support the management of differences and minimize negative friction by understanding the nature of cooperation and the causes of conflicts in our structures and processes. Organizational policies and procedures, work and job design, and other human resource issues must be addressed with this in mind if quality competence is to develop and improve (Shortell et al., 1995a).

Motivation: To bring about improvements in human behavior and, therefore, the behavior of human systems, we must understand why people act as they do and then plan improvements that support positive motivation (Deming, 1993, 1986).

Creativity: To manage and improve quality, we must encourage new and better ideas. To create the sources for these ideas, we must have organizations whose strategy, culture, structure, and processes promote reflection and creativity (Shortell et al., 1995b).

Understanding Knowledge Development. In this fourth improvement science, we are concerned with how best to promote and sustain individual and group inquiry and learning in a changing, dynamic workplace. Berwick (1995) and Nevis et al. (1993) suggest the following:

- Learning must be cyclical, that is, we must realize that things are changing rapidly and that we must continually ask important questions again because the answer may change.
- Learning must be iterative, that is, we must build our knowledge with each new lesson and never assume a fixed solution.
- Learning and action must be joined, that is, gaining knowledge cannot be separated from applying that knowledge, because we learn best by doing.
- Learning for improvement in the real world of action requires both local (specific to the place and issue at hand) and general (and generalizable) knowledge. This requirement is very different from the tenets of scientific research, which require proof of generalizability.
- Learning for improvement must attend to the dimension of time and record events sequentially. Information for improvement must tell the story throughout a process (from beginning to end), not simply take a picture at one point in time.

In summary, managing and improving health care quality is at its best a scientific pursuit that requires the application of both professional knowledge and knowledge for improvement.

Strategic Leverage

Hamel and Prahalad (1994), Senge (1990), and others writing in recent years about organizational performance have stressed the importance of "leverage" in effecting improved strategic organizational performance, including quality. As leverage is essential to effective performance, it must become a central concern of any organization that defines quality as a primary focus of its work. Simply put, leverage is created when the most focused and efficient actions are taken to bring about enduring improvements in organizational structures, processes, and outcomes.

Hamel and Prahalad (1993) emphasize the strategic application of resources (e.g., budgetary and other resource allocations, knowledge, management expertise, community power and connections) and of stretch objectives (e.g., performance objectives that foster high levels of achievement) in creating leverage. According to Senge (1990), leverage is created through learning processes that identify the underlying structure and process related to a situation and then determine the point in the system where the least effort will produce the most positive change. Organizations can leverage quality by (1) focusing on strategy, (2) focusing on evaluating performance in such a way that they are stretched to high levels of achievement, and (3) enhancing their ability to learn (Arrington et al., 1995).

Leverage through Focusing on Strategy.   Strategic alignment is an essential element in quality management and improvement (Shortell and O'Brien, 1994). Strategic alignment is achieved, and leverage created, when strategic effort and resource investment center on a finite portfolio of essential goals *over time* and are deployed throughout the organization on clearly identified performance objectives *at any one point in time* (Hamel and Prahalad, 1993). Quality performance depends on balancing investments on the "essential few" goals that will accelerate success, stretch achievement, create synergy, and add value; quality management and improvement requires long-term concentration of effort and resources.

The choice of strategic orientation is another central element of managing and improving quality. A strategic orientation is the position the organization chooses to take in its environment and the characteristics of that position. Miles and Snow (1978) describe a typology of strategic orientations that include prospectors, analyzers, defenders, and reactors. Each of these orientations represents a particular set of behaviors generally and, specifically, a particular approach to the quality management and improvement.

Prospector organizations are strategically dynamic in their relationships with their environments. Their service mix is diverse, and they are commonly the first to develop a new service or enter a new market. Prospectors are adept at sensing early signs of change in market demand, have the financial and human resources needed to pursue and create new opportunities, and are comfortable with high degrees of risk and ambiguity. According to recent research (Shortell et al., 1995a and 1995b; Shortell and O'Brien, 1994), prospectors like to be considered quality management and improvement leaders and are frequently the first among their peer organizations to try new or minimally tested improvement technologies. Prospectors may take a planned approach to quality management and improvement overall, but they are also likely to emphasize "just in time training" on a day-to-day basis.

> While top management may be given some initial training, the organization might quickly jump ahead to some pilot, and even ongoing, projects and then "backfill" with specific training as the need arises. The prospector approach

emphasizes seizing opportunities as they emerge, albeit within an overall framework of implementation. In this approach, physicians are trained as needs arise . . . (Shortell and O'Brien, 1994, p. 91).

Analyzers are more strategically cautious than prospectors and much less at ease with risk and ambiguity. Although holding on to a established mix of services and a stable market position is a dominant goal of an analyzer organization, this goal is tempered by the analyzer's interest in taking on new service and market opportunities that look promising. Analyzer organizations are likely to be most comfortable managing and improving quality by following a prescribed sequence such as that suggested by Deming (1986) or Juran (1989). Top managers are trained before organizationwide implementation is begun, followed by middle managers, and so on down the organizational hierarchy. Physician training follows a similar maxim: leadership competence is developed before the rank and file are approached. Once the education process is well under way, very focused project work on high-profile issues begins. The success of these first endeavors is carefully evaluated before activities are expanded (Shortell and O'Brien, 1994).

Defender organizations, like analyzers, seek stability in their environments, their services, and their markets. The defender's primary strategic goal is technical efficiency. Innovation is less important to the defender than effective performance using existing services in existing markets. Defender organizations are most likely simply to extend current quality assurance activities to enhance their ability to manage and improve quality. Existing committees, councils, and so on are given added responsibility, and new techniques or methods are "grafted onto or incorporated into existing approaches" (Shortell and O'Brien, 1994, p. 92). The focus is on meeting the requirements of external accrediting bodies such as the Joint Commission on the Accreditation of Healthcare Organizations.

The fourth strategic orientation, reactor, actually represents the absence of a coherent strategic orientation. Reactors may appear to be prospectors, analyzers, or defenders at varying times; over time, their behavior is inconsistent. Reactors may use quality improvement methods and tools as amenable problems arise, but their use is not typically part of a planned approach to change in a reactor organization. Quality management and improvement as processes may occur sporadically throughout a reactor organization, but there is limited physician involvement and no visible leadership commitment (Shortell et al., 1995a, 1995b; Shortell and O'Brien, 1994).

Clearly, the different strategic orientations support very different approaches to quality management and improvement. The organization's approach to managing and improving quality should be congruent with its strategic orientation. Prospectors and analyzers are more likely to manage and improve quality effectively because the goals of their orientations are consistent with an emphasis on quality (Shortell et al., 1995a, 1995b; Shortell and O'Brien, 1994). Because of their limited comfort with risk and ambiguity, however, defender and reactor organizations are less likely to support quality management and improvement (Shortell et al., 1995a, 1995b; Shortell and O'Brien, 1994).

Leverage through Supporting and Evaluating Performance. Quality management and improvement requires organizational and managerial performance to be stretched by and evaluated in terms of key performance objectives that derive from primary strategic goals. Quality management and improvement activities

> challenge some traditional conceptions of human resource activities. Is traditional evaluation of employees a helpful action? How should accountability be structured in the workplace? What rewards should be given? What are the . . . motivators of employees? How is recognition managed? The answers to these questions create a work environment that addresses just wage considerations; power to employees in their area of expertise; recognition of worker contributions; . . . and respect for the contributions of all (Brodeur, 1995, p. 117).

Organizations interested in enhancing their capacity to manage and improve quality must, at the least, review their human resource philosophy and practices and in most cases create and communicate a very different philosophy and very different practices. The changes most commonly called for include the following:

- A philosophy that considers employees as partners and as valuable assets, rather than costs.
- Recruitment, selection, and retention practices that value the internal over the external labor market.
- Performance appraisal systems that are developmentally focused and not linked to compensation.
- Compensation that is externally equitable, balances monetary and nonmonetary rewards, and emphasizes collective rather than individual achievement.
- Training and development programs that are transforming (rather than conforming).
- A strategic as well as operational position for the human resource function within the organization (Haddock et al., 1995).

Leverage through Ongoing Learning. Organizations increase their competence by learning from their own and others' aggregate experiences (Hamel and Prahalad, 1993; Senge, 1990; Argyris, 1990; Argyris and Schon, 1978). The ability to create leverage in an organization is derived from the organization's ability to learn (Senge, 1990), which expands when (1) those conditions that limit learning are removed, (2) knowledge gained in one area is used to improve performance in another area, and (3) collaboration occurs with others trying to improve their own performance (Arrington et al., 1995). The ability to learn reduces the amount of time and effort an organization must expend to develop new services and improve its operations. Experts agree that an organization's learning capacity is critically related to managing and improving quality (Argyris, 1990; Argyris and Schon, 1978; Senge, 1990; Nevis et al., 1993).

An organization's capacity to learn is directly tied to the systems that are in place to direct and support learning. The major components of a learning system are facilitating factors and learning orientations or styles (Nevis et al., 1993). *Facilitating factors* are those normative structures and processes that make it possible and easy to learn. An organization's *learning orientation* is its approach to acquiring, sharing, and using knowledge. Learning orientations are based on the organization's basic cultural assumptions and values supporting those assumptions, its core competencies, and its previous learning experiences. Together, facilitating factors and learning orientations create the patterns of behavior that constitute the organization's learning system.

Why are facilitating factors and learning orientations important in the management and improvement of quality? These characteristics of an organization's learning style suggest which approaches and methods can be used to enhance quality.

Facilitating factors: Three main factors promote organizational learning.

1. The organization must be committed to understanding community need by
   (a) understanding the organization as a system
   (b) scanning and understanding its environments
   (c) involving leadership in vision development and implementation
2. The organization must be committed to developing a culture, structures, and processes that are capable of learning by
   (a) fostering a climate of openness
   (b) promoting diversity in its human resources and internal capabilities
   (c) seeing experimentation as a desirable activity
3. The organization must be committed to creating opportunities for learning by
   (a) making decisions on the basis of measurement and facts, thus providing ongoing continuing education
   (b) developing its ability to initiate learning at all levels (top to bottom)
   (c) using performance gaps to identify new learning opportunities.

These factors are very similar to the attributes described by Deming (1986), Juran (1989), and others as managing and improving quality. Learning will be facilitated and quality improved to the extent that these characteristics exist in the organization. The presence of these characteristics creates the potential for leveraging quality; their absence suggests that there is much work to be done before the capacity to manage and improve quality can be developed.

Learning orientations: Nevis et al. (1993) also describe seven learning orientations that determine how learning will occur in the organization and the character of what will be learned. These orientations are not inherently good or bad; they simply describe a range of states of being. They consist of the following elements:

1. Knowledge source is the relative degree to which the organization develops new knowledge internally as opposed to learning from the work of others external to the organization.
2. Learning focus is the relative extent to which new learning is focused on improving current processes as opposed to searching for new ones.
3. Value chain focus represents those core competencies (e.g., research and development, particular product or service lines) that the organization values enough to invest funds and human resources in them and thereby increase its knowledge and skills in those areas.
4. Knowledge focus is the relative emphasis on understanding organizational or community health status outcomes versus understanding the processes that create those outcomes.
5. Skill development is the relative emphasis on the development of individual knowledge, skills, and competence versus the development of teams or groups that work effectively together.
6. Documentation mode is the relative extent to which knowledge gained through education and experience is seen as personal (something retained by an individual) versus as a collective resource (shared through communication and codification).
7. Dissemination mode is related to documentation mode, that is, the relative extent to which learning is either encouraged to evolve naturally or is induced through controlled structures and processes for education.

Methods and Tools

The methods and tools of quality management and improvement have been developed specifically for improvement activities or borrowed from many fields of endeavor ranging from engineering to group psychology to operations research to statistical analysis. Plsek (1995) identifies three categories of techniques commonly in use: improvement techniques, quality planning techniques, and measurement techniques. Plsek also provides an extensive bibliography of theoretical and applied references for each of the methods and tools.

Improvement Techniques.   These techniques include tools for process description and design, tools for data analysis and synthesis, and tools for supporting group or team activities. These tools are typically the ones introduced when an organization first begins educating its members for quality management and improvement. The primary use of these tools is in the improvement of existing processes.

Quality Planning Techniques.   These techniques include tools both to carry out and support customer need identification, process design, and strategic planning and deployment. Used primarily by teams to organize information and formulate plans for new processes, products or services, these tools are critical in the development of a strategic focus and the deployment of that focus throughout the organization.

Measurement Techniques.   These techniques support the identification of important and appropriate measures of performance, including benchmarking techniques, which not only build on a long history of performance measurement in health care but also push their users to meet three objectives:

1. To highlight the perceptions of customers as valid measures.
2. To focus on cross-functional processes and their measures.
3. To question the use of performance measures in determining rewards and punishments (Plsek, 1995).

Taking into account history and these three objectives, then, any system for managing and improving quality should include, at the least, measures of clinical performance, customer perceptions and satisfaction, process performance, and financial performance.

Figure 9.4 summarizes these techniques. A small but growing number of health care organizations fully comprehend and routinely use these methods and tools in their daily work as well as for improvement projects. They are leading the field in the management and improvement of health care quality.

Use of Consultants.   One of the most commonly considered tools at the beginning and during the development of quality management and improvement competence is the use of consultants: Should outside consultants be used? If so, when? Where and for what purposes can they be most effective? If the organization prefers to develop knowledge internally, it might best support quality management and improvement by forming study groups or internal task forces (e.g., a quality council composed of internal members only), aided—but not driven—by outside consultants. If external knowledge

Figure 9.4   A Basic Tool Kit of Techniques for Managing Quality

Improvement Techniques

Quality improvement projects and teams

Models for improvement

Tools for process description
Flowcharts (chronological)
Cause-effect diagrams (causal)

Tools for data collection
Checksheets
Datasheets
Interviews
Surveys

Tools for data analysis
for categorical data
Pie charts
Bar charts
Pareto diagrams

for continuous data
Average, median (center)
Range, standard deviation (spread)
Histograms (shape)
Line graphs (sequence)

to study relationships between variables
Scatter diagrams

to determine stability of a process
Control charts

Advanced tool: design of experiments(DOE)

Tools for collaborative work
Brainstorming
Boarding
Multivoting
Decision matrices
Composite techniques (e.g., nominal group)

Planning Techniques

Management and planning tools
Affinity diagram
Relationship diagram
Tree diagram
Activity network diagram
Process decision program chart (PDPC)
Failure mode and effect analysis (FMEA)

Models for process improvement

Critical paths, clinical guidelines, & algorithms

Models for strategic planning
The annual quality plan
Hoshin planning/strategic quality management
Organization-as-a-system exercise

Customer needs analysis
Dimensions of quality
Focus groups and surveys
Moments of truth method
Critical incident technique

Advanced tool: **quality function deployment (QFD)**

Measurement Techniques

Traditional approaches in health care

Framework for a comprehensive measurement system
Clinical outcomes
Customer perceptions of quality
Internal process performance
Financial performance

Benchmarking
Internal benchmarking
Competitive benchmarking
Functional (or group) benchmarking
Generic benchmarking

Source: Paul E. Plsek. "Techniques for Managing Quality." *Hospital & Health Services Administration.* 40 (1) , Spring 1995.

is preferred, a consultant might be hired to provide special expertise. Using outside consultants as the principal vehicle for quality management and improvement design and development in an internally focused organization will likely fail, as will not using outside consultants in an externally focused organization. The point is to evaluate and understand organizational learning preferences and use consultants accordingly.

Daily Work Life

Organizations are capable of managing and improving quality to the extent that each person in the organization (1) understands the aim of the organization and its work structures and processes (Nolan, 1994) and (2) is committed to and competent at working collaboratively to build knowledge for improvement as part of the organization's daily work (Plsek, 1995).

Physicians and other clinicians are educated to build new knowledge using the scientific method and typically do so regularly through the practices that they commonly apply in the diagnosis and treatment of patients:

1. They develop a theory (a preliminary diagnosis) concerning the nature of the patient's problem.
2. They test that theory by taking therapeutic action in anticipation of a particular response within a predicted time frame.
3. They evaluate the patient's response in light of their theory.

If the predicted effect of the action and the experienced response are similar, the initial theory is corroborated, that is, the diagnosis is most likely correct and the treatment sufficient. The clinician has developed new knowledge for managing this patient (and future patients), now and in the future, through linking theory and action with prediction and measurement (Batalden, 1995).

The PDSA (Plan-Do-Study-Act) or PDCA (Plan-Do-Check-Act) cycle is a simple method, very similar to that just described, for iteratively building knowledge through experimentation. It also supports continuous learning in daily work. (Deming called the PDSA cycle the Shewhart cycle; the Japanese refer to it as the Deming cycle). Regardless of nomenclature, the method—which is commonly used and has been widely tested—is as follows:

- The *plan* stage is the process of designing a proposed action predicted to be an improvement and developing an approach for investigating its effect on the system.
- The *do* stage consists of instituting a change and formulating a plan for evaluating its effect.

- The *study/check* stage involves measuring and assessing the effect of the change, examining the underlying theory, and evaluating predictions.
- The *act* stage consists of standardizing or dropping the change as indicated by the results. The most crucial consideration here is how to make the improvement enduring (if there is an improvement), that is, deciding what related changes must be made and communicated, what policies must be adapted, and so on. A related concern is how to communicate and share results so that the experience is replicated throughout the organization and/or is used to stimulate further organizational learning.
- Where the change did not result in an improvement, the underlying theory must be revised, and new tests of change for improvement must be designed.

The PDSA cycle allows everyone in the organization to apply a scientific method to the work of improvement, to take reasoned action, and to learn from both successful and unsuccessful experiments. The reader who would like to explore this concept in more detail can refer to any of many works on quality management and improvement available in the general and health care management literature. The recent escalation in the literature and practice of outcomes research, guidelines development, and other clinical process improvement activities may further infuse the principles and practices of quality management and improvement into daily work life (Goonan, 1995; James, 1995; Lengnick-Hall, 1995; Gale, 1994).

Batalden (1995) notes the following problems in regard to using the PDS(C)A cycle iteratively to develop new knowledge and to incorporate learning into work in health care organizations:

- Many people are comfortable with developing theory and with taking action but not with linking the two.
- Health care workers are not accustomed to using prediction and measurement for learning outside the clinical arena.
- Health care organizations are not accustomed to doing small-scale or pilot studies in the process of making changes, nor are they good at replicating successes elsewhere.
- Learning is often viewed as personal, not organizational, and is therefore frequently not communicated or shared.
- There is a prevailing sense that health care work is too urgent and workers too busy for planning and checking related to that planning.

These challenges must be addressed if health care organizations are to continue to increase their competence in managing and improving quality. Implementation of the suggestions recommended earlier in this chapter concerning strategy leadership, learning for improvement, and using the methods and tools of quality improvement has been found to support a culture in which daily work life can and does change (Shortell et al., 1995b).

❧ WHAT IS THE EVIDENCE?

> For those who wish to 'cut to the quick,' the evidence suggests that: (1) the concept is great, (2) design is important, but (3) implementation appears to be everything" (Shortell et al., 1995b).

As the health care system of the United States continues to restructure, health care organizations will increasingly need to produce efficient and effective products and services that meet or exceed customers' needs and expectations and at the same time to be accountable to the communities they serve. Does quality management and improvement provide support in this regard? What evidence do we have that "it works"?

Culture, technology, strategy, and structure are all relevant organizational dimensions to be considered when assessing the evidence for the effectiveness of quality management and improvement in US health care organizations. The literature suggests that the cultural, technical, strategic, and structural dimensions of quality management and improvement may all be associated with positive organizational quality (Shortell et al., 1995a, 1995b). Health care organizations that adopt an orientation to quality as described in this chapter, as opposed to those that do not, appear to experience the following:

- significantly more satisfaction with their improvement efforts
- improved organization-physician relationships
- greater employee empowerment
- greater perceived impact on profitability
- greater perceived impact on productivity
- statistically significant cost savings
- no perceived impact on patient outcomes (Shortell et al., 1995a, 1995b)

Few, if any, health care organizations report significant activity in regard to clinical process improvement, arguably the most strategically important core process of health care organizations. This is a conspicuous shortcoming when one compares the health care literature with the general management literature. Most quality management and improvement in other fields has been directed at organizations' most strategically important core processes. Most reported use of the methods and tools of quality management and improvement in health care organizations has been to improve administrative and patient care support activities, not clinical processes (Shortell et al., 1995a, 1995b).

> This is undoubtedly due to the fact that complex health care organizations are involved in complex and diverse "production processes" that involve the specialized interests of many different professional groups and that make it difficult to reliably measure outcomes of care. Further, many of the key "producers" (i.e., physicians) are not employees of the organization. Nevertheless, the ultimate payoff of quality initiatives lies in the ability to improve the core clinical processes associated with patient care (Shortell et al., 1995b, p. 16).

Many obstacles impede health care organizations from building quality management and improvement (Shortell et al., 1995a, 1995b; Berwick et al., 1990). These can be organized according to the cultural, technical, strategic, and structural dimensions of quality management and improvement. Culturally, the major obstacles are reported as follows:

- The needs of internal customers are emphasized over those of external customers.
- Large health care organizations usually are hierarchical, authoritarian, bureaucratic, relatively inflexible structures.
- Senior leadership is not *really* committed.
- Health care organizations are dominated by command and control and hero/heroine leadership styles.
- Middle management resists processes and structures that minimize the organization's need for middle managers.
- There is limited physician involvement (Shortell et al., 1995a, 1995b).

Technically, the major obstacles are reported as follows:

- There is limited targeted training in team-based problem solving, particularly at the level of skill development.
- Only limited and inferior data and information systems exist to support improvement efforts.
- The ability to understand cause-and-effect relationships clearly is limited.
- Complex, highly interdependent, not fully understood systems are the primary supports for the core process—clinical care.

Strategically, several issues impede capacity development:

- Health care organizations are not particularly capable strategists.
- Cross-functional and interdepartmental coordination is difficult at best.
- Learning is rarely shared and transferred.

Structurally, several barriers arise:

- Few health care organizations have an existing structure that supports quality management and improvement, nor have they significantly developed appropriate structures or processes to focus strategically on such activity.
- Traditional quality assurance and risk management activities are not integrated with quality management and improvement.
- Planning and financial systems are not integrated with, nor are they designed to support, quality improvement efforts.
- Human resource philosophies and practices are at odds with the purposes of quality management and improvement.
- Quality information is not used in decision making at the senior levels of the organization.

What is the evidence? While most would agree that health care's interest in quality management and improvement has outlasted that which would have been accorded something that was simply a fad, the theory's potential to improve the quality of health care and control costs remains essentially unproven. But despite the difficulty that our typically large, bureaucratically organized health care organizations have had in becoming the kind of flexible organizations where quality management and improvement practices seem to have their greatest effect, some modest successes have been reported. Perhaps the transformation of health care delivery through managed care and capitation will create organizations even more capable of reaping the benefits of increased competence through quality management and improvement.

🐾 REFERENCES

Argyris, C. *Overcoming Organizational Defenses: Facilitating Organizational Learning.* Boston, MA: Allyn & Bacon, 1990.

Argyris, C. and D. A. Schon. *Organizational Learning.* Reading, MA: Addison-Wesley, 1978.

Arrington, B. A. , K. Gautam, and W. J. McCabe. "Continually Improving Governance." *Hospital and Health Services Administration* 40 (1), Spring 1995: 95–110.

Batalden, P. B. "Organizing the Production of Health Care as a System." Presentation, Woodstock, VT. 11 July 1995.

Batalden, P. B. and P. K. Stolz. "A Framework for the Continual Improvement of Health Care." *Joint Commission Journal on Quality Improvement* 19 (10) October 1993: 424–444.

Batalden, P. B. , S. D. Smith, J. O. Bovender, and C. D. Hardison. "Quality Improvement: The Role and Application of Research Methods." *Journal of Health Administration* 7 (3) Summer 1984: 577–83.

Berwick, D. M. "Improving as Science." *Improving Clinical Practice*. San Francisco: Jossey-Bass, 1995: 3–24.

Berwick, D. M., A. B. Godfrey, and J. Roessner. *Curing Health Care*. San Francisco: Jossey-Bass, 1990.

Berwick, D. M. "Continuous Improvement as an Ideal in Health Care." *New England Journal of Medicine*. 320 (January 5) 1989: 53–56.

Brodeur, D. A. "Work Ethics and CQI." *Hospital and Health Services Administration* 40 (1), Spring 1995: 111–123.

Crosby, P. *Quality Without Tears: The Art of Hassle-Free Management*. New York: Plume, 1984.

Deming, W. E. *The New Economics for Industry, Government, Education*. Cambridge, MA: Massachusetts Institute of Technology Center for Advanced Engineering Study, 1993.

Deming, W. E. *Out of the Crisis*. Cambridge, MA: Massachusetts Institute of Technology Center for Advanced Engineering Study, 1986.

Donabedian, A. "Evaluating the Quality of Medical Care." *Milbank Memorial Fund Quarterly* 44 (3), Part 2, 1966: 166–203.

Donabedian, A. "Quality Assessment and Assurance: Unity of Purpose, Diversity of Means." *Inquiry* 25, Spring 1988: 173–192.

Donabedian, A. "Continuity and Change in the Quest for Quality." *Clinical Performance and Quality Health Care* 1 (1), 1993: 9–16.

Ferguson, S., T. Howell, and P. Batalden. "Knowledge and Skills Needed for Collaborative Work." *Quality Management in Health Care* Winter 1993: 1–11.

Flood, A. B. "The Impact of Organizational and Managerial Factors on the Quality of Care in Health Care Organizations." *Medical Care Review* 51 (4), 1994: 381–428.

Gale, F. M. (ed.). *Tales in Pursuit of Quality in Health Care.* Tampa, FL: American College of Physician Executives, 1994.

Goonan, K. J. *The Juran Prescription: Clinical Quality Management.* San Francisco: Jossey-Bass, 1995.

Haddock, C. C., C. Nosky, C. A. Fargason, and R. S. Kurz. "The Impact of CQI on Human Resources." *Hospital and Health Services Administration* 40 (1), Spring 1995: 138–153.

Hamel, G. and C. K. Prahalad. "Strategy as Stretch and Leverage." *Harvard Business Review* March–April 1993: 75–84.

James, B. "What Is TURP? Controlling Variation in the Performance of Clinical Processes." *Improving Clinical Practice.* San Francisco: Jossey-Bass, 1995: 167–202.

Juran, J. M. *Leadership for Quality.* New York: The Free Press, 1989.

Kaluzny, A. D., C. P. McLaughlin, and D. Kibbe. "Quality Improvement: Beyond the Institution." *Hospital and Health Services Administration* 40 (1), Spring 1995: 172–188.

Kurz, R. S. "CQI: Expanding the Impact." *Hospital and Health Services Administration* 40 (1), Spring 1995: 1–3.

Lengnick-Hall, C. A. "The Patient as Pivot Point for Quality in Health Care Delivery." *Hospital and Health Services Administration* 40 (1), Spring 1995: 25–39.

Miles, R. E. and C. C. Snow. *Organizational Strategy, Structure, and Process.* New York: McGraw-Hill, 1978.

Mulley, A. G. "Industrial Quality Management Science and Outcomes Research: Responses to Unwanted Variation in Health Outcomes and Decisions." *Improving Clinical Practice.* San Francisco: Jossey-Bass Inc. 1995: 73–107.

Nelson, E. C., J. J. Mohr, P. B. Batalden, and S. K. Plume."Improving Health Care: Part 1. The Clinical Value Compass." Presentation, Woodstock, VT. 13 July 1995.

Nevis, E. C., A. J. DiBella, J. M. Gould. *Organizations as Learning Systems.* Working Paper #3567–93. Sloan School: Organizational Learning Center, 1993.

Nolan, T. "Interview: Pursuing a Common Aim." *Quality Connection* 2 (4), 1994: 4–5.

O'Leary, D. S. "Accreditation in the Quality Improvement Mold—A Vision for Tomorrow." *Quality Review Bulletin* 17 (3), 1993: 72–77.

Paul E. Plsek. "Techniques for Managing Quality." *Hospital & Health Services Administration* 40 (1) , Spring 1995.

Senge, P. M. *The Fifth Discipline: The Art and Practice of the Learning Organization.* New York: Doubleday, 1990.

Shortell, S. M., J. L. O'Brien, J. M. Carman, R. W. Foster, E. F. X. Hughes, H. Boerstler, and E. J. O'Connor. "Assessing the Impact of Continuous Quality Improvement/ Total Quality Management: Concept Versus Implementation." *Health Services Research* 30(2) June 1995a: 377–401.

Shortell, S. M. , Daniel J. Levin, J. L. O'Brien, and Edward F. X. Hughes. "Assessing the Evidence on CQI: Is the Glass Half Empty or Half Full?" *Hospital and Health Services Administration* 40 (1), Spring 1995b: 4–24.

Shortell, S. M. and J. L. O'Brien. "Evaluating New Ways of Managing Quality." Interviewed by A. B. Cohen. *The Joint Commission Journal of Quality Improvement* 20 (2) 1994: 90–96.

US Chamber of Commerce. *The Malcolm Baldrige Award.* 1993.

Young, M. J., Steven Rallison, and Philip Eckman. "Patients, Physicians, and Professional Knowledge." *Hospital and Health Services Administration* 40 (1), Spring 1995: 40–49.

Organizational Processes in Health Care Management

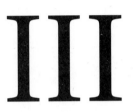

Building Effective Health Care Teams*

10

Donde P. Ashmos, University of Texas at San Antonio

🐚 BUILDING EFFECTIVE HEALTH CARE TEAMS

> Yes, teams have troubles. They consume gallons of sweat and discouragement before yielding a penny of benefit. Companies make the investment because they've realized that in a fast-moving, brutally competitive economy, the one thing sure to be harder than operating with teams is operating without them (Fortune, Sept. 4, 1994).

Health care organizations, like other entities in corporate America, have wasted little time in adopting teamwork philosophies, altering organizational structures to reflect the need for teams, and reorganizing work tasks where teams of interdependent workers share responsibilities for major tasks. US companies in particular have looked to the use of this format as a remedy for quality and performance problems. For a variety of reasons, health care organizations make wide use of teams, with much

*Special thanks to Dennis Duchon and Reuben McDaniel for their help in the development of this manuscript. Thanks also to Laurie Milton for her assistance.

of the basic work of health services organizations now being carried out in this manner. In spite of the popularity of teams and their obvious apparent virtues, there is increasing evidence that teams have resulted in disappointing outcomes (Delbecq and Gill, 1985; Nahavandi and Aranda, 1994).

Why is it, then, that teams make good theoretical sense, yet in practice managers often find team experiences frustrating and their results disappointing? The answer, in part, is that many of the fundamental assumptions behind the use of teams are derived from an organizational paradigm that is no longer appropriate for organizations operating in fast-paced, hyperturbulent environments. This paradigm, referred to by Wheatley (1992) as the Newtonian organization, views organizations as operating in an orderly and predictable world in which they are understood by managers in a scientific way. In this paradigm poor management is the result of ignorance or incompetence. In Newtonian organizations teams are used as a way of (1) exercising control (allowing people to participate in teams will increase their acceptance of solutions and their commitment to decisions) and (2) reducing uncertainty (increasing the amount of information that enhances the chance of finding the right solution). Through exercising control and reducing uncertainty, managers using teams hope to increase organizational stability. When teams don't produce increased stability, or the specific outcomes that are expected to increase stability, we often assume either a failure of leadership or a failure of followership. This chapter argues that conventional assumptions about teams lead organizations to use teams for the wrong purposes, creating expectations that cannot be fulfilled and therefore result in disappointing outcomes. What is needed is an alternative organizational paradigm, leading to different assumptions about teams and, ultimately, more useful outcomes from teamwork.

The chapter's first section defines teams and describes common varieties of teams. The second section presents an old and new organizational paradigm for considering the use of teams. Section three explores several conventional assumptions about teams that need to be discarded in order for organizations to reap the most benefit from the use of teams. The text explicates each of these assumptions and proposes an alternative view. Section four suggests how to build more effective teams. Finally, section five speculates about the kinds of teams that are likely to be prevalent in the future.

❧ Teams—A Definition

Teams are most often promoted as a way of increasing the participation of workers in executing tasks that require the knowledge or expertise of workers from several functional areas (Hirschorn, 1991). Teams are often described as a "coordination device" and are formed around frequently occurring problems. As such, the team is charged with discussing and solving problems appropriate to the team's level in the hierarchy (Galbraith, 1977). In addition to serving the purpose of problem solving, teams are being increasingly formed to carry on some portion of the regular work of the organization (Scott, 1987). Three types of worker-manager teams are particularly common in health care organizations today: problem-solving teams, special-purpose teams, and self-managed teams (Hellreigel and Slocum, 1992).

A *problem-solving* team is a formal group of employees within a department, often volunteers, who meet to discuss ways to improve quality, productivity, and the work setting. This type of group usually has very limited authority, if any, for implementing its ideas and most often disbands upon completion of its task. Mobil Corporation, in an effort to manage health care costs in its Beaumont plant, created the Beaumont Health Care Implementation Team, whose purpose was to serve as an interface between the health care community in Beaumont and the management and employees of the Beaumont plant. The team met with employees and local providers in the community, drafted suggested improvements in the health care plan, and passed them on to the corporate office. The group disbanded after completing its task. In an HMO a team consisting of representatives from the HMO, physicians, and clients might form a team to solve the problem of how to broaden the HMO's appeal to a wider range of physicians. After developing a range of alternatives, the team would disband.

A *special-purpose* team is a formal group of employees from various departments or organizational levels that is responsible for a whole range of potential situations. Their tasks may include designing work reforms, linking separate functions, increasing the number of innovations, and improving the link between strategic and tactical problems. These teams usually operate with more authority than the problem-solving teams. In a nursing home chain, a Total Quality Improvement team that operates across nursing homes for the purpose of developing an organizational policy to respond to changes in state regulations is an example of a special-purpose team. Such a team would typically comprise representatives from several levels throughout the company and would be authorized by management to develop and implement new policy that would govern behavior in individual nursing homes.

A *self-managed* team is a formal group of employees who work together on a daily basis to produce an entire good or service and perform numerous managerial tasks related to their jobs. Such a team has the authority to control the way in which its members perform their jobs, and therefore fundamental changes in how work is organized often result. A surgical team or operating room team are examples of self-managed teams. A case management team in a mental health facility also functions as a self-managed team, with a psychiatrist, social worker, nurse, and family member planning and delivering the appropriate mental health service. In each case, team management occurs within the team as it responds to events.

These three types of teams, while different from one another in their scope and level of responsibility in the organization, share the underlying assumption that allowing organizational members some participation in work decisions will better enable the organization to achieve its goals, thus ensuring predictability. Each of these types of teams is expected to reduce uncertainty by bringing more information to bear on a problem at hand, thereby improving the predictability of the system.

&ent; Old versus New Paradigm for Considering Teams

The issue of teams is most often viewed from two perspectives. The first is a *psychological perspective*, which promotes the use of teams as a motivating mechanism for minimizing workers' resistance to change and increasing their acceptance of team outcomes and commitment to goals and decisions (Locke and Schweiger, 1979). The second perspective is a *cognitive perspective*, which views teams as a way to reduce uncertainty by increasing the information, knowledge, and expertise that their members bring to bear on a particular problem or task (Locke and Schweiger, 1979). From the cognitive perspective, team members may contribute to problem solving or improve their understanding of decisions they are supposed to implement through their involvement in discussing and deciding those issues. Thus, the use of teams is believed to reduce uncertainty either about a problem's solution or about the solution's implementation. Both the psychological and cognitive perspectives make the same assumption: that managers can improve their ability to better match intentions to outcomes through the use of teams, that is, that teams improve the ability to control organizational functioning. From the psychological perspective, managers use teams to gain workers' acceptance and commitment and thus ensure desired outcomes. From the cognitive perspective, managers use teams to obtain information needed to solve problems or to ensure effective implementation of agreed solutions—increasing the likelihood that intentions and outcomes are the same.

These two perspectives about the use of teams are based on the Newtonian view (Wheatley, 1994) in which organizations function largely as machines and the need for control, rationality, and predictability drives most actions. (Chapter 11 of this volume further explains the Newtonian model.) These organizations are held together by clearly stated goals, explicit rules, and highly specified roles. In Newtonian organizations it is organizational structure that creates order based on managerial intentions at a certain moment (Weick, 1993).

The use of teams in Newtonian organizations is popular but its popularity may be waning (Nahavandi and Aranda, 1994). One premise of teamwork is that it is a way of empowering workers, yet in Newtonian organizations managers maintain control over workers. Opponents of teams commonly argue that they are a waste of time, that the effort put into developing trust doesn't translate into creativity, and that top management often fails to support the work of teams (Nahavandi and Aranda, 1994). In addition, although teams are promoted as a way of minimizing pressure from autocratic managers, the pressure workers feel from their peers can be equally coercive. In either case, the underlying motivation for the use of teams in many organizations, while not explicitly stated, is to gain command and control. This view of teams has led to a number of conventional assumptions about teams that are challenged later in this chapter.

If we consider organizations from a perspective other than the Newtonian point of view, our view of teams—and their role and purpose in organizations—will likely change. While organizations are often seen as machines that crave control and predictability, an alternative view is that organizations are in fact complex adaptive systems (Stacey, 1995) operating in an unpredictable world. Complex adaptive systems face unknowable futures (Stacey, 1992) and exhibit dynamic living qualities in which what matters most is not any specific part of the system but the connection between the parts (Wheatley, 1992). (Chapter 11 of this volume further analyzes this paradigm.) From this alternative point of view, organizational teams take on a very different significance, serving rather to reduce equivocality by bringing people together to make sense out of what is happening around them (Weick, 1995). From this perspective, teams offer organizations a way to surface conflict, develop shared meanings, and question prevailing assumptions in the organization's voyage through the unknowable.

From an organizing perspective, Weick (1979, 1995) argues that it is important for organizations to ask—and try to answer—the question, how do I know what I think until I see what I say? Teams, which are often microcosms for the organization, are a mechanism for collectively seeing what the organization thinks. Teams offer the opportunity for an organization to test out ideas, assumptions, and interpretations of events; to argue and question; and to develop shared meaning about the events and the world it is facing. From this perspective, the purpose of teams in health care organizations is not to answer questions or accumulate information to reduce uncertainty; rather, it is to Figure out what questions to ask, to sort through the multiple cues and interpretations that create confusion and ambiguity in organizations. Weick (1995) suggests why it is that teams often cause frustration in organizations.

> My hunch is that many [meetings] prove to be unproductive because they are directed at problems of uncertainty that are better handled by other media that are more efficient. I would also bet that those meetings that are directed at problems of ambiguity fail to handle it because potentially rich media are

squelched by autocratic leadership, norms that encourage obedience, unwill-ingness to risk embarrassment by disagreeing with superiors, reluctance to admit that one has no idea what is going on, and so on (p. 186).

The purpose of teams in organizations that exist in highly turbulent environments, such as health care organizations, is, therefore, to bring different viewpoints together to help reduce equivocality, not to remove ignorance. Until health care managers accept this notion and an alternative paradigm of organizations, teams will continue to be disappointing for most health care organizations, which operate in fast-moving, turbulent environments.

Since the long-term future of health care organizations today is unknowable and unpredictable, leaders of these organizations cannot be expected to lead teams of health care professionals and managers into uncharted waters with old navigational principles (Stacey, 1992). "The trouble with standard maps and traditional navigational principles is that they can be used only to identify routes that others have traveled before: they can make sense only for managing the knowable" (Stacey, 1992, p. 3). Teams can enable managers of health care organizations to create the route while the journey is under way, but only if conventional assumptions about teams are challenged.

❧ CHALLENGING CONVENTIONAL ASSUMPTIONS ABOUT TEAMS

As already noted in the introduction to this chapter, the dominance of the Newtonian view of organizations has led to conventional assumptions about the use of teams. If an alternative view of organizations is adopted that uses teams more for sensemaking and equivocality reduction than to find specific solutions, the conventional assumptions must be replaced with a revised set of assumptions about the usefulness and purpose of teams in organizational life. Following are seven conventional assumptions about teams and suggested revisions.

> *Assumption #1:*   *Teams encourage commitment and acceptance of decisions.*
> *Revision:*   *Effective teams delay commitment and acceptance of decisions.*

The theoretical basis for the use of teams in organizations derives from our under-standing of the literature on participation and involvement (Locke and Schweiger, 1979), which originated in the human relations school of management (McGregor, 1960; Likert, 1967). Based on these earlier views of human behavior, conventional wisdom about teams suggests that participating in them causes workers to *increase their commit-ment* to the organization or to their department and therefore become more motivated to carry out the decisions or the changes that are developed. Lawler (1991) describes high-involvement management, which makes use of teams, as the "commitment approach," because it is based on the notion that if people are going to care about the performance of the organization, they need to know about it and be able to influence it.

Another motivational reason for using teams is that highly involved workers are more likely to *accept the outcomes* of decision processes in which they have been a part. Research has shown that increased participation leads to increased acceptance of decisions (Lawler and Hackman, 1969) and reduced resistance to change (Kahn, 1974; Lawrence, 1971). The Vroom-Yetton-Jago model of leadership styles (Vroom and Yetton, 1973; Vroom and Jago, 1988) emphasizes the need to consider trade-offs between acceptance of a decision by subordinates and the quality of the decision outcome (Vroom and Jago, 1978).

Conventional wisdom about teams also suggests that teams will help make workers happier, thereby helping managers to motivate them and increase their commitment to and acceptance of decisions and changes in the organization. This increased motivation is believed to result in many good outcomes for the organization: improvements in productivity, quality, absenteeism, and turnover (Lawler, 1991).

Most organizations today, and certainly health care organizations, function in highly turbulent environments in which it is difficult to make sense of the events and realities of their worlds. As approaches to competitive advantage change, and the health care industry is continually redefined, few of the environmental conditions remain familiar. Thus, drawing on multiple experts throughout the organization through the use of teams becomes the only way to make sense out of what's happening. When teams are viewed from this perspective, there is no decision to accept, no outcome to commit to. Rather, team members are needed to develop understandings of the ambiguous situations in which organizations find themselves. March describes ambiguous situations as those "that cannot be coded precisely into mutually exhaustive and exclusive categories" (March, 1994, p. 178).

One of the well-documented disadvantages of using teams to make decisions is the resulting tendency toward intragroup cohesion and groupthink (Janis, 1982). Groupthink is the overemphasis on agreement and consensus that occurs in highly cohesive groups because members are unwilling to evaluate one another's ideas. When groupthink occurs, teams limit themselves to the consideration of only a few alternative solutions and fail to think through the implications of the issue before them. Due to the desire of individual group members for group acceptance, teams in this situation often make premature decisions, accepting and committing to solutions that have not been carefully considered.

When managers construct teams as a way of getting workers to buy in to their decisions, or in the hope that workers can be manipulated, they lose the opportunity "to share perceptions among themselves and gradually define or create meaning through discussion, groping, trial and error, and sounding out" (Huber and Daft, 1987, p. 151). This process by its very nature is time-consuming and means that the process of commitment to decisions and acceptance of outcomes is intentionally delayed rather than encouraged. Eagerness to reach a premature conclusion and the assumption of unanimity among team members prohibit sensemaking. If teams take seriously the business of helping to shape the organization's unfolding future, they will resist the urge for quick closure. Weick (1995) describes meeting for the purpose of sensemaking: "Too many cues and too many interpretations and too little closure persist for too long when people try to discover what they really ought to be addressing and what kinds of understanding they need to negotiate. Such gatherings are not for the faint of heart" (p. 186).

Assumption #2: *Teams help the organization by gathering necessary information for making decisions.*

Revision: *Effective teams help the organization "unlearn" and then learn.*

One of the most significant reasons for the popularity of teams is that "organizations are now so complex that it is virtually impossible for an individual to have all the information necessary to make a good decision" (Nahavandi and Aranda, 1994). This understanding is not new; participation researchers have suggested for some time that a major reason to involve organizational members in decision making is to increase the information, knowledge, and creativity that they will bring to bear on problems (Locke and Schweiger, 1979). Thus, teams, particularly problem-solving teams, have been used because the information necessary for solving problems is believed to be distributed throughout the organization. Interdependency therefore creates the need for teams to solve specific problems or to execute certain tasks.

Although it is clear that interdependencies exist and that efforts to coordinate and integrate critical information are necessary, in most turbulent environments teams may do more good when they see themselves as responsible for helping organizations "unlearn" rather than just solve problems. Hamel and Prahalad (1994) describe this process as "learning to forget" or "unlearning the past." Their view is that managerial frames serve as genetic codes that are easily passed on by teams from one generation to the next and actually endanger the organization. Organizations, particularly those experiencing success, find it difficult to alter the frame, since it seems impossible that yesterday's environment could be that much different from today's. Hamel and Prahalad tell the story of an experiment that was done with monkeys (p. 51):

Four monkeys were put into a room. In the center of the room was a tall pole with a bunch of bananas suspended from the top. One particularly hungry monkey eagerly scampered up the pole, intent on retrieving a banana. Just as he reached out to grasp the banana, he was hit with [a] torrent of cold water from an overhead shower. With a squeal, the monkey abandoned its quest and retreated down the pole. Each monkey attempted, in turn, to secure the banana. Each received an equally chilly shower, and each scampered down without the prize. After repeated drenchings, the monkeys finally gave up on the bananas.

With the primates' huts conditioned, one of the original four was removed from the experiment and a new monkey added. No sooner had this new, innocent monkey started up the pole than his companions reached up and yanked the surprised creature back down the pole. The monkey got the message—don't climb that pole. After a few such aborted attempts, but without ever having received a cold shower, the new monkey stopped trying to get the bananas. One by one, each of the original monkeys was replaced. Each new monkey learned the same lesson: Don't climb the pole. None of the new monkeys ever made it to the top of the pole; none even got so far as a cold shower. Not one understood precisely why pole climbing was discouraged, but they all respected the well-established precedent. Even after the shower was removed, no monkey ventured up the pole.

Teams, if properly charged, can keep health care organizations from repeating processes and implementing solutions that have outlived their usefulness. In this way teams can call attention to the need to reenvision the future, invent new strategies, question yesterday's approaches to the delivery of health care, and sustain competitive advantage. Only when this kind of organizational unlearning occurs can real learning take place as well. According to this view, teams are not just gathering information and seeking solutions; rather, they are engaged in questioning and in helping clarify what issues need addressing by the organization.

Assumption #3:	*Teams help create order in organizations.*
Revision:	*Effective teams help create disorder in organizations.*

When teams are used to increase workers' commitment or acceptance or are used to uncover information needed to solve problems already identified, the implicit assumption prevails that a new kind of order will be restored to these organizations. A more motivated work force enables managers to meet organizational goals more easily. The systematic processing of information needed to solve organizational problems is consistent with a rational approach to management and increases the likelihood that organizational intentions will be realized.

However, the use of teams for sensemaking, for developing collective meaning in organizations is a messy process (Weick, 1995). When teams are charged with helping manage the unknowable, conflict occurs, disagreement is evident, and polar assumptions come into plain view. The process of figuring out what events mean and developing a collective understanding of what has transpired is neither orderly nor one with which many managers will be comfortable. It means a lack of closure when we want closure. It means disagreement when we want agreement. But ultimately, it means a better shot at developing a picture of the world and our environment that makes sense. "People argue their way into a new sense of what they confront" (Weick, 1995, p. 145).

Complex adaptive systems are characterized by irregularity and disorder. Because such systems face unpredictable, unfolding futures, they do not respond to intentional, rational approaches to restructuring. Rather, "irregularity and disorder can occur because of the nature of the system itself—individuals are free to disrupt institutions" (Stacey, 1995, p. 480). Teams, in such systems, are subsystems that reflect the characteristics of the larger system. Thus, successful teams will be those skilled in argument, dialogue, and conflict surfacing—all of which are disorderly processes for most organizations.

Assumption #4:   *Teams enable execution of the organization's strategy.*
Revision: *Effective teams alter the organization's strategy.*

Participation in decision making has traditionally been encouraged as a way of ensuring that those employees who are to execute the decisions will understand those decisions better (Lawler and Hackman, 1969; Locke and Schweiger, 1979). This view, lodged in the Newtonian perspective, suggests that the manager's primary job is to ensure that intentions result in outcomes. From this perspective, teamwork is a way of improving the chances of realizing the organization's strategic intentions. Thus, the conversation about the role of middle managers in strategy formulation has taken on significance largely because it is believed that middle managers responsible for implementing strategy will be more successful if they are also involved in formulating the strategy, because they will then have a better understanding of the organization's strategic goals. For example, Floyd and Wooldridge (1992, p. 27) assert that "unsuccessful execution of strategy is caused by middle and operating-level managers who are either ill-informed or unsupportive of the chosen direction." Guth and MacMillan (1986) further warn that middle managers who are left out of the formulation process or are inadequately informed of the strategy may deliberately sabotage its implementation. Approaches to strategic management therefore encourage strategy formulation teams to expand to include the implementers so that the implementers will better understand—and thus be better equipped to implement—strategic decisions.

Beyond their role in formulating strategy, teams have perhaps received the most attention as a way of assuring strategic goals related to quality improvements. Due to American perceptions of the success teams in Japanese companies have achieved in improving quality, American companies have followed the trend toward organizing around teams. Teams are now a common mechanism in many corporate restructuring and reengineering efforts, and in most cases they are charged with improving productivity and processes related to achieving the organization's goals.

Nahavandi and Aranda (1994), however, argue that teams have not done for the United States what they did and still do for Japan. Whereas quality improvements have occurred in US companies, it is not clear that those improvements are attributable to teams. Sitkin et al. (1994) observe that traditional approaches to total quality management (TQM), which advocates the use of teams, emphasize control and do not enable the learning-oriented behavior necessary for the highly uncertain conditions that created the need for TQM in the first place.

The alternative view of organizations as complex adaptive systems allows teams to be seen as playing a role in altering the organization's strategy. When teams are viewed as vehicles for sensemaking, their interpretations and the meaning they uncover will inform the organization's strategy and most likely alter it. Mintzberg argues that "formulation and implementation [should] merge into a fluid process of learning through which creative strategies evolve" (p. 105). In highly turbulent environments, firms will need "an ability to create the future" (D'Aveni, 1995, p. 240). And in the fast-changing world of health care, organizations need to move beyond teamwork as a way of improving strategy execution and rely on them more to develop a collective picture of the organization's ideal future and Figure out how best to bring it about. This highly ambiguous task of helping the organization reinvent itself will not be easy. Argyris (1990) suggests that most management teams may function well for routine concerns, but break down under the pressure created by confronting complex issues that may be embarrassing or threatening.

The world in which health care organizations exist is much too complex for even a top management team to formulate strategy. Yet those health professionals who implement many of their organization's strategies need to be viewed as strategy formulators rather than just implementers. Further, the sensemaking, the development of a shared understanding of what providing high-quality health care now means, will be possible only when it is done by teams comprising a full range of health care professionals. The ongoing assessment and reinvention of the organization's strategy must be seen as a job for multiple teams within most health care organizations.

Assumption # 5:   *Teams support and reinforce the hierarchy.*
Revision: *Effective teams undermine the hierarchy.*

A common prescription regarding the design of teams is that attention be given to the organizational levels they need to represent, the specific managers who will be given responsibility for team outcomes, and their proper reporting relationship (Galbraith, 1977). Teams are often established for the purpose of carrying out the intentions of top management, and care therefore is taken to ensure the appropriate vertical and lateral relations within the organization.

One of the reasons teams have met with difficulties is that they invariably undermine some existing distribution of power. Middle managers often see employee teams as a threat to their authority, while employees see teams as a source of division. A common frustration with matrix organizations, which make significant use of teams, is that the structural difficulties are too great for some. Reporting to a functional leader and a project leader proves difficult. These concerns are real, and organizations using teams would be better off recognizing that teams operate in conflict rather than in harmony with the organization's existing hierarchy. From a Newtonion perspective, this tension is a problem. But according to the view of organizations as complex adaptive systems, this tension is a normal condition, one that in fact encourages the health of the system.

> Teams in business tend to spend their time fighting for turf, avoiding anything that will make them look bad personally, and pretending that everyone is behind the team's collective strategy—maintaining the appearance of a cohesive team. To keep up the image they seek to squelch disagreement; people with serious reservations avoid stating them publicly, and joint decisions are watered-down compromises reflecting what everyone can live with, or else reflecting one person's view foisted on the group (Senge, 1990).

Assumption # 6:   *Teams are guided by the organization's belief systems.*
Revision: *Effective teams challenge the organization's belief systems.*

Most managerial prescriptions for how to get the most out of teams call for a clear and guiding vision by the leader. This vision derives from the organization's belief system or may even contribute to the definition of that belief system.

In highly turbulent environments, teams will challenge the organization's belief systems as they try to make sense of what is happening, which is precisely what effective teams should be doing in such environments. Challenging, questioning, provoking—these are the activities that such organizations need. However, as Senge (1990) argues, most managers find collective inquiry threatening because they are trained never to admit that they don't know the answer.

In the health care industry, where so much of the industry structure has been and continues to be redefined, organizations that were once in one kind of business now find themselves in another kind of business. Hospitals, for example, used to think they were in the medical care delivery business; now they find themselves in the health care delivery business. This fundamental change necessitates an alteration in their belief system. Effective teams can see realignments in the environment and can grasp the ways in which the public thinks differently about health care and the roles of providers have changed. These kinds of changes signal the need for a constantly evolving belief system. Traditional approaches to managing organizations assumed that the organization already had a vision—usually that of its top managers—and that this vision was expressed in the organization's belief system. To accomplish their work, teams took the vision and/or belief system and used it to direct the execution of their tasks. Now, as intended strategies give way to emergent strategies, so too do assumed belief systems give way to evolving ones. Effective teams help define, clarify, and give meaning to the organization's emergent belief system.

> *Assumption # 7:*   *Teams are empowered by top management.*
> *Revision:*   *Effective teams empower themselves.*

Conventional wisdom says that teams have to be empowered by top management (Conger and Kanungo, 1988) in order to function. Such empowerment usually refers to widespread participation, the dispersal of power throughout the organization, and the establishment of teams of employees who are charged with making and implementing the decisions necessary for redesigning their jobs (Senge, 1990; Stacey, 1992). In a common view of empowerment reflected in the words of Ford and Fottler (1995, p. 22), "a manager could choose to provide higher degrees of empowerment for some individuals and teams doing certain tasks than for others." The assumption is that empowerment occurs to the degree that managers allow it to. From a Newtonian perspective, empowerment is still a control mechanism.

Organizations confronting the "unknowable" (Stacey, 1992, p. 196) face everchanging and open-ended issues that are best addressed through teams operating in a spontaneous and self-organizing way. Such teams help top management explore the strategic agenda and enable new visions and possibilities to emerge. These self-organizing teams are necessary so that organizations can innovate and reinvent themselves (Hamel and Prahalad, 1994); they cannot be controlled by top managers. As Stacey (1992) argues:

> A team can be truly self-organizing only if it discovers its own goals and objectives. This means that top managers setting up such a team must avoid the temptation to write terms of reference, set objectives or prod the group to reach some predetermined conclusion. They must limit themselves to presenting the groups with some ambiguous challenge (p. 196).

The participants in such teams empower themselves because power is derived not so much from the organization's hierarchy but from their own ability to influence one another and contribute to sensemaking conversations. The ability to argue, convince, and persuade others is what empowers these teams.

When teams are responsible for specific task execution, managers can "empower" teams. But when the role of teams as complex adaptive systems is to participate in producing the organization's unfolding and unpredictable future, empowerment derives elsewhere. In this alternative role, teams are responsible for recognizing an organizational situation—often in the face of contradictory information—and helping the organization make sense out of what they see. In this arena teams empower themselves in how they talk about contradictions, surface new mental models, and give meaning to what they see. When they serve in this way as interpretation systems for organizations (Daft and Weick, 1984), it is difficult for managers to empower teams to interpret; rather, it is team members' abilities to interpret confusing information that give them power.

𝕰𝕬 MAKING TEAMS MORE EFFECTIVE

Given the variety of ways in which teams can and should be used in organizations, how can managers create an environment in which teams can flourish? How can managers contribute to the building of effective teams? At least five considerations can improve the way in which teams are put together and the way in which they function. First, teams are clearly a way of increasing the amount of participation in either sensemaking or problem solving. Thus, it is important for managers to consider the multiple dimensions of participation and the ways in which teams can affect each of those dimensions. Second, teams—particularly self-managed teams, or those that are going to be ongoing—will go through stages of development as a group. Managers should consider those stages, anticipate the difficulties encountered at each stage, and help facilitate the transition from one stage to another. Third, teams will increasingly serve as the organization's collective mind. Therefore, it is important to consider how teams develop such a collective mind, which may be quite different from the process by which they develop as a group. Fourth, when teams function as decision-making groups, they can use structured approaches to decision making to improve the process. Fifth, as teams serve more and more as sensemaking mechanisms, and as the environments in which health care organizations become increasingly complex, conflict will abound. Effective teams will not shy away from conflict; rather, they will be skilled at surfacing and managing conflict.

Teams as Participation Mechanisms

This chapter has expressed the view that teams are a mechanism for participation in the organization—in particular, to bring about the unfolding future of the organization. Participation is typically defined as a mechanism for joint decision making (Leana, 1987; Locke and Schweiger, 1979). Ashmos and McDaniel (1991) identify several components of participation, based on an information-processing view of participation (see Figure 10.1). Participation in decision making involves the following components: the percentage of the group to be involved, the breadth of the group's participation, and the proportion of decision makers in the group. Participation also includes the timing of the group's involvement, the decision-making activities in which the group played a part, and the organizational mechanisms through which the group participated. More participation is characterized by a higher percentage, greater breadth, higher proportion, earlier entrance into the decision-making process,

Figure 10.1   Format for the Balance Sheet

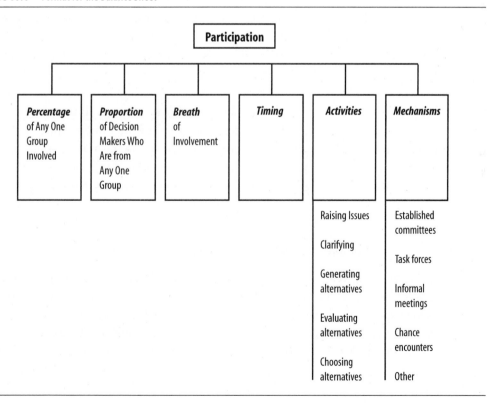

being part of several decision activities, and involvement through several mechanisms (Ashmos and McDaniel, 1996).

Teams are an effective way for managers to increase the percentage of people from any one professional group in health care organizations involved in decision making or sensemaking. When constructing teams in health care organizations, managers should ask themselves the question, what percentage of any one group needs to be involved in sensemaking or solving critical organizational problems? Asking this question is a reminder to push for heterogeneity across teams as a way of complicating the organization's approach to the issues at hand.

Teams are also an effective way of increasing the breadth and proportion of participants outside the top management group. Again, when health care managers consider the breadth and proportion question in establishing teams, the sensemaking "work force" will ultimately be more diverse, yielding a richer picture of what is happening in and around the organization.

In working with teams, it is important for managers to consider when to assemble teams—that is, early or late in the life of an issue. Sabatier (1978), for example, has shown that when organizational members are involved early in the life of a strategic issue, their ability to influence the way the issue is resolved improves.

It is also important to think about which of the decision-making or sensemaking activities are most suited to teams: identifying the problem, clarifying the problem, generating alternatives, evaluating alternatives, or choosing from among alternatives. Organizations may want to use one team for one of these activities and a different team for yet another.

Finally, the participation model can help guide the manager in considering what kind of formal arrangement will best serve the needs of the issue around which the team is being formed. In some cases, for example, the team may need to be constructed as a more or less permanent structural appendage, whereas in other cases the team should be designed with its own sunset clause and schedule for dissolution.

Development of the Team as a Group

Teams that interact on an ongoing basis and are responsible for getting work done or for problem solving will cohere as a group in stages. The development of a team is a dynamic process, which never reaches stability. However, there is strong evidence that most groups experience a pattern of behavior that reflects at least four stages: forming, storming (or differentiation), norming (or integration), and performing (or maturity) (Albanese and Van Fleet, 1983; Tuckman and Jensen, 1977; Hillreigel and Slocum, 1993).

Forming: When a team first comes together, the group members get acquainted, test the waters for what is acceptable group conduct, and begin to identify themselves as part of the team. This stage is characterized by considerable uncertainty as team members try to understand their role and the role of others.

Storming/differentiation: Once team members begin to feel comfortable with their role, conflict inevitably occurs. This stage may involve resistance to the group, emotional responses to the role of the team, and interpersonal hostility. There may be conflict over the group's attempt to constrain individuals or over leadership roles.

Norming/integration: This third stage occurs after some agreement on roles for the group and leaders has been reached and group cohesion starts to occur. Team members begin to identify with a common purpose, share values, and experience camaraderie. This is the stage at which there is most danger of groupthink, because team loyalty becomes important.

Performing/maturity: This final stage occurs when team members are aware of one another's strengths and weaknesses, have accepted individual differences, and function efficiently and effectively. At this stage the group has a structure for dealing with conflict and for moving on.

Development of the Team as Collective Mind

As teams are used for a greater variety of purposes in organizations (some teams may function like permanent workgroups, whereas others are more temporary and focus on trying to make sense out of ambiguous organizational events) and as membership in teams is likely to be more and more fluid, attention to the development of collective mind becomes critical. In particular, if teams are to have responsibility for helping an organization make sense of its world and collectively give meaning to its unfolding future, it is important to consider the development of the team as a collective mind as well as the development of the team as a group. Weick and Roberts describe collective mind as a pattern of heedful interrelations of actions in a social system (1993, p. 357), which is important to organizations because it results in fewer organizational errors. They point out, however, that a group may be in a mature developmental stage as a group and yet undeveloped as a collective mind. When groupthink occurs, it can be said that the group is relatively mature—having moved through the stages of forming, storming and norming—but acts heedlessly, an indication of undeveloped collective mind. Similarly, it is possible for a group to be undeveloped, yet act heedfully, as is the case with temporary aircraft cockpits or jazz improvisation (Weick and Roberts, 1993).

Weick and Roberts suggest three features of heedful interrelating: heedful contributing, heedful representing, and heedful subordinating. Each of these contributes to making the pattern of interrelating more complex, improving the team's ability to sense and understand the complexity created by unexpected events (Weick and Roberts, 1993, p. 366).

Heedful contributing occurs when teams are diverse in membership, when they are loosely coupled to a broad range of other activity systems within the organization, and when communication is intentional and strategic. *Heedful representing* takes place when there is mutual respect among team participants and when action is well coordinated. *Heedful subordinating* occurs when there is trust within the group.

To enable teams to develop as collective mind, health care managers should pay attention to these three factors. Intentionality about the membership of the team, its relationship to other teams, and its method of communication foster the development of the collective mind. Developing respect and trust among members is also essential.

Using Teams for Group Decision Making

Health care organizations face a variety of tasks and rely on varying degrees of interdependency to solve problems. Decision making by teams is likely to be superior to individual decision making when (1) the greater diversity and amount of expertise and knowledge found in a group is relevant to the issue at hand, (2) the collective ability of the group to process information and develop interpretations is greater than that of any one individual, (3) the issue confronting the organization is complex and ambiguous, and (4) the issue affects a wide range of organizational members, many of whom will have some responsibility in implementing solutions to the problem.

Team decision making is not without its difficulties. In addition to there being potential for groupthink among cohesive teams, team members can also easily feel their time has been wasted when it could have been used more valuably on other tasks. Two major considerations for effective team decision making are (1) fostering creativity and (2) surfacing and managing conflict.

Fostering Creativity.   One way of fostering creativity in teams is through *brainstorming*. Traditional brainstorming is usually done with a team of 5 to 12 people, each of whom states as many ideas as possible within a given period, preferably 20 to 60 minutes. In brainstorming sessions (1) the wilder the ideas the better, (2) no one can be critical of others' ideas, (3) members are encouraged to build from other ideas or combine previously stated ideas (Osborn, 1957).

Brainstorming is primarily a process for generating ideas and does not lead to a team consensus. An even more effective approach is the *nominal group technique (NGT)* (Delbecq, Van de Ven, and Gustafson, 1975), a structured process for creative decision making ensuring that everyone on the team is heard and that consensus is reached. Using this process, team members pool their individual judgments in order to solve a particular problem and determine an appropriate course of action. This technique is especially useful for teams that do not have a lengthy history of being together as a group or whose membership changes frequently. It is called "nominal" because it does not require the group to be an ongoing, interacting group with established norms, roles, and patterns of behavior. It is an excellent process for use with a group "in name only." Group members are all physically present, as in a typical committee meeting, but the members function independently. A problem is presented and the following steps are then taken:

1. Before any discussion takes place among the team, each team member silently and independently writes down his or her ideas for solving the problem.
2. Following the silent period, each team member (one at a time, in round-robin fashion) presents one idea to the group . All ideas are recorded for the team to see. No discussion takes place until all ideas have been recorded.
3. After all the individuals have presented their ideas, the group discusses the ideas for clarity and evaluation. Ideas are then merged, eliminated, expanded, or altered.
4. Each team member privately votes on his or her preferred ideas. This could be done by having each person list an order of preference. The final decision is determined by the idea with the highest aggregate ranking.

The primary advantage of the NGT is that it encourages independent thinking in the midst of a formal team meeting. Everyone participates and expresses opinions while building consensus among the members. NGT is considered more effective than brainstorming because in face-to-face brainstorming an individual may get bogged down in generating new ideas by waiting for another person to finish talking. In brainstorming, team members may be concerned about how others will view their ideas. The advantage of NGT is that individuals initially write down their own ideas on paper, so that the act of sharing the idea later seems more objective and less personal (Huber, 1980). As teams become more and more fluid, or in some cases experience a short life and in other cases long life, the benefits of NGT become increasingly important. When teams are undeveloped as a group, NGT is an effective way of maximizing input from individuals in the team in a collective setting.

Surfacing and Managing Conflict.   Conflict is a normal condition of organizational life, and certainly a pervasive aspect of working together in teams. The view of teams presented in this chapter argues strongly for the use of teams for collectively making sense out of what is happening, a process that is laden with conflict. Weick (1995, p. 36) explains that this conflict arises because "divergent, antagonistic, imbalanced forces are woven throughout acts of sensemaking."

Rather than avoid conflict, health care managers should learn how to foster disagreement and surface conflict. Two structured approaches to programmed conflict can help managers surface disagreements and use conflict creatively (Cosier and Schwenk, 1990).

1. **Devil's advocacy**— The devil's advocate method of programmed conflict calls for an individual or small group of individuals to develop a systematic critique of an idea or a set of ideas (Cosier and Schwenk, 1990). The person assigned the role of devil's advocate tries to uncover and articulate weaknesses in the assumptions underlying the idea, internal inconsistencies, and problems that could develop if the idea were pursued. The role of devil's advocate should be rotated so that no one person is identified as the critic on all issues. An advantage of this approach is that when individuals are required to present contrary arguments, others are likely to feel more comfortable disagreeing and the conflict will seem less personal and emotional.

2. **Dialectical inquiry**— Dialectical inquiry is more structured than the devil's advocacy approach because it requires a structured debate between two conflicting courses of action. This method, which can be traced back to Plato and Aristotle, involves synthesizing the conflicting views of a thesis and an antithesis (Cosier and Schwenk, 1990). The advantage of this approach is that organizational members have the opportunity to hear a well-prepared debate of the assumptions underlying two contrary proposals. False and misleading assumptions become apparent, and decisions based on such assumptions can then be avoided.

This chapter suggests that managers can be more successful at building effective teams if they pay attention to participation, the developmental stages of groups, development of the collective mind, ways to enhance group decision making, and conflict management. The question arises, how will I know if the team has been effective or not? Hellreigel and Slocum (1992) offer the following seven criteria for team effectiveness.

1. Members know why the team exists.
2. Members have adopted procedures for making decisions.
3. Members have achieved trust and openness among themselves.
4. Members have learned to receive help from and give help to one another.
5. Members have achieved a sense of freedom to be themselves, while feeling a sense of belongingness with others.
6. Members have learned to accept and deal with conflict within the team.
7. Members have learned to improve their own functioning.

❧ THINKING ABOUT TEAMS FOR THE FUTURE

In response to increasing complexity, many health care organizations have begun using teams, yet as Delbecq and Gil (1985) point out, "recent accounts of teamwork and collaboration efforts in hospitals and medical centers have been noticeably ineffective" (p. 145). Fortune magazine quotes Ed Lawler on teams: "Teams are the Ferraris of work design. They're high performance but high maintenance and expensive" (1994, p. 86). Teams will most likely become an increasingly essential part of organizational life in the future. Whether they are used for accomplishing specific work tasks, or for the more equivocal task described in this chapter of helping the organization make sense out of the future as it unfolds, teamwork requires attention and intentionality. As organizations find themselves facing complex and turbulent environments, as technology continues to develop at a rapid pace, and as it becomes increasingly difficult to develop new and creative ways to create and sustain competitive advantage, the nature of teams in organizations will change. These kinds of changes make it likely that teams will assume any or all of the following forms.

Teams When There Is No Face-to-Face

As health care delivery systems become larger, more complex and more geographically dispersed, it will be more and more common for teams to be formed that seldom meet in person. Within a hospital system, teams will likely be created that rarely meet in a given room at a given time but conduct business throughout the year. Thus, typical approaches to team building focusing on building trust, sharing experiences, developing relationships—and relying on face-to-face contact to achieve these outcomes—will have to give way to other approaches.

Virtual Teams

Given the increasing pace of organizational life and the pressures faced by most managers, there may not be enough time or resources to give teams the longevity that was possible in another time. Thus, it is likely that teamwork in organizations will look more chaotic as teams are constituted, charged, and quickly disbanded. However, managers may need the ongoing contribution of teams long after the team is gone. As Weick (1993, p. 640) observes in describing virtual role systems, "An organization can continue to function in the imagination long after it has ceased to function in tangible distributed activities." The same is likely true of teams. If the team stays intact in the manager's mind, the manager can continue to benefit from the team by simulating team members, their roles, and their perspectives long after the team has dissolved.

Electronic Teams

Access to e-mail and Internet chat rooms have already changed the way people relate to one another at work. The ease of contact brought about by computer technology allows connections that were not previously possible and expands the definition of what it means to be a team. Electronic teams share many of the characteristics of more traditional teams, for example, multiple participants and opinions, access to a broad range of knowledge and expertise, a variety of differing perspectives on a problem. Yet they are also very different. Issues that used to warrant rich media such as face-to-face contact (Lengel and Daft, 1988) may well have to be addressed in the future with less rich media such as e-mail, due to geographical distances between organizational members or shortage of resources for travel. Health care managers will need to pay attention to the nuances of electronic communication and the particular challenges, as well as opportunities, that it poses for building teams in organizations.

Philosophically Diverse Teams

The most critical challenge facing health care organizations today is the sensemaking task described by Weick (1995). Since the future for most health care organizations is unpredictable and unknowable, teams of philosophically diverse people will be the best equipped to envision and understand the future as it unfolds. Diversity ensures the consideration of multiple perspectives, multiple interpretations, and multiple ideas for forging the future. Thus, assembling teams with attention to people's values and perspectives, in addition to their academic disciplines or expertise, will be very important for health care managers.

෭ CONCLUSION

Yes, teams have troubles, as the *Fortune* writer notes. I have tried to suggest that some of the trouble is created by the use of an outdated organizational paradigm, the Newtonian organization, which insists that success comes to managers who command and control their organizations. A command and control approach to the use of teams leads to disappointing outcomes—particularly for organizations operating in extremely turbulent, uncertain times, as many health care organizations are. The view of organizations as complex adaptive systems requires conventional assumptions about teams to give way to a different set of assumptions, which have been explored in this chapter. In this new kind of organization, managers should be specific about the use of teams, considering them mechanisms for increasing participation and recognizing the similarities and differences in how teams develop as groups and as collective minds. There are specific ways in which teams can function better as decision-making groups or as sense-making groups in which conflict and argument abound. Finally, there are a number of possible forms that teams may adopt in the future.

Is teamwork a high-performance possibility? The answer is yes, particularly if used in the right way. Is teamwork a high-maintenance proposition? Undoubtedly it is. Maintaining well-running teams requires rethinking assumptions about their purposes and what it means to work collectively to help organizations navigate the uncharted waters in which they find themselves.

REFERENCES

Albanese, R. and Van Fleet, D. D., 1983. *Organizational Behavior: A Managerial Viewpoint*. Hinsdale, IL: Dryden.

Argyris, C., 1990. *Overcoming Organizational Defenses*. New York: Prentice-Hall.

Ashmos, D. P. and McDaniel, R. R., 1991. Physician participation in hospital strategic decision making: The effect of hospital strategy and decision content. *Health Services Research*, 26 (3), 375–401.

Ashmos, D. P. and McDaniel, R. R., Jr., 1996. Understanding the participation of critical task specialists in strategic decision making. *Decision Sciences*, 27 (1), 103–121.

Cosier, R. A. and Schwenk, C. R., 1990. Agreement and thinking alike: Ingredients for poor decisions. *Academy of Management Executive*, 4 (1), 69–74.

D'Aveni, R. A., 1994. *Hypercompetition: Managing the Dynamics of Strategic Maneuvering*. New York: The Free Press.

Daft, R. L. and Weick, K. E., 1984. Toward a model of organizations as interpretation systems. *Academy of Management Review*, 9 (2), 284–295.

Delbeq, A. L., and Gil, S. L., 1985. Justice as a prelude to teamwork in medical centers. *Health Care Management Review*, 10 (1), 45–51.

Delbeq, A. L., Van de Ven, A. H., and Gustafson, D. H., 1975. *Group Techniques for Program Planning: A Guide to Nominal and Delphi Processes*, Glenview, IL: Scott, Foresman.

Floyd, W. W. and Woolridge, B., 1992. Managing strategic consensus: The foundation of effective implementation. *Academy of Management Executive*, 6 (4), 27–39.

Ford, R. C. and Fottler, M. D., 1995. Empowerment: A matter of degree. *Academy of Management Executive,* 21–31.

Fortune, The Trouble with Teams. Sept. 5, 1994, 86–92.

Galbraith, J. R., 1977. *Organization Design.* Reading, MA: Addison-Wesley.

Guth, W. D. and Macmillan, I. C., 1986. Strategy implementation versus middle management self-interest. *Strategic Management Journal,* 7 (4), 313–328.

Hamel, G. and Prahalad, C. K., 1994. *Competing for the Future.* Boston: Harvard Business School Press.

Hellreigel, D. and Slocum, J. W., 1992. *Management.* Reading, MA: Addison-Wesley.

Hirschorn, L., 1991. *Managing in the New Team Environment: Skills, Tools, and Methods.* Reading: MA: Addison-Wesley.

Huber, G. P., 1980. *Managerial Decision Making.* Glenview, IL.: Scott-Foresman.

Huber, G. P. and Daft, R. L., 1987. The information environments of organizations. In F. M. Jablin, L. L. Putnam, K. K. Roberts and L. W. Porter (eds.), *Handbook of Organizational Communication.* Newbury Park, CA: Sage, 130–164.

Janis, I. R., 1982. *Victims of Groupthink,* 2nd ed. Boston: Houghton Mifflin.

Lawler, E. E., 1988. Choosing an involvement strategy. *Academy of Management Executive,* 2 (3), 197–204.

Lawler, E. E. and Hackman, J. R., 1969. Impact of employee participation in the development of pay incentive plans: A field experiment. *Journal of Applied Psychology,* 53, 467–471.

Leana, C., 1987. Power relinquishment versus power sharing: Theoretical clarification and empirical comparison of delegation and participation. *Journal of Applied Psychology,* 1987, 72(2), 228–233.

Lengel, R. H., and Daft, R. L., 1988. The selection of communication media as an executive skill. *Academy of Management Executive,* 2 (3), 225–232.

Likert, R., 1967. *The Human Organization.* New York: McGraw–Hill.

Locke, E. A. and Schweiger, D. M., 1979. Participation in decision-making: One more look. In B. Staw (ed.), *Research in Organizational Behavior,* Vol. 1. Greenwich, CT: JAI Press, Inc., 265–339.

March, J. G., 1994. *A Primer on Decision Making.* New York: The Free Press.

McGregor, D., 1960. *The Human Side of Enterprise*. New York: McGraw-Hill.

Mintzberg, H., 1987. Crafting strategy. *Harvard Business Review*, 65 (4) July-Aug., 66–75.

Nahavandi, A. and Aranda, E., 1994. Restructuring teams for the re-engineered organization. *Academy of Management Executive*, 8 (4), 58–68.

Osborn, A. F., 1957. *Applied Imagination*, rev. ed. New York: Scribner.

Sabatier, P., 1978. The acquisition and utilization of technical information by administrative agencies. *Administrative Science Quarterly*, 23 (3), 396–417.

Scott, W. R., 1987. *Organizations: Rational, Natural and Open Systems*. Englewood Cliffs, NJ: Prentice-Hall, Inc.

Senge, P. M., 1990. The Fifth Discipline: *The Art and Practice of the Learning Organization*. New York: Doubleday.

Sitkin, S. B., Sutcliffe, K. M., and Schroeder, R. G., 1994. Distinguishing control from learning in total quality management: A contingency perspective. *Academy of Management Review*, 19 (3), 537–564.

Stacey, R. D., 1992. *Managing the Unknowable: Strategic Boundaries Between Order and Chaos in Organizations*. San Francisco, CA: Jossey-Bass.

Stacey, R. D., 1995. The science of complexity: An alternative perspective for strategic change processes. *Strategic Management Journal*, 16 (6), 477–495.

Tuckman, B. W., and Jensen, M.A., 1977. Stages of small group development revisited. *Group and Organizational Studies*, 2, 419–427.

Vroom, V. and Yetton, P. 1973. *Leadership and Decision–Making*. Pittsburgh: University of Pittsburgh Press, 1973.

Vroom, V. and Jago, A., 1988. *The New Leadership: Managing Participation in Organizations*. Englewood Cliffs, NJ: Prentice-Hall.

Weick, K. E., 1979. *The Social Psychology of Organizing*, 2nd. ed. New York: Random House, Inc.

Weick, K. E., 1993. The collapse of sensemaking in organizations: The Mann Gulch disaster. *Administrative Science Quarterly*, 38 (4), 628–652.

Weick, K. E., 1993. Organizational redesign as improvisation. In George P. Huber and William H. Glick (eds.), *Organizational Change and Redesign: Ideas and Insights for Improving Performance*. New York: Oxford University Press, 346–379.

Weick, K. E., 1995. *Sensemaking in Organizations.* Thousand Oaks, CA: Sage Publications, Inc.

Weick, K. E. and Roberts, K. H., 1993. Collective mind in organizations: Heedful interrelating on flight decks. *Administrative Science Quarterly,* 38 (3), 357–381.

Wheatley, M. J., 1992. *Leadership and the New Science: Learning About Organization from an Orderly Universe.* San Francisco, CA: Berrett-Koehler Publishers, Inc.

Strategic Leadership: A View from Quantum and Chaos Theories*

11

Reuben R. McDaniel, Jr., The University of Texas at Austin

ᔕ LEADING IN UNCERTAIN TIMES

Uncertain times in health care are not the result of economic and political pressures, as real as these may seem. Rather, they are the result of the quantum and chaotic nature of the world. This nature is sometimes expressed as economic uncertainty, sometimes as political uncertainty, sometimes as technological uncertainty, and sometimes as the uncertainty that emerges from the fragile nature of the human condition. However, today's science teaches us that these expressions of uncertainty are rooted in a deeper and more fundamental uncertainty: the uncertain state of nature and the uncertain unfolding of the world over time.

* Special thanks to Diane Rhodes and Michelle Walls for their contributions to the development of this chapter. Thanks also to Ruth Anderson, Donde Ashmos, Elena Mota, and anonymous reviewers for useful comments on earlier drafts. The remaining errors are my own.

❧ The Leadership Problem in Health Care

> "In a changing world, it is not just the old answers that are suspect. It is also the old questions" (Weick and Roberts, 1995, p. 186).

The existing health care system is designed to solve an old set of problems. People used to be willing to spend increasing sums of money to avoid taking responsibility for their own health or the way the health care system was delivered. While the health care system, designed primarily to address acute care of a relatively young population, increasingly relied on highly technical interventions controlled by health care providers. When Aaron Wildavsky (1979, p. 285) suggested that we were "doing better and feeling worse," he was not optimistic about the existing medical model's ability to contribute much to resolving this paradox. "Most of the bad things that happen to people's health are at present beyond the reach of medicine. . . . Current medicine has gone as far as it can" (p. 284). Alice Rivlin (1983), in a commencement address at the Rand Graduate Institute, suggested that politicians were moving toward a solution to these problems. "It's pretty simplistic, but may be the only thing to do: put an arbitrary limit on the amount of available money and its rate of growth, and just tell the practitioners to do the best they can. Put the money on the stump and run" (p. 6).

It certainly seems as though health care resources are limited and dwindling. This situation will require significant leadership in the health care community as choices are made about who gets what share of the pie. New insights are required about how to attack behavioral issues such as smoking cessation, weight control, and careless activity leading to the communication of sexually transmitted diseases; and these new insights are likely to require the creation of new kinds of health care organizations. It will not be possible for strategic leaders in health care simply to wait for people—perhaps politicians—or outside forces—perhaps markets—to fix problems.

Comprehensive, government-initiated health care reform may not happen in the United States because political institutions may be structured in ways that make this impossible (Steinmo and Watts, 1995). Some analysts suggest that it is now economics, not politics, that is driving change (Lamm, 1994). However, because of the skewed set of incentives, normal rules of competition may not apply (Teisberg, Porter, and Brown, 1994). People may not trust the private sector and competition to guide change, because sometimes a segment of the private sector of the health care industry makes promises to reform that do not always appear to be fulfilled. For example, the pharmacy industry, according to some studies, has failed to keep its promise to hold drug cost increases at or below the rate of inflation (Families USA Foundation, 1995). Simply depending on the free market to encourage reform may not lead to satisfactory health care solutions.

Managed care is offered as an appropriate strategy. However, it is not always clear that managed care organizations provide acceptable solutions. "The facet of managed care that physicians appear to object to most is the feeling that they have lost control over how they practice medicine" (Richardson, 1992, p. 44). In addition, some are suspicious that managed care reallocates, rather than saves, money. As reported in the *Wall Street Journal*, HMOs seem to have considerable cash, with little idea how to spend it (Anders, 1994). "All told, nine of the biggest publicly traded HMOs are sitting on $9.5 billion of cash, calculates Margeo Vignolla, a health-industry analyst at Salomon Brothers, Inc." (Anders, 1994, p. A1). Of course, some HMOs have developed creative investment strategies, namely, investing in the tobacco industry according to tobacco companies' filings with the Securities and Exchange Commission (Hilzenrath, 1995; Inglis, 1995). It seems doubtful that simply depending on a managed care system for reform will lead to any more satisfactory solutions.

Given reservations about the possibility of markets alone, or managed care alone, to resolve issues in health care, strategic leaders of health care organizations face greater responsibility than ever. They have an opportunity to invent new strategies, perhaps even new organizations, to provide the leadership that health care organizations need in order to be successful. Yet even identifying the meaning of success and the role of managerial factors in achieving these successes will be difficult (Flood, 1994). While new techniques and technologies will be developed, such as improved information systems (Samuelson, 1995) and systems integration (Goldsmith, 1994), the appropriate use of these technologies will require significant strategic leadership. Because the changes in health care will be fundamental, there will be a need for equally fundamental changes in the way health care managers attempt to provide strategic leadership, which will in turn require radically new ways of thinking about health care organizations. Before such new ways of thinking can be explored, it is necessary to understand the existing set of beliefs that still guide many managerial leadership efforts. This understanding will enable one to contrast traditional paradigms with the more modern paradigms essential for providing effective strategic leadership in health care.

❧ TRADITIONAL PARADIGMS FOR MANAGEMENT

Many understandings of organizations are based on Newtonian physics (Capra, 1982; Wheatley, 1992; Stacey, 1992; Keil, 1994; Begun, 1994; Stacey, 1995). In the Newtonian view, in the beginning God created the material particles, the forces between them, and the fundamental laws of motion. In this way the whole universe was set in motion and has continued to run ever since, like a machine, governed by immutable laws. The world is a mechanical system that can be described objectively, without reference to the observer.

Based in part on his understanding of Newton's physics, Locke developed an atomistic view of society, describing it in terms of its basic building block, the human being (Capra, 1982). Locke was guided by the belief that there were laws of nature governing human society similar to the laws governing the physical universe. The function of a social system such as a health care organization, therefore, would not be to impose its laws on people but to discover and enforce natural laws that existed before the social system was formed.

Traditional paradigms of management have relied on Newton and Locke's complementary visions of an orderly and predictable world governed by natural laws. Organizations, according to this view, operate in a deterministic and predictable way, with stability being the dominant mode. Managers seek to discover and enforce natural laws that existed before organizations came into being. Change in organizations will be orderly and regular unless management is flawed. Guided by these philosophical underpinnings and this prescription of an ideal organization, most managers use static models of work and assume that any failure to manage correctly is the result of incompetence or ignorance.

A major role of health care managers in this Newtonian world is decision making, which requires an ability to predict possible outcomes of alternative courses of action (Duncan, Ginter, and Swayne, 1995). Based on these predictions, strategic leaders make and communicate plans. If the expected does not happen, it is because prediction or planning is incorrect. Therefore, management is improved by improving prediction and planning skills. This view leads to the development of ever more sophisticated information systems and ever more sophisticated algorithms for manipulating this information (Owens, Fairchild, and Goldberg, 1994). "Objective information builds consensus and drives good decisions" (Griffith, 1994, p. 265). Prediction and planning lead to success.

The following assumptions are among those that guide the behavior and education of health care leaders using these traditional paradigms:

- Large effects have large causes.
- If a given tactic works once, it can be counted on to work again.
- If managers identify worker needs, then managers can use this knowledge to manipulate workers on behalf of organizations.
- Each person should have a clearly defined role, or job description, and confine himself or herself to the prescribed behavior for that role.
- Organizational structure is fixed, and lines of authority and lines of information flow are the same.

We now understand that these Newtonian-based assumptions are in error and that following them will lead to organizational disaster (Capra, 1982; Stacey, 1992; Wheatley, 1992; Kiel, 1994). Perhaps the most important thing we are learning today about organizations is that if they are going to survive, they must give up their obsession with retaining control, knowing what is going on, and seeking stability (Vaill, 1989; Stacey, 1992; Wheatley, 1992; Bergquist, 1993). The scientific basis for new ways of looking at organizations is not Newtonian physics but quantum theory (Herbert, 1985; Rae, 1986) and chaos theory (Prigogine and Stengers, 1984; Gleick, 1987). These newer understandings of nature, which have long since replaced classical mechanics in physics (Jones, 1992), are now providing significant insights into the design and management of organizations (Stacey, 1992; Wheatley, 1992; Bergquist, 1993; Kiel, 1994; Begun, 1994). The critical nature of the problems facing the current health care system demands that leaders in health care management take advantage of these insights.

❧ EMERGING PARADIGMS FOR MANAGEMENT

In the 20th century, physicists for the first time faced a serious challenge to their ability to understand the universe. Every time they asked nature a question in an atomic experiment, nature answered with a paradox; and the more they tried to clarify the situation, the sharper the paradoxes became (Capra, 1982, p. 64). In contrast to the mechanistic Cartesian view of the world, the world view emerging from modern physics can be characterized by words like organic, holistic, and ecological. The universe is no longer seen as a machine, made up of a multitude of objects, but as one indivisible, dynamic whole whose parts are essentially interrelated and can be understood only as patterns of a cosmic process (Capra, 1982, p. 66).

If we believe that there is a solution to all problems and that the only concern is how smart we are or how hard we are willing to work, we will make fundamental errors in how we approach the world. *On the other hand, if we believe that the world is unknowable, our approach to management and organizations will be fundamentally different.*

Quantum Theory

Quantum theory tells us that the world is unpredictable—not just that we do not have enough information to understand what is going on but that the world is *fundamentally* unknowable. It also tells us that any measurement of a phenomenon affects the phenomenon itself and that relationships between elements are more important in understanding a system than the elements themselves. Because these insights are so far from our traditional beliefs, they are difficult to comprehend. Quantum theory forces us to reconsider our deepest convictions about reality.

Unpredictability. The basic conclusion of quantum theory is that the future behavior of a system is not predictable, regardless of one's certainty about its present state (Rae, 1986, p. 24). Newtonian physics led us to believe that if we knew with sufficient accuracy the present state of a system, we could determine both its complete history and its complete future (Capra, 1982). The quantum world offers no such possibility. In the quantum world the problem is *not* that we do not have enough information about the present state of affairs, or even the past state of affairs, to predict the future. No matter how accurate or complete our information is, the world is fundamentally unknowable. "Indeterminacy is not a matter of our inability to do better" (Rohrlich, 1987, p. 147).

Measurement. When we try to know the world, particularly through measurement of its states, we come face to face with the Heisenberg principle, which states that if one measures position accurately, one must sacrifice an accurate knowledge of momentum (Herbert, 1985, p. 68; Hey and Walters, 1987, pp. 16–18). The more we emphasize one aspect in our description of any phenomenon, the more uncertain the other aspects become (Capra, 1982, p. 68). Therefore, every attempt to know one attribute of a system reduces our ability to understand its other attributes.

The world is not independent of the observer (Herbert, 1985). No longer can we study anything as separate from ourselves. What we see in the quantum world depends on what we are looking for. We now know that measurement of one property of a system (its position) destroys the other property of the system (momentum). When we attempt to describe an electron, if we look for waves, we see waves; but if we look for particles, we see particles. An electron is thus a particle or a wave depending on what one is looking for. It is the intention of the observer that determines what is observed.

Obtaining some knowledge about an object excludes the possibility of simultaneously obtaining certain other knowledge about it. For example, it is impossible to make calm and complete observations of a patient's mental state while trying to perform highly technical diagnostic or treatment procedures. The very act of checking a person's blood pressure or weight creates anxieties that make it difficult to get other information from that person. Likewise, patient satisfaction surveys call attention to certain aspects of the client's experience and fail to notice other aspects. These difficulties are the result not of bad measurement but of the very nature of measurement processes. We must therefore look carefully at the things we think we know through measurement, because in fact we may not know the truly important things about a situation.

Relationships.   In modern physics, the image of the universe as a machine is superseded by a view of the universe as one indivisible, dynamic whole whose parts are interrelated in truly fundamental ways. All events are connected, but these connections are not causal in a classical sense. A classical view of connections is expressed in terms of mechanical linkages, where things are pushing and pulling on each other and each element is trying to resist the influence of the other. When these connections are considered, they are thought of in terms of causes and effects. The fundamental questions in classical physics are concerned with the properties of each element; connections take a back seat to individual elements. But in a quantum world, it is connections or relationships between things that count, not the things themselves. Each thing derives its meaning from its relationships with other things, not from its fundamental local properties (Herbert, 1985, especially pp. 210–31).

Relationships are all there is to reality, and nothing exists independent of its relationships with the environment. According to Niels Bohr, "Isolated material particles are abstractions, their properties being definable and observable only through their interactions with other systems" (Herbert, 1985, p. 161).

One example of the importance of relationships in health care is the nature of nursing work. Nursing functions in a health care setting are defined in part by the relationship of nursing to both medical and housekeeping functions. These relationships contribute to the definition of what constitutes appropriate work for nursing staff. Another example of the importance of relationships is the fact that patient health is sometimes understood relative to a previous physical state ("I am so much better than I was") and sometimes relative to what a physician thinks is possible ("You are so much better off than some of my other patients with this disease"). Patient satisfaction surveys, often used to assess the quality of a health care system, are greatly influenced by the particular relationship the patient has in mind when filling out the survey. Failure by strategic leaders to recognize the critical importance of relationships may lead to misallocation of nursing staff and misinterpretation of patient surveys.

Chaos Theory

A basic concern in chaos theory is the way in which nonlinear systems change over time. Nonlinear dynamic systems are those in which the relationships between time-dependent variables are nonlinear. These interactions have three types of outcomes (Kiel, 1994): (1) stability, the dampening of effects through negative feedback; (2) instability, small changes that accumulate and explode because of positive feedback; and (3) chaos, randomness within constraints, because the interaction of positive and negative feedback in the system causes a point attractor to develop that is independent of time.

Chaos theory provides insights into the nature of complex adaptive systems such as health care organizations that respond both to feedback and feedforward and are operating in turbulent environments.

Unknowability.   A fundamental insight of chaos theory is that the unfolding of the world over time is unknowable. One reason that the future state of a chaotic system is unknowable is its sensitive dependence on initial conditions (Kellert, 1993; Thiétart and Forgues, 1995). Any error in measurement of a system's initial state, no matter how small that error is, will eventually "become comparable to the predicted values— and from that moment on, your prediction will bear no useful relation to the actual behavior" (Cohen and Stewart, 1994, p. 191). In addition, chaotic systems are unknowable because of the nonlinear, time-dependent relationships between system elements (Prigogine and Stengers, 1984). "Chaotic systems scrupulously obey the strictures of differential dynamics, unique evolution, and value determinateness, yet they are utterly unpredictable. Because of the existence of these systems, we are forced to admit that the world is not totally predictable: by any definition of determinism that includes total predictability, determinism is false" (Kellert, 1993, p. 62).

Therefore, strategic leaders cannot control long-term outcomes for organizations. While new patterns of behavior are likely to fall within recognizable sets, they are never exactly the same as previous behaviors. Leaders cannot determine future states of organizations. For example, the emerging role of primary care providers as gatekeepers in health care is reshaping the patterns of behavior among physicians and between primary care physicians and hospitals. Because strategic leaders cannot control the direction of these new patterns of behavior, they cannot determine the future state of physician-hospital relationships. No matter how successful or unsuccessful previous managerial actions were in establishing good physician-hospital relationships, the new situation is indeterminate and the strategic leader is not in control.

Small Causes.   Small (very small) differences in initial conditions can quickly (very quickly) lead to large (very large) differences in the future state of a system. This understanding suggests that it is extremely unlikely that one health care organization will be able to follow the example of another and achieve the same results. This means that management techniques such as benchmarking need to be very carefully evaluated. Even if organizational situations look alike, they are not; and the small difference in initial conditions may lead to radically different outcomes of any management action. Changes in small places create large systems change, not because they build one upon the other but because they share in the unbroken wholeness that has united them all along (Waldrop, 1992). A seemingly small adjustment in the scheduling of nursing staff may completely disrupt physician-nurse relationships or completely upset a previously smoothly running emergency room. Quantum theory and chaos theory each suggest that more attention in organizations needs to be given to little things—in particular, those little things that are generating positive feedback in the system. "The changing relationships between cause and effect often defy management's best efforts at control and lead to unintended consequences" (Kiel, 1994, p. 33). Information flows across space and time in unpredictable ways, creating new structures and forms as the situation requires. Managing these information interactions requires a new understanding of the oneness of the universe, even as the parts create their own uniqueness.

❧ LEADERSHIP TASKS

What leadership tasks do these emerging paradigms suggest for health care managers? Clearly, the old standards of planning, organizing, controlling, and decision making are inadequate for the world of quantum relationships and chaotic, time-dependent organizational development. Nor is leadership simply a question of motivation and communication. Rather, strategic leadership in health care will require attention to sensemaking, learning, and designing.

Sensemaking

Organizations are social structures seeking meaning. Because the world is unknowable, meaning cannot be gained through efforts at rational behavior. Rather, meaning must come through the making of sense. The problem is not the bounded rationality of decision makers but the fundamental unpredictability of the world. Sensemaking is not a "stopgap" measure but a strength of organizations. "The goal of organizations, viewed as sensemaking systems is to create and identify events that recur to stabilize their environment and make them more predictable" (Weick, 1995, p. 170). Note that the goal is not to find predictability but to make predictability. Sensemaking is enhanced through paying attention, complicating yourself, and developing collective mind.

Paying Attention.   The nature of reality as we now understand it through the new sciences requires strategic leaders to pay attention to and carefully observe the world as it unfolds. Organizational survival is often a struggle for alertness (Weick and Roberts, 1993, p. 374); and the valuable item in short supply in organizations is not information but attention (Simon, 1994). Right now, most health care leaders have too much information on their desks. What they don't have is the time to pay close attention to the world around them so that they can notice, in a thoughtful way, important changes and developments that are occurring (Senge, 1990; Argyris, 1992).

Beyond creating time for attention, leaders must create a greater variety of ways to pay attention. Leaders can structure patterns of relationships within organizations that enable all stakeholders to become more careful observers and to be more attentive to the world around them. Conversely, leaders can organize in ways that block the ability to observe and limit the range of attention. Being careful is a social act. To act with care, people must see how their behavior relates to that of others and must understand their behavior in the context of joint action with others. This suggests that the notion of dual hierarchies as a strategy for simplifying the management of clinical and administrative functions in health care organizations may be extremely dysfunctional for the overall health of the system because it limits the range of attention and obstructs people from truly acting with care.

Complicate Yourself. Traditional views of organizations focus on ways to simplify things in an effort to gain control (La Porte, 1975). In complex adaptive systems, however, oversimplification leads to errors, because if an organization is simple, it misses and/or masks the complexity that is out there in the environment (La Porte, 1975; Weick, 1979). Health care executives must therefore complicate their organizations so that they are in a position to cope with complicated environments as they unfold over time. Complexity is something to be applauded, not shunned; it is simplifying organizations in order to gain control that is dysfunctional. Rather, leaders must seek to develop complicated sets of relationships within organizations, networks of information-driven connections that enable organizations to create order from a chaotic world (Senge, 1990; Freedman, 1992). The purpose of organizing, therefore, is to complicate things rather than simplify them—and to complicate things in organized ways that enable people, with their bounded rationality, to function and contribute.

A key strategy for complicating organizations is to make them more diverse. "Complicated observers take in more. They see patterns that less complicated people miss, and they exploit these subtle patterns by concentrating on them and ignoring everything else" (Weick, 1979, p. 193). Some ways of thinking about the world see homogeneity as desirable, whereas others favor heterogeneity (Glick, Miller, and Huber, 1993). If leaders focus on homogeneity, they will try to make everybody like everyone else, and their organizations will make little contribution. Groupthink and decreased decision-making effectiveness represent very real dangers for organizations where newcomers behave and think like those who have always been a central part of the organization (Janis, 1989). Oversocialization or socialization that occurs too quickly reduces people's potential contribution to organizational growth and development. It also increases the probability that people will change to fit organizations rather than change organizations so that they can cope with developing situations (March, Sproull, and Tamuz, 1991). It is only when diverse groups focus on heterogeneity and their own unique characteristics that they generate the energy required for survival. Health care executives should therefore encourage heterogeneity in their organizations by de-emphasizing socialization behaviors and emphasizing the value of diverse points of view.

Here are some other ways in which organizations complicate themselves:

- They engage in parallel information processing.
- They use more real-time information.
- They use multiple advisers.
- They increase the number of goals.
- They broaden the number of strategic activities.
- They deepen the involvement of workers.
- They increase decentralization.
- They decrease formalization.
- They expand the number of scanning activities.
- They increase the number of people with external contacts.
- They pursue multiple generic strategies.

Successful adaptive systems tend to move toward increasing complexity because of selection pressures favoring complexity. Systems with the highest complexity tend to increase in complexity (Gell-Mann, 1994, p. 371), and more complex organizations tend to be more successful. The death of organizations is not random but reflects a preference for young organizations, namely, those that are not yet complex enough to be adaptable. Older organizations are less likely to die. This difference suggests that the adaptive mechanisms are not constant and that a state of equilibrium may not exist for adaptive systems, nor for real organizations in a dynamic environment.

Develop Collective Mind.　In a world defined by quantum theory and chaos theory, there are significant strategic advantages to be gained by concentrating on the development of collective mind. A well-developed organizational mind is a social element built of ongoing interrelating and dense interrelationships (Weick and Roberts, 1993). Reliable performance requires a well-developed collective mind in the form of a complex, attentive system, tied together by trust.

A smart system does the right thing regardless of its structure and regardless of whether the environment is stable or turbulent. We suspect that organic systems, because of their capacity to reconfigure themselves temporarily into more mechanistic structures, have more fully developed minds than do mechanistic systems (Weick and Roberts, 1993, p. 377).

Do not confuse the idea of a well-developed group mind with that of a well-developed group. *Undeveloped group—developed mind* suggests "coordination of actions over alignment of cognitions, mutual respect over agreement, trust over empathy, diversity over homogeneity, loose over tight coupling, and strategic communication over unrestricted candor" (Eisenberg, 1990, p. 160). Overestimation of group power, morality, and invulnerability lead to *developed group—undeveloped mind*. It is the well-developed collective mind that enables organizations to invent new solutions and see new opportunities as the uncertain world of health care unfolds. Members in developed groups may be too committed to the group and its present way of doing business to be able to function in an environment in which careful sensemaking is a necessary condition of organizational success.

Learning

Both quantum theory and chaos theory lead to the conclusion that future states of an organization are unknowable. Because the future is unknowable, success for health care organizations comes through organizational learning. Learning replaces control as complex adaptive systems anticipate the future (Senge, 1990; Stacey, 1992; Zimmerman, 1993). Strategic leaders, therefore, should help organizations focus on *learning* rather than *knowing*, since it is through the former process that leaders and organizations can successfully cope with the turbulent unfolding of the health care world.

Learning in Real Time.   Chaos theory suggests that future states of an organization are unknowable because of sensitive dependence on initial conditions and properties of feedback in nonlinear systems. Because the future is unknowable, most organizational success comes through learning. This learning is not the learning that takes place before action is undertaken, but learning in real time. As noted by Stacey (1992, p. 17), "The most important learning we do flows from the trial-and-error action we take in real time and especially from the way we reflect on those actions as we take them."

Health care organizations are constantly making predictions about the future based on various internal models of the world. For example, models of relationships among health care professionals determine which professional groups are involved in each decision situation. They then learn as a result of using these models to make sense out of their encounters with the world (Waldrop, 1992). Strategic leaders help organizations take advantage of what the world is saying. Through the intelligent use of both feedback and feedforward, leaders help organizations develop sensible views of the world and act accordingly. Health care organizations cannot expect to *know* the world through learning, but they can expect to *make sense* of the world through an ongoing learning and interpretation process (Daft and Weick, 1984; Thomas and McDaniel, 1990).

The dominant logic of an organization is a primary determinant of organizational intelligence and is one emergent property of complex organizations as they try to adapt to unpredictable, changing environments (Bettis and Prahalad, 1995). Strategic leaders attend to the development of a dominant logic because they understand that this logic forms the grounding for organizational learning in real time. A key to emerging strategy in self-organizing systems is to deal effectively and creatively with what comes, not to secure something known and fixed; no competitive advantage is sustainable, and the route to success is innovation and organizational learning (D'Aveni, 1994). Organizations need to engage in learning processes that enable a pattern of action to emerge as the organization interacts with its environment (Wheatley, 1992; Kiel, 1994; Bettis and Prahalad, 1995).

Learning Skills.   A convenient way to categorize organizational learning skills is in terms of exploration versus exploitation (March, 1991). Health care organizations learn through exploring new possibilities—search, variation, risk taking, experimentation, play, flexibility, discovery, innovation. This kind of learning is unreliable but tends to lead to systems improvement. Health care organizations also learn through exploitation of old certainties—refinement, choice, production, efficiency, selection, implementation, execution. This kind of learning tends to be more reliable, and organizations often prefer refining existing competencies because it seems less risky. Exploitation increases reliability of performance at the expense of average performance level. Exploitation also degrades organizational learning in situations where organizations and individuals are learning from each other (March, 1991). These observations suggest that health care organizations should make special efforts to focus on exploring new possibilities in recognition of the fact that health care right now needs qualitative improvements in systems performance rather than incremental adjustments to existing behaviors.

Because critical experiences in organizations do not occur very often, organizations must become skilled at learning from samples of one. Each experience must become an opportunity for learning. As March, Sproull, and Tamuz (1991) suggest, in their investigation of how organizations can learn when history offers only meager samples of experience, "They attempt to experience history more richly, to formulate more interpretations of that experience, and to supplement history by experiencing more of the events that did not occur but could have" (p. 9). Recalling that future states of chaotic systems are sensitive to small differences in initial conditions, they consider it improbable that many experiences will repeat. Therefore, the capacity to learn from a single event is crucial.

The central role of strategic leaders attempting to promote learning in health care organizations is to present members with ambiguous challenges that inspire them to search for innovative ways to respond. Creative tension in organizations enables members to learn (Senge, 1990). It is not leaders' responsibility to find answers and teach them to others. Rather, they are responsible for creating environments in which learning is expected and rewarded and organizational members develop the content of learning as they respond to new challenges.

Designing

Positive feedback and disequilibrium are forces that accomplish growth and adaptation. We no longer think about the design of organizations as finished. Organizations are in a constant state of becoming, and in order to grow, they must have sources of new information about both internal and external situations. Strategic leaders in health care must avoid overreliance on single sources for information. For example, sometimes an organization will maintain a long-term relationship with a single marketing firm. While this may be comfortable, it is likely to lead to a limited view of the world.

As health care organizations exchange information with their environment, they learn more about themselves and develop greater freedom from environmental demands. This can happen only if sources of information are rich and varied. Health care organizations should not simply be taking in information; they should seek to change their environments. Traditional management theory suggested that an environment was "out there" and that the task of strategic leaders was to design organizations to match environmental needs. Self-organizing systems interact with their environments, creating change "out there" as well as "in here." Organizations and their environments are thus involved in a mutual adjustment process to achieve better harmony between them. Organizations do not have a stable, fixed design, but strategic leaders are continually in the process of designing an organization as the world unfolds.

Connections.   Leaders sometimes feel responsible for figuring out what is needed and then inspiring others to accomplish organizational goals. However, once one recognizes the real complexity of problems in health care, it becomes clear that no leader working alone can resolve these issues. Leaders need to develop and manage connections among people so that they can work together to identify organizational goals, develop organizational action alternatives, and choose which alternatives to implement (Wheatley, 1992; Stacey, 1992, 1995; Hirsschhorn and Gilmore, 1992; Ambrose, 1995). "No matter how visionary, or smart or forward looking or aggressive that one brain may be, it is no match for conditions of interactive complexity" (Weick and Roberts 1993, p. 378). When managers overlook interrelating and connecting, key people are left out of decision making, and key tasks are neglected. One issue in designing information systems for health care organizations is exactly how to involve clinicians in the design process to achieve an appropriate balance of considerations and produce an information system that they view as a help rather than a hindrance as they try to do their jobs. Failure to make key connections results in a more limited understanding of events as they unfold and less potential for learning while doing. This in turn will cause heedful behavior to decrease and collective mind to cease functioning well. Small gaps will grow into disasters if strategic leaders do not pay attention to interrelationships and connections.

Looking at organizations through the lens of quantum theory and its revelations about the importance of relationships in the physical world offers new insights into the importance of connections in organizations. Organizational theorists traditionally focus on people's roles in organizations, but roles are simply intermediate states in a network of interactions (Weick, 1993a). People in health care organizations do not have jobs; they have multiple, dynamic roles that are constantly changing and evolving over time. This changes strategic leadership tasks from managing people to managing connections between people. The important thing is the set of relationships; the quality of connections between people is more important than the quality of the people themselves.

One way to think about the connections in organizations is to think about who participates in sensemaking and decision-making activities (Ashmos and McDaniel, 1991; Ashmos and McDaniel, 1996). It is not true that everybody should participate all of the time. Research by McDaniel and Ashmos (1995), has shown, for example, that group participation by internal stakeholders in hospital strategic decision making is affected by strategic content and the nature of hospital strategy. Those hospitals with the appropriate level of participation by a larger number of different groups had lower costs. As Wheatley (1992, p. 64) noted, "Participation, seriously done, is a way out from the uncertainties and ghostly qualities of this nonobjective world we live in. We need a broad distribution of information, viewpoints, and interpretations if we are to make sense of the world." Visionary strategic leaders hold lots of meetings because they are opportunities for participation. This participation creates collective mind and the opportunity to make sense of the deeply unknowable world. Strategic leaders should ensure that people in these meetings do not simply focus on the routine and bring to the table information needed to reduce uncertainty. Rather, they should plan meetings so that they focus on the development of shared meanings that can serve to reduce ambiguity and equivocality (Weick, 1995).

Diversity.   Because the health care world is becoming ever more complicated as information moves quickly through cyberspace, health care organizations must develop complicated patterns of relationships if they are to make sense out of their world. This is a simple law of systems, Ashby's law of requisite variety: "[O]nly variety in [one element] R can force down variety due to [another element] D; only variety can destroy variety" (Ashby, 1956, p. 207). The only way to conquer variety is with variety; therefore, if strategic leaders wish to succeed in the high-variety environment of health care, they must have great variety in their organizations. Anderson and McDaniel (1992) have shown that in effective nursing homes, the participation of RNs in decision making was higher when managers perceived high levels of environmental turbulence. Top hospital managers who use more information in decision making, thereby complicating their worlds, are more likely to interpret their environments as positive (Thomas and McDaniel, 1990; Thomas, McDaniel, and Anderson, 1991) and are therefore more likely to see greater opportunities for strategic action (Smircich and Stubbart, 1985). Leaders and their organizations must complicate themselves rather than seek stability and simplicity (Weick, 1979).

Increasingly, it seems that frontline managers understand the complexity out there but that top managers are less able to sense the complexity of current issues (Ghoshal and Bartlett, 1995). One might theorize that because top executives in America are such an uncomplicated bunch—mostly elderly white men—they have great difficulty in seeing the world outside their historic frame of reference. Additionally, top management has a tendency to isolate itself from the environmental turbulence in which the organization functions. Because frontline managers are more diverse and closer to all the action, they see more of the complications organizations face. Tom Peters (1988) recognized this situation when he indicated that enhancing American competitiveness requires the development of more flexible, porous, adaptive, and fleet-of-foot organizations whose communications patterns and organizational relationships are not tightly constrained but are constantly in flux as the global environment in which American organizations must operate changes over time.

This approach leads to the assertion that if health care organizations are going to survive, strategic leaders must create complex sets of relationships among people who are different from one another, in which each person has an important role to play as a source of critical information for organizational sensemaking and learning. There are many different types of health care professionals, all with differing views of the health care world and unique contributions to make in the emerging health care environment (Begun and Lippincott, 1993). Strategic leaders must ensure that each has an appropriate avenue of participation in decision making. "By intentionally creating a diverse workforce, management generates cultural pluralism in the organization. This is not succumbing to political correctness but recognizing that the fluctuations generated by multiculturalism help to ensure the levels of instability that may generate organizational renewal" (Kiel, 1994, p. 188). Managers must create environments that attract variety and bring in new information that can be used to understand the world as it unfolds. 3M recognized the potential of Post-It notes when it accepted the value of an adhesive that doesn't stick very well. Honda captured a market for small motorcycles when it recognized that its intended product, a large motorcycle designed to compete in the traditional market, was not the only kind of motorcycle that people wanted. In each case an alternative view of the world led to frame-breaking change and economic success.

Thes examples help us to see that if strategic leaders are going to be successful in hyperturbulent environments, they must create diverse organizations in which people of diverse backgrounds have important seats at decision-making tables (Herriot and Pemberton, 1995).

If organizations are going to use exploration as a key learning strategy, they need to contain people who are not overcommitted to existing ways of doing things. The organization also needs a diverse set of stakeholders to enhance the probability that frame-breaking learning can occur (Argyris, 1992). If organizations are going to learn from samples of one, they must be able to engage in rich interpretations that can squeeze all of the possible learning from the fragile fragments of information in their experiences. When people who are very much alike observe the same phenomenon, they see the same thing and are likely to interpret it in the same way. When people who are unalike observe an event, they are likely to see and interpret it very differently. When a variety of clinical and nonclinical people examine population health status and seek ways to improve that status, the probability increases that the organization will detect consequential events in the environment and develop more creative responses to situations.

If organizations are viewed from a Newtonian perspective, where elements of systems behave in a deterministic fashion and managerial problems include command and control along with prediction and planning, diversity in the organization can be seen as a barrier to managerial success. For example, in their recent textbook *Human Resource Management: The Strategic Perspective*, Miner and Crane (1995) suggest, "Demographics and individual differences in the labor force are important to a firm strategically because they can create opportunities, but also they set limits on what can be done at a feasible cost. Labor force changes are creating increasing diversity and this, too, is something with which companies must cope" (pp. 72–73). The thrust of Miner and Crane's argument is that the opportunities created by diversity are a way to deal with labor shortages and the problems involved in how to get those who are diverse to look like typical workers.

On the other hand, if the natural world is seen as quantum in nature and chaotic in its unfolding, then a diverse work force constitutes not just a response to public policy directives or even a belief in the justice of diversity. Rather, organizational diversity is an objective sought as a source of strategic advantage. Because diverse organizations are better able to cope with complexity in relationships they face, and because diverse organizations are better able to learn to cope with the unknowability of the world, diverse organizations are more likely to survive and prosper.

It is easy to talk to someone who is just like yourself because the assumption sets are clear, implicit meanings are obvious, and so it is easier to build trust (Fernandez, 1993). However, levels of understanding in work groups made up of people who are very much alike are much lower than those that exist in diverse work groups (March, 1994). Improvement in understanding requires that people interact in rich and meaningful ways, and strategic leaders must be sensitive to the fact that people may not have the skills required to interact in these ways. This view suggests that all groups need training in how to exchange information and understandings so that they not only communicate facts and rules but also achieve a richer level of understanding and sensemaking. Health care organizations cannot tolerate internal wars between physicians and nurses, nor can they allow destructive relationships between nonclinical staff and clinical staff. Strategic leaders must take responsibility for establishing lines of communication between diverse groups, or the groups are likely to resist establishing the connections required for a rich exchange of critical information.

Self-Organization.   Organizations are complex, self-organizing, adaptive systems governed by nonlinear relationships (Thiétart and Forgues, 1995).

Although the behavior of organizations is unpredictable and unknowable, it is not random. There is order in chaotic systems because of their emergent properties (Cohen and Stewart, 1994) and self-organization capabilities (Prigogine and Stengers, 1984; Waldrop, 1992). The richness of interactions among parts and between the system and its environment allows the system as a whole to undergo spontaneous self-organization. "[F]orm and function engage in a fluid process where the system may maintain itself in its present form or evolve to a new order. The system possesses a capacity for spontaneously emerging structures. It is not locked into any one form but instead is capable of organizing information in the structure that best suits the present need" (Wheatley, 1992, p. 91).

Self-organizing occurs when interactions and dialogues between group members produce coherent behavior regardless of whether or not there is a hierarchy. Informal groups and networks of managers within an organization coalesce, and no central authority organizes them. This network of informal contacts and coalitions that develops in an organization is critical to its well-being. These networks behave in a controlled way and are a vital part of the organization (Stacey, 1992).

Strategic leaders must therefore see that one of their responsibilities is to get people together and help them engage in the conversations that enable them to self-organize. Self-organization leads to long-term patterns of action that emerge from convergent behavior and collective action in the absence of prior central intention, grand designs, or continuing central control (Wheatley, 1992; Freedman, 1992; Zimmerman, 1993; Stacey, 1995). Strategic leaders must not think about deterministic sets of relationships between intent and outcomes. Rather, the self-organizing nature of complex adaptive systems means that leaders must think in terms of continually developing agendas of issues, aspirations, challenges, and individual intentions (Stacey, 1992).

Self-organization occurs when there is a rich dialogue among organizational actors (Wheatley, 1992). Included in the communications must be stories about the nature of the organizations. "Stories of an organization are critical conversations between the present and the past . . . [and] the organization's future is found in current conversations about the future" (Bergquist, 1993, p. 146). It is easy for newcomers, especially those systematically excluded in the past, to miss stories that define an organization. Strategic leaders can be important levers in ensuring that diverse groups come to share stories that help organizations define themselves. However, it is not only organizational stories that are important but also newcomers' stories, which are a source of new energy and information required for organizational survival (Wheatley, 1992).

Leading in Uncertain Times

There are 12 key leverage points for strategic managers in the health care industry. This view of leadership suggests that a major purpose of strategic leadership is to move health care organizations to the edge of chaos, where the creative forces required to meet the complex strategic issues facing the industry can be developed.

Strategic leadership in uncertain times leaves little room for heroic autonomous individuals. In such circumstances the manager cannot *be in command, have control, predict the future,* or *plan for success.*

The current mental model for management focuses on equilibrium, but health care organizations are quantum systems operating in chaos. Indeed, chaos is the true state of any successful business, because the constant creativity and innovation necessary for success can occur only in this state. The fact that times are uncertain in health care is not a phenomenon that will go away when political questions are settled but rather the result of the nature of the world. Strategic leaders need to shift their behavior and adopt new ways to approach leadership roles. Noted below are several specific suggestions for managers as they try to provide strategic leadership in uncertain times.

Give Up Planning and Control. Strategic leadership cannot be a matter of cookbooks or formulas. Strategic leaders' jobs are more intellectual and scholarly in the best sense of these words. They require high-quality thought and action and an experimental frame of mind (Vaill, 1989). Planning is a defense against anxiety (Stacey, 1995, p. 491). Control is a way to attempt to bring stability to a dynamic system. However, the key message of the dynamic systems model is that a continual preoccupation with order, stability, and consistency damages organizational creativity and ability to cope with the unknowable. Leaders who are in touch with alternative ways of thinking about organizations will reduce their anxiety by paying attention to learning, connections, and emergent strategies.

Move to the Edge of Chaos. Organizations are able to exist on the edge of chaos, on the boundary between order and disorder. Here, things are fluid; and pushes and pulls keep systems at once on balance and off balance. It is at the edge of chaos that organizations find creativity. Systems in this state create their own environment and their own future. The role of top managers here is to enable strategy to emerge by creating conditions in which key groups of stakeholders can discover new directions. Strategic leaders must strive to present groups with ambiguous challenges. These challenges should be chosen to provoke the kind of emotion and conflict that leads to an active search for new ways of doing things. Managers must take organizations to the boundary of chaos, where creativity and complexity combine to generate new opportunities for organizational growth and development within the boundaries of an organization's integrity or self-reference.

Create New Organizations with New Forms. "It is the ability to combine old resources in new ways to reduce new uncertainties that determines organizational effectiveness. Thus designs don't determine resource distribution; it's the other way around. Further, it is not resources per se that determine design, but the capacity to create resources from the residue of past experience" (Weick, 1993b, p. 355). We are part of what we lead, and we do not lead independent of ourselves. We cannot stand apart from what we lead. We do not lead, then follow, as leading and following are closely tied together. This is a derivation from the Heisenberg principle, according to which observers are part of measurement. Leadership, therefore, can and must come from everywhere in the organization. The strategic leadership task in organizations is to create an environment where lots of people can lead, and this distinguishes vibrant organizations from stagnant ones.

Develop Self-Referent Organizations. Because details of long-term futures are completely unknowable, managers must adopt a style of management that relies on processes of self-organizing, participation, and complex learning. Complex adaptive systems operating in this way have a capacity for self-reference; and it is this capacity that strategic leaders must promote and nourish. Through high levels of interaction within organizations and between organizations and their environments, people come to have a shared idea of who they are and what they are trying to do. They develop a self-reference that provides the boundaries for organizational action. Self-reference facilitates orderly change in turbulent environments. In response to environmental disturbances that signal a need for change, systems with a strong sense of self change in ways that remain consistent with themselves in that environment. Health care organizations must be helped to focus their activities on what is required to maintain their own integrity.

Self-referent systems encourage autonomy and allow small fluctuations and changes as people strive to adjust to dynamic local conditions. In these ways organizations are able to preserve global stability and integrity in the environment. As organizations gain experience in allowing fluctuation within boundaries, they develop even greater levels of autonomy and integrity.

Enhance the Quality of Connections. Because the quality of connections between workers is more important than the quality of each individual worker, strategic leaders must be better at managing systems of connections between workers than in managing workers themselves. One key characteristic of good connections in an organization is the capacity to carry rich exchanges of information, which can be accomplished by using a wide range of information media and by a willingness to experiment with new ways of communicating (Daft and Lengle, 1984). Channels of information flow do not necessarily follow channels of authority. Rather, information is delivered directly to those who can use it without going through a chain of command (Huber and McDaniel, 1986, p. 584). Aggressively led health care organizations use more networks to get work done, and these networks extend across multiple health care professionals and multiple organizational units.

Teach People What Other People Are Doing. People at all levels need to be taught what other people are doing so that they can help each other more effectively and efficiently. When strategic leaders hire people, they should hire those who can help them do their job rather than just carry out assigned job functions. Workers must see the overall direction of the organization, and they must be aware of their responsibility for the whole product or service. The excuse "that's not my job" is not acceptable. Training programs should focus on the overall organizational goals and on the leader's job rather than the worker's job. If strategic leaders are clear that they are more interested in the outcomes of health care systems than in the specific performance of individual actors, and if people in the organization are rewarded for helping each other, the organization will be better able to develop effective responses to the complexity it faces.

Create Learning Organizations.   Organizations must learn to do old things better, and they must learn to do new things. Organizations must learn not only new ways to achieve existing goals but also what new goals they should pursue. Managers must be able to develop creative tensions between organizational visions and current reality, because it is through these creative tensions that the drive for learning takes place.

Strategic leaders should not be expected to know what is going on and then tell others what to do. Rather, the manager's task is to create an organizational environment in which learning is highly valued, and in which people listen to and respect insights and understandings that are different from their own. The development of creative tension, rather than its suppression, is a key function of strategic leaders, because this tension is a prerequisite for organizational learning.

As different people in the organization examine issues, they will discover their own intentions and provide boundaries around instability. Self-referent insights will emerge as people work together to look at open-ended issues from many angles and perspectives. The group dynamics conducive to complex learning has no place for highly competitive win-lose polarization but involves open questioning and public testing of views and assertions. Consensus and commitment are not the norm; instead the group alternates between conflict and consensus, between confusion and clarity. Given good strategic leadership, people can become skilled at handling ambiguous issues, revealing differences, and generating new perspectives.

Think About Organizational Design as an Ongoing Process.   Strategic leaders must think about organizational redesign as well as design, because rethinking work processes is an ongoing fact of life in health care organizations. Crucial decisions about what goes on must be made closer to the actual work itself, and the responsibility for organizational well-being must therefore be more widely distributed. Reliance on work rules for obtaining compliance must be reduced in order to gain the flexibility required to deal with rapid environmental changes. Work units must be smaller, because it is difficult to manage interdependencies when they are large.

Don't Be Responsible for Setting Goals for Workers or for Organizations.   Managers are not responsible for setting goals for workers or for organizations, even though goal setting has historically been considered a major task of strategic leadership. Managers are responsible for enabling organizational stakeholders, including workers, to discover goals. Health care organizations—with their diverse set of professionals, their multiple stakeholders, and their rapidly developing complexity—need to have goal setting widely dispersed. This does not mean that there is no coordination but rather that coordination occurs through a dynamic exchange of information rather than through leaders' heroic efforts. Organizations are required to identify opportunities as they emerge in real time.

Decrease Emphasis on Competition and Increase Emphasis on Cooperation. Emphasis on competition must decrease and emphasis on cooperation must increase. Strategic leaders must develop both internal joint ventures and strategic partnerships with other organizations. Alliances cannot depend on hierarchical authority or legal relationships to enable cooperation; shared interests must be successfully negotiated on an ongoing basis (Thomas, Ketchen, Trevino, and McDaniel, 1992). Individual workers or subunits are not motivated by setting up internal systems of competition, because such competition is a barrier to the teamwork that is necessary to achieve organizational aims.

Work Smarter. Managers are often told to work smarter, not harder. Working smarter does not mean knowing a lot about situations, because they are changing much too rapidly. Vaill (1989) suggests alternative conceptions of working smarter—working collectively smarter, working reflectively smarter, and working spiritually smarter.

> To work collectively smarter is to remain in touch with those around us, both with their ideas and with their energy. [To work reflectively smarter is] to reconsider what the world is presenting to us, to examine the grounds on which an idea rests, and the assumption that must hold true if a proposal is to work as intended. To work spiritually smarter is to pay more attention to one's own spiritual qualities, feelings, insights and yearnings. It is to reach more deeply into oneself for that which is unquestionably authentic (Vaill, 1989, pp. 30–31).

This prescription for working smarter fits the quantum, chaotic world of health care organizations and provides guidance for strategic leaders.

Provide for the Emergence of Visions and Values. Strategic leaders in health care organizations must help these organizations to develop a vision of who they are and where they have been. They must also help organizations identify, through tough interaction, values that will guide organizations to the future. A vision of the future is impossible because of fundamental uncertainty in the system. Therefore, positive action designed to move organizations along emanates from a clear vision of organizational history, a clear vision of where the organization is now, and a clear set of values. Strategic leaders cannot impose these visions and values but must let them emerge from the organization itself.

🕊 CONCLUSION

Often, change in health care brings a reallocation of scarce resources with little or no improvement in the general welfare. There is a growing need to reach beyond a single institution to the health of the community or population. Who should be better off if the health care system improves? Whom should health care leadership represent? These difficult questions must be addressed. Rather than avoid these challenges, strategic leaders need to embrace them.

People working in health care organizations sometimes want stability because they do not understand the positive value of change. They fail to grasp the inevitability of not knowing with certainty what is going on in the world. Therefore, the work of strategic leaders is difficult. They must keep confronting people with ambiguous challenges that will keep the system far from equilibrium and at the edge of chaos. There is an implicit order within chaos where system behavior is highly complex and unstable. It is certainly difficult for managers to "trust that something as simple as a clear core of values and vision, kept in motion through continuing dialogue, can lead to order" (Wheatley, p. 147). However, it is this method that is appropriate for keeping health care organizations moving in sensible directions.

❧ References

Ambrose, D. 1995: Creatively Intelligent Post-Industrial Organizations and Intellectually Impaired Bureaucracies. *Journal of Creative Behavior*, 29(1), 1–15.

Anders, G. 1994, December 21: HMOs Pile Up Billions in Cash, Try to Decide What to Do with It. *Wall Street Journal*, A1, A12.

Anderson, R. A. and McDaniel, R. R. 1992: The Implication of Environmental Turbulence for Nursing-Unit Design in Effective Nursing Homes. *Nursing Economics*, 10(2), 117–125.

Argyris, Chris 1992: *On Organizational Learning*. Malden, MA: Blackwell Publishers.

Arrington, B., Kurz, R. S. and Haddock, C. C. 1994: Leadership Development. In Myron D. Fottler, S. Robert Hernandez and Charles L. Joiner (eds.), *Strategic Management of Human Resources in Health Service Organizations*, 2nd ed., Albany, NY: Delmar Publishers, Inc., 224–245.

Ashby, W. Ross 1956: *An Introduction to Cybernetics*. London: Chapman and Hall Ltd.

Ashmos, D. P. and McDaniel, R. R., Jr. 1991: Physician Participation in Hospital Strategic Decision Making: The Effect of Hospital Strategy and Decision Content. *Health Services Research*, 26(3), 375–401.

Ashmos, D. P. and McDaniel, R. R., Jr. 1996: Understanding the Participation of Critical Task Specialists in Strategic Decision Making. *Decision Sciences*, 27 (1), 103–121.

Begun, J. W. 1994: Chaos and Complexity: Frontiers of Organization Science. *Journal of Management Inquiry,* 3(4), 329–335.

Begun, J. W. and Lippincott, R. C. 1993: Meeting the Challenges: Change and Adaptation in Five Health Professions. In James W. Begun and Ronald C. Lippincott, *Strategic Adaptation in the Health Professions,* San Francisco: Jossey-Bass, 195–223.

Bergquist, William 1993: *The Postmodern Organization: Mastering the Art of Irreversible Change.* San Francisco: Jossey-Bass.

Bettis, R. A. and C. K. Prahalad 1995: The Dominant Logic: Retrospective and Extension. *Strategic Management Journal,* 16(1), 5–14.

Capra, Fritjof 1982: *The Turning Point: Science, Society, and the Rising Culture.* Hammersmith, London: Flamingo.

Cohen, Jack and Ian Stewart 1994: *The Collapse of Chaos: Discovering Simplicity in a Complex World.* New York: Penguin.

D'Aveni, Richard A. with Robert Gunther 1994: *Hypercompetition: Managing the Dynamics of Strategic Maneuvering.* New York: The Free Press.

Daft, Richard L. 1994: *Management,* 3rd ed. Orlando, FL: The Dryden Press.

Daft, R. L. and Lengel, R. H. 1984: Information Richness: A New Approach to Managerial Behavior and Organization Design. In Barry M. Staw and L. L. Cummings (eds.), *Research in Organizational Behavior,* Vol. 6, Greenwich, CT: JAI Press, 191–233.

Daft, R. L. and Weick, K. E. 1984: Toward a Model of Organizations as Interpretation Systems. *Academy of Management Review,* 9(2), 284–295.

Duncan, W. Jack, Ginter, Peter M. and Swayne, Linda E. (1995). *Strategic Management of Health Care Organizations,* 2nd ed. Boston: PWS-Kent Publishing Company.

Eisenberg, E. 1990: Jamming: Transcendence Through Organizing. *Communications Research,* 17, 139–164.

Families USA Foundation 1995, March: Worthless Promises: Drug Companies Keep Boosting Prices. Washington, DC: Families USA Foundation.

Fernandez, John P. with Barr, Mary 1993: *The Diversity Advantage: How American Business Can Out-Perform Japanese and European Companies in the Global Marketplace.* New York: Lexington Books.

Flood, A. B. 1994: The Impact of Organizational and Managerial Factors on the Quality of Care in Health Care Organizations. *Medical Care Review,* 51(4), 381–428.

Freedman, D. H. 1992: Is Management Still a Science? *Harvard Business Review,* 70(6), 26–27, 28, 30, 32–33, 36–38.

Gell–Mann, Murray 1994: *The Quark and the Jaguar: Adventures in the Simple and the Complex.* New York: W. H. Freeman and Company.

Ghoshal, S. and Bartlett, C. A. 1995: Changing the Role of Management: Beyond Structure to Process. *Harvard Business Review,* 73(1), 86–96.

Gleick, James 1987: *Chaos: Making a New Science.* New York: Penguin.

Glick, W. H., Miller, C. C. and Huber, G. P. 1993: The Impact of Upper–Echelon Diversity on Organizational Performance. In George P. Huber and William H. Glick (eds.), *Organizational Change and Redesign: Ideas and Insights for Improving Performance.* New York: Oxford University Press, Inc., 176–214.

Goldsmith, J. C. 1994: The Illusive Logic of Integration. *Healthcare Forum Journal,* 38(5), 26–31.

Griffith, J. R. 1994: Principles of the Well-Managed Community Hospital. In Anthony R. Kovner and Duncan Neuhauser (eds.), *Health Services Management: Readings and Commentary,* 5th ed. Ann Arbor, MI: Health Administration Press, 257–269.

Herbert, Nick 1985: *Quantum Reality: Beyond the New Physics.* New York: Doubleday.

Herriot, Peter and Pemberton, Carole 1995: *Competitive Advantage Through Diversity: Organizational Learning From Indifference.* London: SAGE Publications, Ltd.

Hey, Tony and Walters, Patrick 1987: *The Quantum Universe.* Cambridge: Press Syndicate of the University of Cambridge.

Hilzenrath, D. S. 1995, July 7: Health Insurance Firms Found to Often Hold Tobacco Company Stocks. *The Washington Post,* C1–C2.

Hinton, Bernard L. and Reitz, H. Joseph 1971: *Groups and Organizations: Integrated Readings in the Analysis of Social Behavior.* Belmont, CA: Wadsworth Publishing Company, Inc.

Hirschhorn, L. and Gilmore, T. 1992: The New Boundaries of the "Boundaryless" Company. *Harvard Business Review,* 70(3), 104–115.

Huber, G. P. and McDaniel, R. R. 1986: The Decision–Making Paradigm of Organizational Design. *Management Science,* 32(5), 572–589.

Inglis, T. 1995: HMOs Investing in Tobacco Industry Represents Conflict of Values. *Texas Nursing,* 69(8), 3.

Janis, Irving Lester 1989: *Crucial Decisions: Leadership in Policymaking and Crisis Management*. New York: The Free Press.

Jones, Roger S. 1992: *Physics for the Rest of Us: Ten Basic Ideas of Twentieth-Century Physics That Everyone Should Know. . . and How They Have Shaped Our Culture and Consciousness*. Chicago: Contemporary Books, Inc.

Kellert, Stephen H. 1993: *In the Wake of Chaos: Unpredictable Order in Dynamical Systems*. Chicago: The University of Chicago Press.

Kiel, L. Douglas 1994: *Managing Chaos and Complexity in Government: A New Paradigm for Managing Change, Innovation, and Organizational Renewal*. San Francisco: Jossey-Bass.

Lamm, R. D. 1994: The Ghost of Health Care Future. *Inquiry*, 31(4), 365–367.

La Porte, T. R. 1975: Complexity and Uncertainty: Challenge to Action. In Todd R. La Porte (ed.), *Organized Social Complexity: Challenge to Politics and Policy*. Princeton, NJ: Princeton University Press, 332–356.

March, J. G. 1991: Exploration and Exploitation in Organizational Learning. *Organization Science*, 2(1), 71–87.

March, James G. 1994: *A Primer on Decision Making*. New York: The Free Press.

March, J. G., Sproull, L. S. and Tamuz, Michal 1991: Learning From Samples of One or Fewer. *Organization Science*, 2(1), 1–13.

McDaniel, R. R., Jr. and Ashmos, D. P. 1995: Internal Stakeholder Group Participation in Hospital Strategic Decision Making: Making Structure Fit the Moment. *Journal of Health and Human Resources Administration*, 118 (3), 304–327.

Miner, John B. and Crane, Donald P. 1995: *Human Resource Management: The Strategic Perspective*. New York: HarperCollins College Publishers.

Owens, R., Fairchild, P., Pierce, A. and Goldberg, R. 1994: Simplified Manual Systems for Clinical Management: The Internal Management Report. In Anthony R. Kovner and Duncan Neuhauser (eds.), *Health Services Management: Readings and Commentary*, 5th ed. Ann Arbor, MI: Health Administration Press, 154–170.

Peters, T. 1988: Restoring American Competitiveness: Looking for New Models of Organizations. *The Academy of Management Executive*, 2(2), 103–109.

Prigogine, Ilya and Isabelle Stengers 1984: *Order out of Chaos: Man's New Dialogue with Nature*. New York: Bantam Books.

Rae, Alistair 1986: *Quantum Physics: Illusion or Reality?* Cambridge: Cambridge University Press.

Richardson, M. 1992: Can Managed Care Control Costs Without Controlling You? *Texas Medicine*, 88(10), 36–44.

Rivlin, A. M. 1983. An Intelligent Politician's Guide to Dealing with Experts. *The Rand Graduate Institute Commencement Addresses: 1974–1983*. Santa Monica, CA: Rand Graduate Institute, 1–7.

Rohrlich, Fritz 1987: *From Paradox to Reality: Our Basic Concepts of the Physical World*. Cambridge: Cambridge University Press.

Samuelson, D. 1995: Diagnosing the Real Health Care Villain. *OR/MS Today*, February, 26–28, 30–31.

Senge, Peter M. 1990: *The Fifth Discipline: The Art and Practice of the Learning Organization*. New York: Doubleday.

Simon, Herbert A. 1994, February 4: Information, Technology and Computers in Management. Lecture at the Graduate School of Business, The University of Texas at Austin.

Smircich, L. and Stubbart, C. 1985: Strategic Management in an Enacted World. *Academy of Management Review*, 10(4), 724–736.

Sorrentino, E. A. 1991: Codependency: Management and Administrative Policy Implications. *Health Care Management Review*, 16(4), 49–54.

Stacey, Ralph D. 1992: *Managing the Unknowable: Strategic Boundaries Between Order and Chaos in Organizations*. San Francisco: Jossey-Bass.

Stacey, R. D. 1995: The Science of Complexity: An Alternative Perspective for Strategic Change Processes. *Strategic Management Journal*, 16(6), 477–495.

Steinmo, S. and Watts, J. 1995: "It's the Institutions, Stupid! Why Comprehensive National Health Insurance Always Fails in America," *Journal of Health Politics, Policy and Law*, 20(2), 329–372.

Teisberg, E. O., Porter, M. E. and Brown, G. B. 1994: Finding a Lasting Cure for U. S. Health Care. *Harvard Business Review*, 72(5), 45–47, 50, 52, 54, 56, 58, 60, 62–63.

Thiétart, R. A. and Forgues, B. 1995: Chaos Theory and Organization. *Organization Science*, 6(1), 19–31.

Thomas, J. B, Ketchen, D. J., Jr., Trevino, L. K. and McDaniel, R. R., Jr. 1992: Developing Interorganizational Relationships in the Health Sector: A Multicase Study. *Heath Care Management Review*, 17(2), 7–19.

Thomas, J. B. and McDaniel, R. R., Jr. 1990: Interpreting Strategic Issues: Effects of Strategy and the Information Processing Structures of Top Management Teams. *Academy of Management Journal*, 33(2), 286–306.

Thomas, J. B., McDaniel, R. R., Jr., and Anderson, R. A. 1991: Hospitals as Interpretation Systems. *Health Services Research*, 25(6), 859–880.

Vaill, Peter B. 1989: *Managing as a Performing Art: New Ideas for a World of Chaotic Change*. San Francisco: Jossey-Bass.

Waldrop, M. Mitchell 1992: *Complexity: The Emerging Science at the Edge of Order and Chaos*. New York: Simon and Schuster.

Weick, Karl E. 1979: *The Social Psychology of Organizing*, 2nd ed. New York: Random House, Inc.

Weick, K. E. 1993a: The Collapse of Sensemaking in Organizations: The Mann Gulch Disaster. *Administrative Science Quarterly*, 38(4), 628–652.

Weick, K. E. 1993b: Organizational Redesign as Improvisation. In George P. Huber and William H. Glick (eds.), *Organizational Change and Redesign: Ideas and Insights for Improving Performance*. New York: Oxford University Press, 346–379.

Weick, K. E. 1995: *Sensemaking in Organizations*. Thousand Oaks, CA: Sage Publications, Inc.

Weick, K. E. and Roberts, K. H. 1993: Collective Mind in Organizations: Heedful Interrelating on Flight Decks. *Administrative Science Quarterly*, 38(3), 357–381.

Wheatley, Margaret J. 1992: *Leadership and the New Science: Learning About Organization from an Orderly Universe*. San Francisco: Berrett-Koehler Publishers, Inc.

Wildavsky, Aaron 1979: *Speaking Truth to Power: The Art and Craft of Policy Analysis*. Boston: Little, Brown & Co.

Yukl, G. 1989: Managerial Leadership: A Review of Theory and Research. *Journal of Management*, 15(2), 251–289.

Zimmerman, B. 1993: The Inherent Drive Towards Chaos. In Peter Lorange, Bala Chakravarthy, Johan Roos and Andrew Van de Ven (eds.), *Implementing Strategic Processes: Change Learning and Co-operation*. Oxford: Blackwell Publishers, 373–393.

Organizational Change and Innovation

12

Beaufort B. Longest, Jr., University of Pittsburgh

❧ INTRODUCTION

Organizational change is a constant in health care organizations. The existence of such change in any organization is observable whenever a measurable modification in "form, quality, or state over time" (Van de Ven and Poole, 1995, p. 512) in its purpose or objectives, culture, strategies, tasks, technologies, people, or structures occurs. Organizational change takes place because managers, in their roles as change agents, perceive some sort of performance gap—a discrepancy between a desired and actual state—in their areas of responsibility and take actions to address the gap.

Health care organizations are not random groups of people and other resources assembled by chance interactions. Instead they are formed, operated, and changed by conscious and formal efforts for the purpose of accomplishing certain objectives that the participants in the organizations could not do as well when acting solely as individuals. From this fact stems the central purpose of management work and of all managers in organizations: to contribute to organizational performance by helping achieve organizational objectives (Longest, 1996). Not all organizations experience the same results in achieving their objectives. A relatively higher-performing organization meets more of its organizational objectives than a lower-performing organization.

Managers can properly be judged by their contribution to organizational performance because they occupy positions that permit them to make unique contributions to it. One of their most important contributions is to be able to know when organizational change is needed and to be able to implement the necessary changes smoothly and effectively.

In addition to the changes managers must make in response to performance gaps in their areas of responsibility, pressures to make changes are imposed on them from outside their domains of responsibility. Some of the pressure comes from inside the organizations. For example, a new strategic plan that includes diversifying into new services or merging with another organization is a potent internal driving force for change that will impact on many parts of the organization attempting to carry out this plan. Such a plan might stimulate personnel changes: New people may need to be hired, current employees retrained, or perhaps layoffs required under new organizational arrangements intended to implement new strategies. Such a plan might also stimulate changes in accounting systems or marketing programs. An internal driving force for change that is routinely seen in health care organizations is the arrival of a new chief executive officer (CEO). A new CEO almost invariably portends significant organizational changes, sometimes bordering on upheaval. Leadership changes are usually followed by shifts in strategic direction and in organizational structure. They are typically powerful internal driving forces for change.

The dynamic external environments of most health care organizations form another continuing set of driving forces for change for these organizations. For example, growing, declining, or aging populations in their market areas or the plans and actions of competitors have significant implications for health care organizations, usually requiring them to change in a variety of ways in response. Public policies and the regulations required to implement them also exert strong and direct external pressures for change on these organizations (Longest, 1994). For example, changes in reimbursment policy for the Medicare and Medicaid programs routinely drive changes in health care organizations. Similarly, National Labor Relations Board rulings can instantly change how these organizations relate to unionized employees. Because they are so dependent on technologies, technological advances exert a strong force for change on health care organizations. The dramatic shift from inpatient to outpatient surgery in the past two decades, for example, is largely attributable to better anesthesia, improved surgical techniques, and advanced postoperative care technologies.

The continuing internal and external pressures for organizational changes, coupled with managers' responsibilties to maximize organizational performance—including implementing changes when necessary—mean that skill in the implementation of organizational changes is among the most important capabilities a manager can possess. This chapter next defines and clarifies organizational change and innovation. It then presents and discusses a four-stage model of the complex process of managing organizational change, with actual applications to managerial practice in health care organizations.

❧ DEFINITIONS OF ORGANIZATIONAL CHANGE AND INNOVATION

As was noted in the opening paragraph, organizational change is a discernible modification in any aspect of an organization. It is "any modification in operations, structure, or ends of the organization" (Hernandez and Kaluzny, 1994, p. 296). This means that organizational changes span a very broad spectrum, ranging from a fundamental shift in a health care organization's purpose or strategic direction to the smallest refinement in a single job description within the organization. The possible focus of organizational changes can include all of those shown in Table 12.1.

It is important to distinguish between organizational change and innovation. Organizational change occurs when there is any modification in an organization's

Table 12.1   The Foci for Organizational Changes, with Examples

Points of Focus	Examples of Organizational Changes
Purpose and Objectives	Changes in an organization's mission statement; addition or deletion of organizational objectives; modification of existing objectives
Cultures	Changes in values that drive the organization; new emphasis on entrepreneurial behaviors
Strategies	Changes in strategic plans or in means to operationalize their accomplishment
Tasks	Changes in job designs; use of cross-functional teams
Technologies	Adoption of new technologies
People	Training of personnel in new techniques; changes in the hiring criteria in use; clarification of roles
Structures	Redesign of reporting relationships; downsizing of the organization; addition of new units

purpose or objectives, culture, strategies, tasks, technologies, people, or structures (Schermerhorn, Hunt, and Osborn, 1991). Most organizational changes occur through the adoption of concepts or ideas, practices, or physical things that have been developed elsewhere by people in other organizations as they were making changes. However, innovation is a special kind of change. An innovative change occurs within an organization when someone within it invents or develops—and is the first user of—a *new* concept or idea, practice, or physical thing. Innovation involves both the invention of new ideas or concepts—or of some new practice or physical thing—and their application or use (Roberts, 1988).

Pelz and Munson (1980) expand the distinction between organizational change and innovation into three types of change based on the source of the particular concepts or ideas, practices, or physical things involved in a change. They point out, on one hand, that concepts or ideas, practices, or physical things involved in organizational changes can be borrowed, directly and without modification, from somewhere else; or they can be adapted from things that have been used elsewhere, that is, borrowed but then modified to fit the adapting organization. On the other hand, concepts or ideas, practices, or physical things involved in an organization's changes can also originate there. Origination, obviously, involves more creativity than borrowing or adapting. This is not to say, however, that origination is necessarily better than borrowing or adapting when organizational changes are being made. A suitable borrowed or adapted concept, practice, or thing is in fact generally easier to implement (another's experience can be very informative) and usually less costly than its original equivalent, because someone else has already borne the development costs.

Adaptation and borrowing are the most common sources of concepts and ideas, practices, and physical things involved in organizational changes in health care organizations—indeed, in all organizations—and reflect the ready diffusion of innovations developed elsewhere. In fact, widespread diffusion of useful innovations characterizes the health care industry. The diffusion of medical technologies such as those involved in imaging, surgery, and diagnostic laboratory procedures has received a great deal of attention, but changes of all kinds are routinely spread by adaptation or borrowing throughout this industry. For example, concepts of corporate restructuring have been widely adapted and borrowed by health care organizations in recent years, as have the concepts of total quality management (TQM) and continuous quality improvement (CQI) (Berwick, 1991; Berwick, Godfrey, and Roessner, 1990; Kaluzny, McLaughlin, and Kibbe, 1992; Rakich, Darr, and Longest, 1993; Rakich, Longest, and Darr, 1992).

The best way to understand the complex concepts of organizational change and innovation is to consider what managers actually do when they engage in managing organizational change. The next section presents the elaborate process of managing organizational change as a four-stage model, with each stage incorporating several tasks that must be successfully accomplished if organizational change is to be well managed.

ও THE PROCESS OF MANAGING ORGANIZATIONAL CHANGE

In order to effectively manage organizational change, managers must accomplish an extensive series of interrelated tasks (Dunham and Pierce, 1989; Rakich, Longest, and Darr, 1992). Their first task is to recognize situations and circumstances that require an organizational change to be made. Then they must identify the nature of the change that is needed in a particular situation. These two closely related tasks are triggered by the internal and external pressures for change discussed in the introduction to this chapter.

After identifying the need for change and the nature of the change that is needed in a particular situation, managers must perform other tasks to assure effective planning to implement the change that is being contemplated. The tasks involved in implementation planning are (1) developing alternative changes for consideration; (2) choosing the change that is to be implemented from among the alternatives; (3) shaping a general strategy for making the change; and (4) developing the techniques that will be used to build support for the change and to minimize resistance to it. Only after an effective implementation planning stage has occurred in this overall process can managers be certain they are prepared for actually implementing change.

Implementing an organizational change is accomplished through three additional tasks, descriptively labeled as unfreezing, changing, and refreezing (Lewin, 1952). Unfreezing the status quo is the task through which managers disturb the status quo of a situation and convince those involved of the necessity of a change. If they cannot be convinced that change is needed, then managers must at least make them fully aware of the impending change and prepare them for it as much as possible. The unfreezing task is followed by the actual change. Some concept or idea, practice, or physical thing—or some combination of these—is introduced that results in some modification in the organization's purpose or objectives, culture, strategies, tasks, technologies, people, or structure. The actual change is followed by yet another task: refreezing the situation in order to stabilize the context and circumstances surrounding the change. This task is necessary if the newly implemented change is to have any chance of stability and durability.

The effective and systematic management of organizational change does not end with implementation. Managers who have the most success with the complex process of managing organizational change evaluate the results of the changes they make and use the information they obtain while carrying out this task to provide feedback for future iterations of the change process. The task in this stage is essentially one of comparing actual with projected results, exploring the reasons for any differences, and using this information wisely to inform and guide future changes.

Figure 12.1 contains a schematic model of the process of managing organizational change. The model shows the four stages involved in managing organizational changes: identification, planning, implementation, and evaluation/feedback (Dunham and Pierce, 1989; Rakich, Longest, and Darr, 1992). Each stage contains a set of tasks that must be accomplished if the stages are to be successfully managed in the overall change process. Both the stages and the sets of tasks involved in them are discussed in the following sections.

Stage 1: Identifying the Need for and Nature of Necessary Organizational Changes

As can be seen in Figure 12.1, the first stage of managing the organizational change process requires that two interrelated tasks be performed. Managers must first recognize the need for an organizational change. Change in organizations, merely for the sake of change, is a very misguided idea. Organizational changes incur a variety of costs and should never be undertaken without a compelling reason. Information that is developed while managers are engaged in routine functions and activities of managing, especially in the functions of planning and of controlling, often help them identify the real need for change. Deviations from the planned operational objectives that have been established for a health care organization, for example, can be an important indication of the need for an organizational change. Generally, such a need is identified when organizational performance along any important parameter falls below established or desired target levels.

Managers routinely monitor actual performance in their domain as a fundamental part of the managerial role (Longest, 1996). Where clear, concrete objectives and standards exist, monitoring outcomes and comparing them with the standards is straightforward. However, to monitor organizational performance effectively, managers must observe more than mere operating results, although these are always important in judging ultimate success or failure. One problem with relying on final outcomes as the basis for determining the need for a change is that these outcomes often occur too late to permit changes that can prevent a negative final result. In addition to this problem, observation of final results alone may not explain why deviations occurred. And if the outcomes do not really suggest why a change is needed, they will give little information about what kind of changes might be needed. To overcome such problems, managers must design their monitoring systems and techniques carefully.

Figure 12.1 A Model of the Process of Managing Organizational Changes

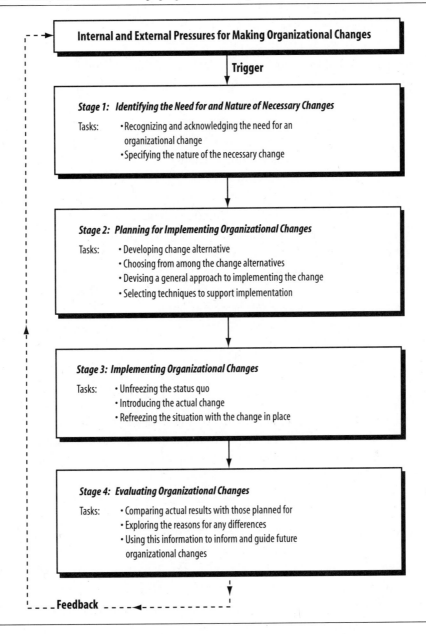

For example, Management Information Systems (MISs) can be designed to collect, format, store, and retrieve in a timely way information useful in identifying when organizational change is needed.

If MISs are to be as useful as possible in helping to identify the need for changes, and especially if they are to help determine the nature of the changes that are necessary, several factors should be considered:

- Managers should match the elements of information covered by their MISs to the actual organizational purposes or objectives, cultures, strategies, tasks, technologies, people, and structures that they might need to change in order to improve organizational performance.
- The elements of information in a MIS should point up exceptions at critical points. To manage organizational change effectively managers must concentrate on the issues and activities most critical to organizational performance.
- The MIS should report deviations promptly. The ideal MIS for helping managers identify when change is needed detects deviations soon after they actually occur. Only if information reaches managers promptly can they know in a timely manner that change is actually needed.
- The MIS should be forward looking. When relying on MISs to help them determine when a change is needed, managers usually prefer a forecast of what will probably happen next week or next month—even though this projection contains a margin of error—to a report, accurate to several decimal points, on the past, about which nothing can be done.

When change is indicated, no matter what the source of the information upon which this indication is based, the next step in the first stage of managing organizational change is to identify the nature of the change that is needed. Again, this depends on information. Often, the information necessary to determine exactly what change is needed is more detailed than the data signaling that a change is required. The following example will clarify how information is used both to recognize a need for change and, more extensively, to identify what kind of the change is actually indicated.

The incident described here occurred at Butterworth Hospital (Berwick, Godfrey, and Roessner, 1990, pp. 94–97). The hospital's respiratory therapy department had to make a change because its MIS indicated that the department was not able to meet all the requests for services that it was receiving. Information on the number of missed respiratory therapy sessions was sufficient to reveal the need for change, but more information was required to determine what kind of change should be made.

To obtain this information, a multidisciplinary team that included members of the respiratory therapy department and other departments that interacted with it was formed and undertook a series of activities intended to determine why the department could not meet the demand for its services. The team first held a brainstorming session to identify all possible reasons why respiratory therapy could not meet demand. Team members organized the list of possible explanations into eight categories and developed the cause-and-effect, or "fishbone," diagram shown in Figure 12.2.

To move their analysis beyond mere speculation regarding possible reasons for the missed respiratory therapy sessions, the team then asked members of the respiratory therapy department to prioritize the possible explanations that had been identified in the brainstorming session. The results of this survey were displayed in a Pareto diagram (see Figure 12.3), showing the six most frequently mentioned reasons why members of the department missed service appointments.

Upon examining their Pareto diagram, the team realized that three of the top six reasons for missed service appointments given by people who delivered respiratory services at Butterworth Hospital related to equipment: equipment unavailable, equipment misstocked, and equipment out of order. The team decided to look at this equipment problem more specifically. By surveying members of the respiratory therapy department again, the team learned that the specific problems were flowmeter and oximeter unavailability and oxygen analyzer downtime. Armed with this information, the team was now easily able to identify what specific organizational changes needed to be made.

This example illustrates both steps in the change identification stage of the process of managing organizational change. At first, managers knew only that an organizational change was needed. This conclusion was based simply on the information that the respiratory therapy department was not fully meeting the demand for its services. Additional, much more detailed information then showed them the specific nature of the changes that were needed to address their organizational performance problem. In other words, the managers who were involved in this situation accomplished both the task of identifying the need for an organizational change and the task of determining the nature of the change that was needed. They had successfully completed the first stage in the complex process of managing organizational change in this instance. However, their task of completely managing this organizational change had only just begun.

Stage 2: Planning for Implementing Organizational Changes

As Figure 12.1 shows, this stage in the overall process of managing organizational changes contains four interrelated tasks. The first task is to develop a set of viable alternative changes for consideration. Usually, when there is an indication that something in an organization needs to be changed, a variety of possiblities for change exist. Even when the nature of the change that is needed is known, there may still be multiple possibilities. Developing this set of possibilities for consideration is the first task in planning for implementation of an organizational change. The second task is selecting

Figure 12.2 Reasons for Missed Respiratory Therapy Sessions: A Cause-and-Effect Diagram

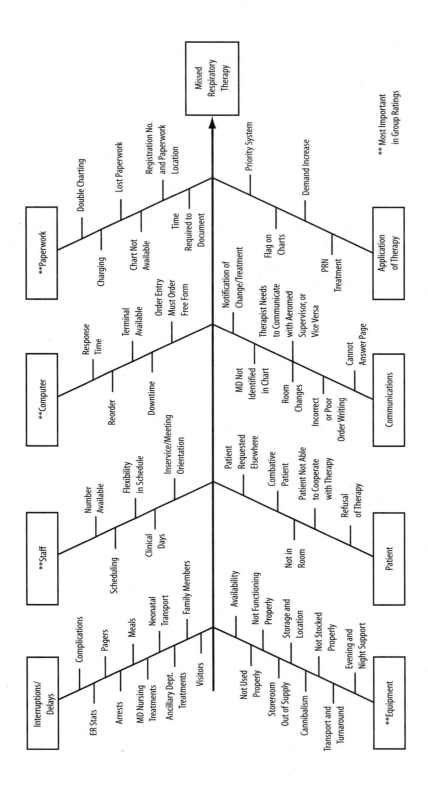

Source: D. M. Berwick, A. B. Godfrey, and J. Rossner. *Curing Health Care: New Strategies for Quality Improvement.* San Francisco: Jossey-Bass, 1990, p. 95. Reprinted with permission.

Figure 12.3   Reasons for Missed Respiratory Therapy Sessions: A Pareto Diagram of Survey Results

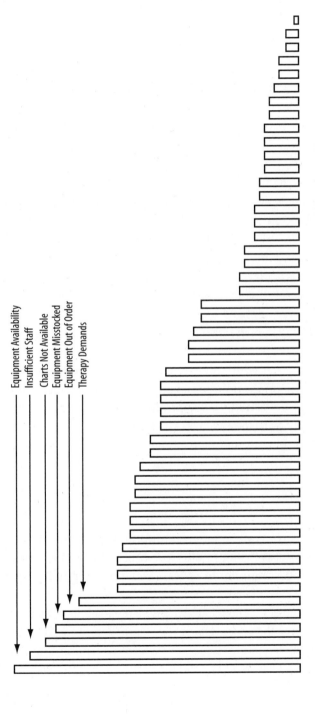

Equipment Availability
Insufficient Staff
Charts Not Available
Equipment Misstocked
Equipment Out of Order
Therapy Demands

Source: D. M. Berwick, A. B. Godfrey, and J. Rossner. *Curing Health Care: New Strategies for Quality Improvement.* San Francisco: Jossey-Bass, 1990, p. 96. Reprinted with permission.

from among these alternatives, after which a general approach to implementing the change can be devised or determined. The final task in this stage of the change process is the selection of techniques that can be used to support the actual implementation of the change being planned and reduce resistance to it within the organization. The planning stage is a crucial precursor to successful implementation. Each of the four tasks within this stage must receive careful attention.

Developing a Set of Viable Alternative Changes for Consideration. It is important to remember when carrying out this task that organizational changes can be borrowed, adapted, or originated. They may or may not involve true innovation. The essence of this task is to search for and develop alternative changes that might work and thus can be actively considered.

Alternative changes can come in ready-made or custom-made forms (Alexander, 1979). Ready-made alternatives are based on ideas that the manager has tried before or have been recommended by others who have introduced similar organizational changes; they can be borrowed or adapted from other contexts. Custom-made alternatives, in contrast, are innovations; they represent something created or invented to bring about a particular change. Obviously, these generally take more time and effort to develop and are thus less likely to appear on a list of viable alternatives than are ready-made alternatives.

In considering the possible changes they might make in a given situation, managers should not necessarily try to think in terms of one best choice. More realistically, several options, each with both positive and negative features, are likely to exist as possible responses to the need for an organizational change. The challenge in carrying out this task of developing relevant alternatives for consideration is to suggest as many potentially satisfactory choices as possible.

During this process, innovative organizational changes can emerge, but only if a new idea or concept, practice, or physical thing is created or invented, which is no small accomplishment. Managers who want their organizations to benefit from innovative organizational changes, therefore, must stimulate and support this process. Senior managers can do this by establishing innovation as a strategically important objective, fostering organizational cultures that value innovation, facilitating creativity and inventiveness (using small, cross-functional teams, for example), and placing a high priority on creativity in at least some of their staffing selections (Schermerhorn, 1993).

In effect, managers who wish to increase the likelihood that their organizations will be able to originate the concepts and ideas, practices, and physical things necessary for innovative organizational changes must devote attention to establishing an organizational climate in which creativity and innovation are stimulated and facilitated. Robbins

(1991) points out the following characteristics of a creative and innovative organizational climate:

- Risk-taking is tolerated, even encouraged. People are encouraged to take risks, and mistakes are treated as learning opportunities.
- Rules, procedures, policies, and similar organizationally imposed controls are kept to a minimum.
- Cross-training and participation in diverse teams is encouraged. There is a recognition that narrowly defined jobs create myopia, whereas diverse job activities give people a broader perspective.
- There is a widespread acceptance of ambiguity in the organization. People and units within the organization are given the opportunity to express their individualities through work.
- A healthy degree of conflict is permitted. Differences of opinion concerning how to do things are tolerated, even encouraged, as a means to increase creativity. Harmony and agreement between individuals and/or units are not seen as necessary to high performance.
- There is a high degree of tolerance for the impractical. People who offer improbable or even foolish answers to "what if" questions are not penalized. There is a recognition of and appreciation for the fact that what seems impractical at first might lead to innovative changes.
- The focus is on ends more than on means. If goals are made clear but people are encouraged to consider alternative routes toward their attainment, innovation might result.
- Communication flows freely. Communication flows laterally as well as vertically, facilitating the cross-fertilization of ideas.

Just as some organizational characteristics encourage innovation and creativity in health care organizations, thus improving the chances of developing innovative organizational changes within them, there are certain behaviors that managers who wish to stimulate creativity and innovation should avoid. Schermerhorn, for example, points out that the isolation of senior managers from the rest of their organizations "fosters misunderstandings about conditions and people in the organization and contributes to a risk-averse climate" (1993, p. 663). He also notes that a focus on short-time horizons and short-term organizational performance can reduce the chances of developing truly innovative solutions to problems and that in many organizations, the incentive and reward systems do not support innovation. He notes that reward systems typically "reinforce regularity and routines, and dislike the surprises and differences that often accompany the process of innovation" (Schermerhorn, 1993, p. 663).

Kanter (1983, p. 101) cautions, only slightly tongue in cheek, that managers who want to foster creativity should avoid the temptation to "regard any new idea from below with suspicion—because it's new, and because it's from below" or to "assign to lower-level managers, in the name of delegation and participation, responsibility for figuring out how to cut back, lay off, move people around, or otherwise implement threatening decisions you have made."

Relying upon their own insights and experiences, as well as those of others, and upon the creative processes available to them, managers who successfully carry out this task will develop a set of possible alternatives to consider. The existence of various alternatives in a situation of impending change requires that each be judged against the others. The question of which of the available options in a particular situation will be best must be addressed.

Choosing from Among the Change Alternatives.

Selecting from among the possible changes under consideration is easy if one alternative is clearly superior to the others. The purpose of selection is, after all, quite straightforward: to pick the alternative that has the greatest number of desired, and least number of undesired, consequences. Most often, however, choosing from among the viable alternatives for change is not easy for managers. Such situations are often gray rather than black or white; in addition, they tend to be quite dynamic. What appears to be the most appropriate alternative may not remain the most desirable choice as circumstances change. Complicating matters even further is the fact that although there are several bases for choosing a particular course of action (experience, intuition, advice from others, experimentation, and scientific or analytical decision making), no basis is best in all situations.

Indeed, choosing from among the available alternatives for change is usually a challenging task. There is no way to ensure that managers will make the best choice, or even select an adequate alternative. However, by comparatively assessing three factors in regard to each alternative, they can often considerably improve the quality of their choices.

First, the manager should assess how well each alternative under consideration supports the organization's stated objectives. This implies that the change alternatives are but the means to an end—an end that has been clearly thought out and stated in the form of an organizational performance objective. If an alternative under consideration does not support the achievement of stated performance objectives better than other available alternatives, it should be scrutinized very carefully. And to be selected over others, it must have some additional very positive features.

Second, the manager should assess the relative cost-effectiveness of each alternative under consideration. Which one makes the maximum use of available resources? There will be times, of course, when economic considerations should not be used as a criterion for making these choices, especially in health care organizations where quality considerations are so important. Usually, however, they are a useful guideline in choosing among change alternatives.

Finally, the manager should compare available choices along the dimensions of their inherent feasibility and the organization's ability to implement them effectively. In making these comparisons, managers must think very practically about how each possibility will actually be implemented in view of the resources available and the particular circumstances of the organizational change. Consideration of these three factors does not guarantee that the best choice—or even a good one—will always be made. It does, however, increase the chances that managers will make their selections wisely.

Devising a General Approach to Implementing Organizational Changes. The third task in the implementation planning stage of managing organizational change is to devise a general or overall approach through which to make the desired change. It is important that managers consider the whole range of general approaches to change in their implementation planning. Although there are many possible approaches to making organizational changes, all of them fit into one of two broad categories. One set of approaches to implementing change is based on the use of power, wherein managers use coercion or sanctions to bring about change. Such approaches are also called force-coercion approaches (Chinn and Benne, 1969) and are top-down in nature. Alternatively, the general approach to change can rely upon reason and rational persuasion. In this kind of approach, managers make organizational changes by convincing those involved of the need for change and explaining the rationale for the changes.

In the power, or force-coercion, approach to implementing organizational changes, managers determine and announce the changes they wish to make; other participants in the organization are expected simply to accept them. There is usually some sort of penalty associated with not accepting top-down directives to make organizational changes.

Changes in the strategic direction of organizations often require top-down, power approaches, as do quick responses to important environmental changes. For example, a change in the reimbursement policy of a major insurance carrier might require an immediate change in affected health care organizations, leaving little time for anything but a top-down edict. As Holt notes, the top-down approach to change offers the advantage of speed by "requiring only a few people to make timely, comprehensive decisions that can be communicated quickly to lower levels. A top-down change (approach) carries great weight and usually reaches deeply into the organization" (1990, p. 618).

Approaches that rely upon reason and persuasion to implement organizational changes come in many forms, but although they are all participative in nature, the degree of participation by managers and other employees in implementing the designated changes can vary widely. In general, increasing the level of participation or involvement of employees in decisions about design and management of organizations—including decisions about organizational changes—can reap substantial rewards, including "higher quality products and services, less absenteeism, less turnover, better decision making, and better problem solving—in short, greater organizational effectiveness" (Lawler, 1988, p. 197). Approaches to implementing organizational change that rely upon participation are very different from top-down approaches. Participation suggests the complete opposite of top-down edicts from senior managers who direct what and how change will be made.

Lawler (1988) has identified three types of approaches to increasing employee participation or involvement in organizations: parallel suggestion involvement, job involvement, and what he terms high involvement. These approaches to involvement or participation vary in the degree to which the following four features are moved downward in an organization: (1) information about organizational performance, (2) rewards that are based on organizational performance, (3) knowledge that enables employees to understand and contribute to organizational performance, and (4) power to make decisions that influence organizational performance (Lawler, 1988).

When information, rewards, knowledge, and power are concentrated at the top of an organization, little opportunity for meaningful involvement or participation in change exists elsewhere in the organization. In contrast, when these factors are moved downward, opportunities to participate actively in managing change increase greatly throughout the organization.

Parallel suggestion involvement encourages employees to suggest what changes are needed as well as how to implement and manage them. Their participation is encouraged, although they are given power only to recommend or suggest changes. Decisions are reserved for managers.

Job involvement focuses on enriching people's work so that they have more influence over it. In effect, employees are empowered to make changes in their own work, although not elsewhere in the organization. These approaches do not give employees power to change the structures or operations of the organizations within which they work, nor to change their strategic directions. However, they do permit a much greater degree of involvement than the parallel suggestion approaches.

High-involvement approaches permit employees not only to decide about changes in their work but also to have meaningful input into decisions to change the organization's purpose or objectives, culture, strategies, tasks, technologies, people, and structures. In some instances of high-involvement approaches to implementing changes, employees, typically working in small groups such as cross-functional teams or quality circles, actually devise the means of implementing an organizational change. For such bottom-up approaches to work effectively in health care organizations, senior managers must encourage and facilitate their use. The primary advantage of using a high-participation, bottom-up approach to organizational change is that it stimulates creativity in the organization (Lawler and Mohrman, 1985). This approach also fosters commitment to implementing changes on the part of those who have played a role in deciding how to approach making changes. Frequently, health care organizations use bottom-up approaches to organizational change when the changes either involve small parts of the organization, such as single departments, or are of a modest operational nature.

Organizational circumstances determine which approach to increased involvement is best in particular situations. "Because they position power, information, knowledge, and rewards differently, these approaches tend to fit different situations and to produce different results. It is not that one is always better than another, but that they are different and, to some degree, competing" (Lawler, 1988, p. 197).

Managers must exercise care when determining how much responsibility to delegate to employees in their approach to implementing organizational changes. For example, parallel suggestion involvement is often quite appropriate in an organization, or a part of one, with a traditional hierarchical structure; well-developed and entrenched management systems; and independent, relatively simple, and repetitive work. However, in a new organization, or a new unit in an existing health care organization involving complex and highly interdependent work and managers who value employee involvement, a high-involvement approach may be much better.

Whether the general approach to implementing change that is selected is based on power or persuasion, managers faced with organizational change must think in terms of how best to convince others that a change is needed and that a suitable change alternative has been chosen for implementation. Beyond this, as agents for change, managers in these situations must influence others to make the decisions and take the actions required to implement the change. In thinking about how to exert this influence, managers have five different bases or sources at their disposal (French and Raven, 1959).

One base from which managers can exert influence over change is the formal power and authority derived from their organizational position. This formal source of influence or authority exists because organizations find it advantageous to assign certain powers to individuals so that they can do their jobs effectively. All managers have some degree of formal power or authority that flows from their position. Of course, managers at different levels of health care organizations possess different amounts of this kind of influence.

Another source of managers' ability to exert influence over organizational change is their power to reward desirable behavior. This source stems partly from the positional source noted above. In other words, by virtue of their positions, managers control certain rewards that buttress their positional power and authority. Rewards include pay increases, promotions, work schedules, recognition of accomplishments, and status symbols such as office size and location. Managers can use these and many other rewards as a source of influence in a period of change. Conversely, managers also have the ability to punish or prevent others from obtaining desired rewards. This, too, can be a source of influence as managers seek to implement organizational changes.

Another important source of managers' ability to influence change is their knowledge or expertise. The ability to exert influence can derive from having knowledge that is valued by the organization and enhances one's ability to influence the thinking of others. This source of influence is personal to the individual with the expertise, in contrast to the positional sources of influence, which are granted to managers by virtue of their positions.

A related source of influence is the ability of some managers to engender admiration, loyalty, and emulation to the extent that they can exert influence. At the senior level of management, this quality is sometimes called charisma. Charismatic managers typically have a vision for their organization, possess strong convictions about the correctness of the vision, exude great self-confidence about their ability to realize the vision, and are perceived by others in their organizations as legitimate agents of change in their pursuit of the vision (Conger et al., 1988).

Once the tasks of identifying available change alternatives, choosing from among them, and devising a general approach to implementing the change have been accomplished, managers can turn to the final task in this stage of managing the change process: determining how to build support for the change and reduce resistance to it so as to maximize the likelihood of its successful implementation.

Selecting Techniques to Support Implementation.   This fourth and final task in the implementation planning stage involves selecting the techniques that will be used to develop support for the change and reduce resistance to it (Dunham and Pierce, 1989). There is no way for managers to assure absolutely that an organizational change, no matter how necessary it may be or how carefully its implementation is planned, will be successfully implemented. However, they can take certain steps to increase the likelihood of a successful outcome. Perhaps the most important is to ensure that the individuals involved in the change fully understand the situation. People who understand the necessity of a change and its details are more likely to adjust to it than those who do not. Managers should provide information about the change as far in advance as possible—including specific details concerning the reasons for it, its nature, its timing, and its expected impact on the organization and the people in it.

When possible, it may be useful for a change to be introduced on a trial basis. Familiarity gained through experience of a change, as well as assurances that it is not irrevocable, can reduce initial insecurity and increase the likelihood of acceptance. Allowing time for a change to be digested by those involved will almost always increase their ultimate acceptance of it.

When implementing organizational changes, managers should also try to minimize disturbances to customs and informal relationships. The culture developed by people at work has real value because it helps them adjust to the workplace and to their roles in it. Change almost invariably disrupts the culture of an organization, but such disturbance can be reduced by facilitating widespread participation in planning and implementing the change. People feel less pressure from changes that they help plan, because they understand them better. They are also likely to be more committed to the success of a change if they are involved in planning for and implementing it.

In considering what support techniques they might find useful in implementing organizational changes, managers must remember that people respond to change in predictable, often negative, ways. Managers, viewing change as the logical response to problems or opportunities, may be surprised to find that others have a very different view of the situation. Employees and perhaps other managers may not support the changes a manager thinks are important; they might might even overtly resist them. While a manager contemplating a change might view such resistance as irrational, it may seem perfectly rational to affected employees, especially if their past experiences with change were negative. These workers each judge change according to their attitudes and feelings, which in turn determine how they respond to change. These attitudes and feelings are not the result of chance but are caused by numerous factors.

One of the underlying reasons a person may view change in a negative way and resist it is that individual's personal history—including biological processes, background, and social experiences away from work—in other words, what the employee brings to the workplace. A second cause is the work environment itself. For example, if an organization has been very stable for a long time, it may be especially difficult to introduce organizational changes. When organizational participants have adjusted to the status quo and believe it is permanent, the introduction of even minor changes can be disruptive. Conversely, in organizations with a history of frequent changes that are seen as part of the organization's culture, people expect change and much more readily accept it.

The many reasons for the often encountered resistance to change among people in organizations include: insecurity, possible social and economic losses, inconvenience, resentment of control, union opposition, and threats to the influence that people have in their organizations (Mondy, Gordon, Sharplin, and Premeaux, 1990). Each of these bases for resistance to change is explored briefly below.

Insecurity is a major source of resistance to change. For many people, there is great comfort in the status quo, and any change is therefore viewed as undesirable because it introduces a degree of uncertainty. Even a seemingly simple change such as moving the photocopying machine can have far-reaching repercussions. To some, it may symbolize management's lack of concern for inconvenienced employees. To others it means more traffic, noise, and interference around their work area. A third group may see such a change as further evidence of the autocracy of managers. Change, then, can reduce the current level of satisfaction. People affected by change often do not know what will happen, but past experience may have taught them to expect the worst. In addition, change suggests to employees that they or their performance in the workplace may have been unsatisfactory.

Possible social losses of various kinds can result from change, and even the fear of such losses can cause people to resist change. Following an organizational change, close friends may have to work in separate rooms or not be able to interact during work. Complex informal relationships are affected by any organizational change involving people. Established status symbols may be destroyed in the process of reorganizing a health care organization, for example. Social acceptance by coworkers may be jeopardized if someone cooperates in a change inaugurated by management that these coworkers have rejected. In such circumstances a person may be forced to choose between cooperating with management and retaining the friendship of coworkers. Thus, what may seem a desirable and logical change can meet heavy resistance because the price in social relationships is too high.

In addition to possible social losses, real economic losses can accompany organizational changes. In many cases new technology allows more work to be done by the same or even fewer people. Resistance by those affected is understandable. Even if employees do not lose their jobs or face reduced earnings, a change may require them to work faster or contribute more in other ways. Such economic losses frequently concern people who face changes in their workplaces.

Inconvenience is a real part of almost all organizational changes, even when they do not involve significant economic or social losses. Any change causes some inconvenience, and extra effort is required to adjust to it. When old habits and ways of doing things must be replaced with new practices, inconvenience stimulates resistance, although if this is the only factor present, the degree of resistance may be minor.

Resentment is a normal human reaction to close control of the actions and behaviors of people. The degree of control exerted by managers is never more clear-cut than during the implementation of changes. In such situations people are made sharply aware that they do not fully control their own destinies in the organizations within which they work.

Unions can be an especially difficult source of resistance to some organizational changes, and health care organizations with unions often encounter opposition to changes that managers would like to make. Unions, after all, do not exist to cooperate with management; their role is to protect the interests of their members.

Threats to individuals' positions and influence within organizations are another reason certain people fear and resist organizational changes. In fact, changes that threaten the power base or influence of individuals, groups, or departments or units of organizations go to the heart of their organizational role and thus stimulate some of the strongest resistance to change. For example, physicians in health care organizations routinely and vigorously resist changes that threaten their power and influence.

All of these factors can cause people to resist change in organizations. Furthermore, they often operate in combination, thus strengthening the resolve of those opposed to change. One of the important aspects of effective planning in this respect is for managers who are about to implement a change to consider in advance how they might usefully address the resistance to it. Fortunately, a number of options are available. Several of the most important options for dealing with resistance to change are outlined in Table 12.2 and discussed below.

Education and communication are among the most common and useful tools available to managers as they seek to overcome resistance to organizational changes. These techniques involve communicating with the people who will be affected by a change to educate them about the nature of the change and inform them about its implications before it is made. Effective communication about a change and education regarding its implementation and implications can turn resistance into support.

Similarly, participation or involvement by those affected in planning for and implementing change can help overcome their resistance, especially when the people most likely to resist it are encouraged to be involved. Such involvement reduces uncertainty and misunderstanding about a change and its implications and reduces resistance to the change. Participating in decisions about a change provides an opportunity for people to gain a clearer picture of the change and enhances their commitment to its successful implementation.

Managers can help people to accept change by facilitating and supporting their adaptation to it. They can accomplish this step through, for example, arranging training programs that teach the new techniques, granting requests for leave during a painful transition period, or even offering special counseling sessions for people affected by a change.

Negotiation and seeking agreement among those involved and affected by a change are additional techniques for reducing resistance to organizational changes. In using

Table 12.2 Techniques for Reducing Resistance to Organizational Changes

Approach	Situational Use	Advantages	Drawbacks
Education + Communication	Where there is a lack of information or inaccurate information and analysis.	Once persuaded, people often will help with the implementation of the change.	Can be very time-consuming if many people are involved.
Participation + Involvement	Where the initiators do not have all the information they need to design the change, and where others have considerable power to resist.	People who participate will be committed to implementing change, and any relevant information they have will be integrated into the change plan.	Can be very time-consuming if participators design an inappropriate change.
Facilitation + Support	Where people are resisting because of adjustment problems.	No other approach works as well with adjustment problems.	Can be time-consuming, expensive, and still fail.
Negotiation + Agreement	Where someone or some group will clearly lose out in a change, and where that group has considerable power to resist.	Sometimes it is a relatively easy way to avoid major resistance.	Can be too expensive in many cases if it alerts others to negotiate for compliance.
Manipulation + Cooptation	Where other tactics will not work or are too expensive.	It can be a relatively quick and inexpensive solution to resistance problems.	Can lead to future problems if people feel manipulated.
Explicit + Implicit Coercion	Where speed is essential, and the change initiators possess considerable power.	It is speedy and can overcome any kind of resistance.	Can be risky if it leaves people feeling angry at the initiators.

Source: J. P. Kotter and L. A. Schlesinger. "Choosing Strategies for Change." *Harvard Business Review,* Vol. 57 (March–April 1979): 111. Reprinted by permission. Copyright © 1979 by the President and Fellows of Harvard College. All rights reserved.

these techniques, managers negotiate with opponents of the change and exchange something of value for reduced resistance. If resistance centers on a few people or a department, it may be possible to negotiate reduced resistance by allocating additional resources or promising to make a desired change at a later date. In the case of unions, collective bargaining agreements often require negotiations over changes. A change in how work is performed might mean a new round of negotiations with the union. If a mutually acceptable agreement is reached, the health care organization may implement a change but grant union members added compensation or other concessions.

Some managers do use manipulation and cooptation techniques as a means of reducing resistance to organizational changes they wish to make, although these techniques raise serious ethical concerns if they are taken to an extreme. Devious manipulative techniques include withholding information about changes from people who might resist, releasing false or misleading information, and playing the interests of one person or group off against others. Cooptation is a form of manipulation, but it is usually less devious than other forms. It may be as simple as bringing a person who is resisting change, or one who might resist it, into the planning process so that these individuals then become proponents of the change. However, cooptation may also involve deceit, which is of course clearly unethical.

At the most devious end of the continuum of techniques for overcoming resistance to organizational changes as shown in Table 12.2 is the use of explicit or implicit coercion. Because of the positional power held by managers in organizations, such techniques are available to managers as a way of getting people to accept changes. People can be threatened with the loss of their jobs or reduced promotion opportunities in an effort to stop them from resisting change. Acceptance of significant changes in an organization can be forced on people by the threat of yet more drastic measures (up to and including closing the organization, for example) if these changes are resisted. Coercion strategies, like manipulation strategies, can easily and often do lead to unethical behavior. The potential for unethical behavior, added to the inevitable anger of people forced into accepting change, makes techniques based on coercion extremely inappropriate and an unethical means of overcoming resistance to change.

Typically, the techniques that managers use to overcome resistance to organizational changes form a "package" of techniques aimed at different people. The selection of appropriate and effective support techniques, as well as the choice of a suitable overall approach to implementing organizational changes, bears directly on the success of implementing any change in a health care organization.

Stage 3: Implementing Organizational Changes

The implementation stage of managing organizational change as presented in Figure 12.1 involves the introduction of a new concept or idea, practice, or physical thing—or some combination of them—into an organization. Whether using a general approach to implementing change that is based on power or one that relies on persuasion, and whatever supportive techniques they plan to employ, managers must accomplish three things in sequence in order to implement any organizational change. They must first disrupt or "unfreeze" the status quo of the situation, then introduce the actual change, and finally stabilize or "refreeze" the modified organizational situation

(Lewin, 1952). These three steps involved in the implementation stage of an organizational change are illustrated in Figure 12.4.

In the first step, the status quo of a situation in which an organizational change is to be made is disrupted or, in Lewin's (1952) terminology, "unfrozen." In this stage the manager prepares those who will participate in or be affected by the change. The manager's efforts at this point are aimed at making others aware of the impending change and reducing or minimizing their resistance to it. If a power approach is being used, this may involve little more than announcing the change and directing those involved as to their roles in it. If a persuasion approach is being taken, preparing people for the change involves providing adequate information about the need for it and

Figure 12.4   Lewin's Three Steps to Implementing Organizational Changes

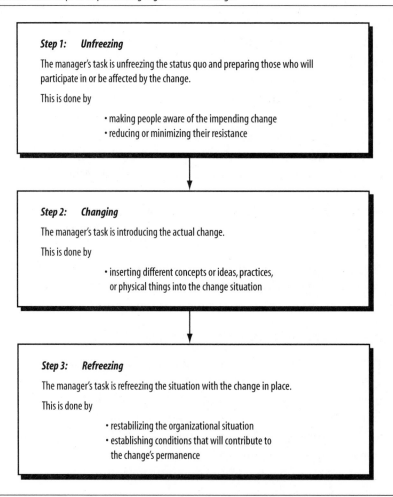

Step 1:   Unfreezing

The manager's task is unfreezing the status quo and preparing those who will participate in or be affected by the change.

This is done by

- making people aware of the impending change
- reducing or minimizing their resistance

Step 2:   Changing

The manager's task is introducing the actual change.

This is done by

- inserting different concepts or ideas, practices,
  or physical things into the change situation

Step 3:   Refreezing

The manager's task is refreezing the situation with the change in place.

This is done by

- restabilizing the organizational situation
- establishing conditions that will contribute to
  the change's permanence

may also require soliciting their participation in its implementation. As noted in the discussion of stage 2 in the process of managing change, people are far more likely to be receptive to change and to help implement it if they understand the advantages of a change and their part in it, especially if they are allowed to participate in its planning and implementation. They are also more likely in this case to fulfill their responsibilities associated with or growing out of the change.

Once the status quo of an organizational situation is broken, whether through a simple, top-down announcement or a much more elaborate participatory approach, the change can actually take place. This second step in implementation is the actual application or insertion of different concepts or ideas, practices, or physical things in the organization. As shown in Table 12.1, organizational changes can be directed at modifying any aspect of an organization—including its purpose or objectives, culture, strategies, tasks, technologies, people, or structures. In this step, some aspect of the organization is actually changed. If the change involves the use of a physical thing that is different in the situation, such as a piece of equipment, it is put in place and people begin using it. If the change involves the introduction of a different concept or practice, such as new reporting relationships, a revised marketing strategy, or a modified accounting system, use of the concept or practice is actually initiated.

In the third step of implementing an organizational change, the change is incorporated into the routines of those responsible for and otherwise involved in its implementation. Ideally, a new equilibrium is established as people adapt to the change and accept it as the norm. The manager's efforts in this step are aimed at restabilizing the situation in the organization and establishing conditions that will make the change permanent. The most important thing a manager can do to ensure the long-term stability of an organizational change is to have overcome the resistance to the change before its implementation. Following implementation, a manager can offer appropriate rewards to those who have successfully implemented the change, positive reinforcement intended to maintain the change, and adequate resources to ensure its continuation. Most important, of course, is the constant vigilance of the responsible manager to make certain that the change sticks.

In effect, again using Lewin's (1952) word for this step, the organizational situation is "refrozen" with the modification in place. Refreezing conditions in the organization around a change is intended to make that change permanent—at least until a future circumstance leads to a decision that the change is inadequate or flawed in some way and should be modified or abandoned. Such determinations are made through managers' systematic efforts to evaluate the organizational changes they have implemented, as will be seen in the discussion of the fourth and final stage in the process of managing an organizational change.

Stage 4: Evaluating Organizational Changes

The fourth and final stage in the process of managing organizational change, evaluation, is often given inadequate attention by managers and may even be overlooked altogether. However, evaluation of the changes that have been implemented is a vitally important stage in any manager's efforts to manage organizational change effectively. In fact, managers should evaluate all of their decisions and actions, including those related to organizational changes, because they have a responsibility to use the resources entrusted to them optimally. All organizational changes involve expending organizational resources such as money and time, which have alternative uses. Systematic evaluation permits managers to determine whether or not the resources used in implementing change have yielded sufficient benefits such as improved or enhanced quality, efficiency, satisfaction, adaptiveness, and organizational survival potential to justify the changes.

Evaluating an organizational change involves collecting adequate data upon which to base a thorough evaluation. The information base must be sufficient to permit managers to determine whether a change has been effectively implemented, whether the objectives established for the change were achieved, and what other related changes or modifications might be needed. Information that a change led to the actual desired outcome or to outcomes that do not match the original objectives provides important input into the overall process of managing organizational change.

When the evaluation stage shows that the results of a change are as desired, managers can turn their attention to other matters. However, when they are not, the original change must be modified. This feedback can also lead to the realization that further change is needed.

As can be seen in Figure 12.1, the feedback loop goes all the way back to stage 1 of the process. When changes do not accomplish their purposes, the process begins again, although this time the manager has more information, new insights into what might or might not work, and more experience of the challenging process of managing organizational change.

❧ CONCLUSIONS AND FUTURE DIRECTIONS

The people involved in health care in the United States, including managers, have achieved some marvelous successes. Among these achievements are diagnostic and therapeutic capabilities that are the most advanced in the world; biomedical research that has brought us to the brink of understanding disease at the molecular level and intervening in diseases at the genetic level; the widespread availability of the latest technology and most sophisticated clinical facilities; and the provision of significant levels of choice for most citizens about who their physicians are and about when and where they obtain health care services (Longest, 1996).

Yet, coexisting with a justifiable sense of pride and accomplishment about these achievements is a growing awareness that the nation faces some fundamental problems regarding health care. Creating, at least in part, its own most serious problem, the health care system has generated decades of rapidly escalating costs, costs that threaten the capacity of the nation to keep pace and exacerbate the problems of those who lack adequate financial resources to gain access to the health care system.

In addition to, and contributing to, the central cost problem, the health care system continues simultaneously to create both excesses and shortages of various capabilities and facilities. We grossly underutilize primary care and preventive services, while overutilizing certain high-technology services (Bodenheimer and Grumbach, 1995). Some of our citizens lack access to even basic health care services, while others are chronically overtreated. These problems have significant ethical implications.

One of the consequences of these problems is an inexorable pressure for change. As is so often the case in the United States, pressure for change in important institutions leads to new attempts to solve problems through changes in public policy (Longest, 1994). But the pressure for change also falls directly on the health care system itself and on the people who manage this system (Longest, 1996). Indeed, if the problems of cost and access are ever to be successfully addressed, improved management in the health care system will be a key part of the solution. Beyond their desire to solve the access and cost problems, many health care managers envision a much improved health care system. Such visions create their own pressure for change. Thus, knowledge of how best to manage the complex process of change is vitally important for the managers of health care organizations—and it will be even more so in the future.

As defined in this chapter, organizational change is a discernible modification in any aspect of an organization's purpose or objectives, culture, strategies, tasks, technologies, people, or structures. Most organizational changes occur through the adoption of concepts or ideas, practices, or physical things—either borrowed directly or adapted and modified to fit the borrower's needs—that have been developed by people who were making changes elsewhere. However, organizational changes can also involve innovation. Innovation is a special kind of change that occurs in an organization when someone within it invents or develops, and is the first user of, a new concept or idea, practice, or physical thing.

The complex process of managing organizational change is presented in this chapter as a four-stage model (Figure 12.1) comprising identification, planning, implementation, and evaluation/feedback. Each stage incorporates several tasks that must be successfully accomplished if organizational change is to be well managed. The first task is for managers to recognize situations and circumstances that require an organizational change to be made. They must then identify the nature of the change needed in a particular situation. These two tasks are closely related and can be triggered by a wide variety of pressures for change.

Identification of the need for change and the nature of the change needed in a particular situation is followed by other tasks that are intended to assure effective planning to implement the change under consideration. The tasks involved in implementation planning are (1) developing alternative changes to be considered in a change situation; (2) choosing the change that is to be implemented from among viable alternatives; (3) shaping a general strategy for making the change; and (4) developing the techniques that will be used to build support for the change and to minimize resistance to it.

The actual implementation of an organizational change is accomplished through three additional tasks: unfreezing the status quo, introducing the actual change, and refreezing the organizational situation with the change in place. Unfreezing the status quo is the task through which managers disrupt the status quo of a situation and prepare those involved for the change. It is followed by the task of actually making the change. Some concept or idea, practice, or physical thing—or some combination of these—is inserted into a situation so that modification occurs in the organization's purpose or objectives, culture, strategies, tasks, technologies, people, or structure. The actual change is followed by the third task of refreezing the organizational situation to give the change a chance of stability and durability.

The management of organizational change does not end with implementation, however. Managers who have the most success with implementing organizational changes evaluate the results of the changes they make and use the information they obtain through carrying out this task to provide feedback into future iterations of the change process. The task at this stage is essentially one of comparing actual results with those that were planned for, exploring the reasons for any differences, and using this information wisely to inform and guide future changes.

‰ REFERENCES

Alexander, E. R. "The Design of Alternatives in Organizational Contexts: A Pilot Study." *Administrative Science Quarterly*, 24: 382–404, 1979.

Berwick, D. M. "Blazing the Trail of Quality: The HFHS Quality Management Process." *Frontiers of Health Services Management*, Vol. 7, No. 4 (Summer 1991): 47–50.

Berwick, D. M., A. B. Godfrey, and J. Roessner, eds. *Curing Health Care: New Strategies for Quality Improvement*. San Francisco: Jossey-Bass, 1990.

Bodenheimer, T. S., and K. Grumbach. *Understanding Health Policy: A Clinical Approach*. Stamford, CT: Appleton and Lange, 1995.

Chinn, R., and K. D. Benne. "General Strategies for Effecting Changes in Human Systems." In W. G. Bennis, K. D. Benne, R. Chinn, K. E. Correy, eds., *The Planning of Change*, 3rd ed., 22–45. New York: Holt, Rinehart, 1969.

Conger, J. A., R. Kanungo, and associates. *Charismatic Leadership: The Elusive Factor in Organizations*. San Francisco: Jossey-Bass, 1988.

Dunham, R. B., and J. L. Pierce, *Management*. Glenview, IL: Scott, Foresman & Company, 1989.

French, J. R. P., and B. H. Raven. "The Basis for Social Power." In D. Cartwright, ed., *Studies of Social Power*, 150–167. Ann Arbor, MI: Institute for Social Research, 1959.

Hernandez, S. R., and A. D. Kaluzny. "Organizational Change and Innovation." In S. M. Shortell and A. D. Kaluzny, eds., *Health Care Management: Organization Design and Behavior*, 3rd ed., 294–315. Albany, NY: Delmar Publishers, Inc., 1994.

Holt, D. H. *Management: Principles and Practices*, 2nd ed. Englewood Cliffs, NJ: Prentice Hall, 1990.

Kaluzny, A. D., C. P. McLaughlin, and D. C. Kibbe. "Continuous Quality Improvement in the Clinical Setting: Enhancing Adoption." *Quality Management in Health Care* 1 (1992): 37–44.

Kanter, R. M. *The Change Masters: Innovations for Productivity in the American Corporation*. New York: Simon and Schuster, 1983.

Lawler, E. E., III. "Choosing an Involvement Strategy." *Executive*, Vol. 2, No. 3 (August 1988): 197–204.

Lawler, E. E., III, and S. A. Mohrman. "Quality Circles After the Fad." *Harvard Business Review,* Vol. 63, No. 1 (January–February 1985): 65–71.

Lewin, K. "Group Decision and Social Change." In G. E. Swanson, T. M. Newcomb, and E. L. Hartley, eds. *Readings in Social Psychology*, 459–473. New York: Holt, Rinehart, 1952.

Longest, B. B., Jr. *Health Policymaking in the United States*. Ann Arbor, MI: Health Administration Press, 1994.

Longest, B. B., Jr. *Health Professionals in Management*. Stamford, CT: Appleton and Lange, 1996.

Mondy, R. Wayne, Judith R. Gordon, Arthur Sharplin, and Shane R. Premeaux. *Management and Organizational Behavior*. Boston: Allyn & Bacon, 1990.

Pelz, D. C., and F. C. Munson. "A Framework for Organizational Innovating." Paper presented at the Academy of Management Annual Meeting, 1980.

Rakich, J. S., K. Darr, and B. B. Longest, Jr. "An Integrated Model for Continuous Quality Improvement and Productivity Improvement in Health Services Organizations." *Clinical Laboratory Management Review,* Vol. 7, No. 4 (1993): 292–303.

Rakich, J. S., B. B. Longest, Jr., and K. Darr. *Managing Health Services Organizations*, 3rd ed. Baltimore: Health Professions Press, 1992.

Robbins, S. P. *Management*, 3rd ed. Englewood Cliffs, NJ: Prentice Hall, 1991.

Roberts, E. B. "What We've Learned: Managing Invention and Innovation." *Research-Technology Management*, Vol. 31, No. 1 (January–February 1988): 11–29.

Schermerhorn, J. R., Jr. *Management for Productivity*, 4th ed. New York: John Wiley and Sons, Inc., 1993.

Schermerhorn, J. R., Jr., J. G. Hunt, and R. N. Osborn. *Managing Organizational Behavior*, 4th ed. New York: John Wiley and Sons, Inc., 1991.

Van de Ven, A. H., and M. S. Poole. "Explaining Development and Change in Organizations." *Academy of Management Review,* Vol. 20, No. 3 (July 1995): 510–540.

Designing Effective Health Care Organizations for the Future

13

James E. Rohrer, University of Iowa

M arket change in health care delivery is proceeding at a breathtaking pace, which should cause the reader to approach this essay with a certain degree of skepticism. Turbulent times are always rife with risk for those who would advise others how to prepare for the future. During the 1980s and 1990s, health care managers were advised to approach their roles in as businesslike a fashion as possible. Intense competition was the justification for this sagacity, and, possibly, at least partly a result of it. Regardless of cause and effect, health care delivery has been very competitive, and managers have been businesslike.

Properly viewed, this recent period in our history is clearly an aberration. Health care is a local affair, and in most local markets competition, at least in primary care, requires unnecessary duplication of resources. More important, perhaps, competition among health care providers causes the public to view health care managers with a certain degree of cynicism. After all, if health care providers will aggressively combat each other over revenues, what might they do to the unsuspecting patient if the opportunity for profit presents itself?

Communities would rather trust their health care delivery systems. Often, they view them as essential public services, like the school system, fire departments, and police protection. This attitude, where found, is a cultural imperative dictating that a sincere community service mission be adopted by the delivery system. Economic realities in the form of production efficiencies associated with natural monopoly reinforce this conclusion.

Grounding the local health care system in community service has important implications. These include the following:

1. The delivery system should seek to enhance community health.
2. The system should be frugal, because communities do not appreciate ostentatiousness or wasted resources in their public services.
3. The critical health care delivery organization is not a physical institution such as a hospital, nursing home, or group practice but a local system of primary care (i.e., community health network). The traditional approach designing health care organizations focuses on the structure of institutions, drawing on formulations such as that offered by Mintzberg (1983). By focusing on the system rather than on an institution, this chapter is proceeding in a different direction.
4. The mission of the local health care system is not a matter of strategic choice. Instead, the mission must be optimization of community health. This requires an emphasis on primary care, health promotion, and prevention.
5. Alternative structures for community-based health systems are more similar than they are different. Key concepts are vertical integration, community-oriented primary care, community governance, population-based planning, and information systems that demonstrate accountability.

The effective health care organization of the future will embrace a mission of community service. Primary care and prevention will be the services around which production processes will be organized. Collaboration among providers will be vital to successful performance. Achieving all this will require substantial change, but there are models to follow. Hopefully, the discussion to follow will provide some ideas on how to proceed.

?■ MISSION

The strategic management literature is replete with discussions of strategic behavior. Some organizations are prospectors, frequently searching for new market opportunities. Others are analyzers that stick to their core operations but will watch for new opportunities. Defenders rarely innovate, and reactors make changes only when forced to do so (Shortell, Morrison, and Friedman, 1990; Miles and Snow, 1978). This body of literature implies that the leaders of health care organizations are largely free to decide what the organization will do.

While descriptions of strategic behavior are of academic value, what practicing managers require is a set of prescriptions. Prescriptions are assertions about what to do. Once they are on the table, along with the rationale that supports them, managers can accept, modify, or reject them.

In keeping with this perspective, let us observe that the first goal of every health services system is to optimize the health of the population by employing the most advanced knowledge about the causation of disease, illness management, and health maximization (Starfield, 1992). This goal is not a matter of strategic choice. Health care organizations that choose to do otherwise declare themselves peripheral to the health care system and risk losing both legitimacy and community support. That some health care providers have ignored this reality in the pursuit of patients, prestige, or profit is irrelevant. After all, the health care system in our country is widely understood to be dysfunctional. The socially responsible manager will seek to optimize community health. In a properly structured health care organization, this will also constitute good performance in the eyes of its governing board.

An example may help clarify this point. Mr. Jones, CEO of Jonesville Medical Center, has aggressively worked toward growth in his organization. Against all odds, he has recruited and retained a full range of specialists and supplied them with equipment. Aggressive marketing has found patients for these physicians. Prenatal care and other types of primary care and prevention have not developed much at all. Cost per case, hospitalization rates per capita, and rates of avoidable health problems are all higher than state averages. As the market shifts toward capitation, Mr. Jones discovers that his revenues are dropping precipitously and his fixed costs are high. His hospital is perceived to be in trouble. He might ask himself why he did not focus his mission on community health from the outset. Doing so would have prevented overinvestment in specialty care while demonstrating a commitment to serving the community. Getting a bond issue passed to subsidize the hospital would be easier today if he had done this.

Given that the purpose of a health care organization is to optimize community health, its mission statement can be expected to emphasize primary care, health promotion, and disease prevention. Specialty care is essential, but it cannot optimize health because preventing illness and promoting optimal functioning require a broader perspective than can be achieved by the disease specialist (Starfield, 1992). Effective medical care must take into account the contexts in which the patient lives and works and the full spectrum of health problems he or she has. A generalist, rather than a specialist, is required to integrate specialty services, understand what services the patient requires, and plan prevention strategies.

Primary care includes appropriate treatment of common diseases and injuries, provision of essential drugs, and coordination of specialty care. It also includes maternal and child health programs, prevention of diseases, promotion of sound nutrition, health education, and environmental sanitation. This mix of services is included in the definition of primary care because a good mix will achieve the maximum impact on community health per dollar invested. Thus, it is clearly consistent with the goal of the health system and should feature prominently in the mission statement.

❧ TYPES OF LOCAL PRIMARY CARE SYSTEMS

Horizontal integration occurs when providers of the same type of service join together, thus capturing a larger market. When providers of different services in the continuum of care join together (e.g., physicians, hospitals, nursing homes, emergency services, and home health), they gain greater control over an entire market area. This process is called vertical integration.

Local primary care systems can be confused with some other types of health care organizations. The term "primary care network" is often used to mean a horizontally integrated collection of primary care physician practices. Primary care networks could spread over regions comprising several communities. A physician-hospital organization (PHO) is a partnership between a hospital and its medical staff. The PHO is community-specific but may not have a mission oriented toward community health. Since PHOs and primary care networks are often formed so that their members can compete for managed care contracts, it is likely that both will eventually organize and deliver services under capitation financing. Capitation payment, from a theoretical perspective, contains incentives that encourage providers to minimize inappropriate care and emphasize prevention programs. However, until providers explicitly adopt optimization of community health as their primary mission, PHOs and horizontal primary care networks will not evolve into local primary care systems.

In the 1980s, four basic types of organizational designs could be identified for primary care organizations, based on whether they were sponsored by a community board, the public sector, physicians, or a hospital (Kaluzny and Konrad, 1982). A community-sponsored organization might be a free clinic, a hospice, or an AIDS program. Typically, these organizations are established because of a perceived failure on the part of health care providers to meet an important need for services, and they tend to be small and informal.

A public sector primary care program typically has what is known as a machine structure. Clear job descriptions exist for personnel and organizational units. For example, the primary care physician does not do community health nursing, and the nurse does not worry about environmental sanitation. This division of labor reduces flexibility but can increase effectiveness in specialized areas. Attention must be directed to coordinating the separate units. This, of course, is the role of the professional administrator (if the organization can afford one), who reports to a governing board such as the board of health.

In a typical, physician-sponsored primary care program the administrator (often an office manager) reports to the medical staff. Support staff, such as registered nurses, nurse practitioners, physician's assistants, laboratory technicians, and clerical personnel, are all accountable to the medical staff either directly or through the administrator. In its most traditional guise, this structure maximizes clinical oversight but does not achieve the benefits possible from a team of health professionals.

Finally, the hospital-sponsored primary care program may consist simply of an outpatient department into which specialty visits are scheduled; an emergency department, which handles patients who do not have a personal physician; or a branch clinic, established to generate inpatient referrals. Naturally, these programs will not begin to achieve the performance of a proactive organization truly committed to optimizing the health of the community.

The four types of primary care organizations described above still predominate in most local health care systems. Many communities have all four types, sometimes several of each. Smaller communities may have less than the full set. Since the limitations of each type do not offset each other with any degree of reliability, many local health systems are uncoordinated, inefficient, and ineffective.

Another perspective on types of primary care organizations was developed by investigators from the Health Services Research Center, University of North Carolina (Sheps et al., 1983). These researchers were focusing on subsidized rural programs, but their ideas are relevant to the general questions of how to organize primary care. They asserted that three relatively stable program characteristics were most important: (1) sponsorship or governance, (2) size and mix of staff, and (3) number of sites. Five forms emerged for them:

1. *Traditional solo or other forms of practice.*
2. *Satellite Practices* (called extension practices by the investigators), controlled by a larger institution such as a health department, private medical practice, hospital, or medical school.
3. *Primary Care Centers*, independent of larger institutions and supported by community groups.

4. *Organized Group Practices*, having at least two full-time physicians and not providing any outreach services.

5. *Comprehensive Health Centers*, having a community governing board and at least three full-time primary care providers, and providing outreach services.

As communities struggle to develop coordinated primary care systems, they will be faced with decisions regarding affiliation with vertically integrated networks, which can be defined as self-governing organizations composed of participants that are themselves autonomous organizations or individuals (Moscovice, Christianson, and Wellever, 1995). Complete vertical integration includes secondary and tertiary care and encompasses large geographic areas. Relationships between primary care systems and regional networks will be discussed in a later section. Their relevance to this discussion lies in the typology of organizational structures used to classify them, since similar dimensions may be relevant to primary care systems.

Moscovice, Christianson, and Wellever (1995) use three dimensions to categorize vertically integrated networks: level of integration, complexity, and assumption of risk. Level of integration is the degree to which the component members function as a single unit. Opposite extremes would be informal networks lacking any basis for action other than mutual interest, versus creation of a single corporation in which all members are subsumed.

Complexity relates to the scope of services and the number of partners whose efforts must be coordinated. The simplest primary care system might be a country doctor, working alone to deliver all of the primary care needed in a community. At the opposite extreme would be an inner-city community served by a hospital, physicians of several different specialties, public health professionals (including community health nurses), a variety of nontraditional health care providers (such as acupuncturists, massage therapists, and chiropractors), and private providers of publicly funded services for vulnerable populations (such as substance abuse treatment programs, community mental health centers, and community health centers). The complexity of the second type of primary care system is much greater (see Figure 13.1).

Networks also vary in the degree to which they share financial risk. In an informal network, the losses of one partner are not shared by the others. Greater risk sharing occurs when the partners agree that losses and profits will be distributed according to some predetermined formula. Each is motivated to cooperate so as to avoid large losses. The maximum in shared risk is achieved when the partners agree to share the net profit or loss from serving an enrolled population. Providers will each be motivated to achieve a balance of services that avoids use of costly services. Each will seek to maintain patient care volume and control production costs.

Physical integration is another dimension of importance in primary care systems. When partners are separately housed, overhead costs are substantially higher.

Figure 13.1   The Community Health Network

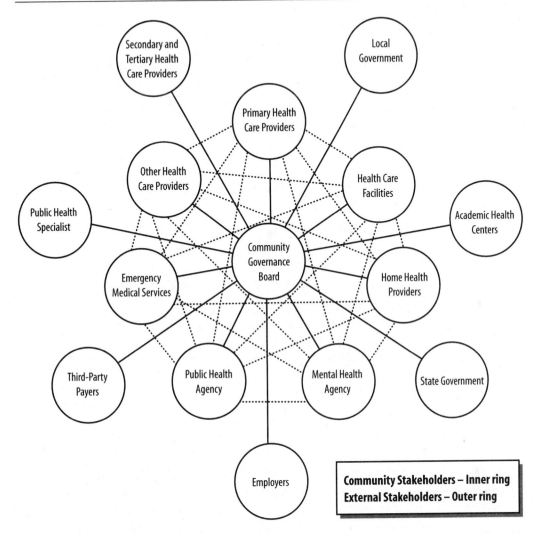

Source: Merchant, James A., Rohrer, James E., Walkner, Laurie M. and Urdaneta, Marta E. 1994: *Provision of Comprehensive Health Care to Rural Iowans in the 21st Century*, PEW/RWJ Health of the Public Report.

Furthermore, the ability of each partner to support skilled administrators is more limited than when resources are pooled. Maximum physical integration is achieved when all partners colocate, perhaps on the premises of the local hospital.

The various dimensions identified above that describe how primary care systems are organized include sponsorships, organization integration, complexity, risk sharing,

Figure 13.2   Typology of Primary Care Systems

Ownership/Sponsorship
  Hospital
  Physician
  Government
  Community

Physical Integration
  Each partner remains on own premises
  Several partners colocate
  Partners physically merge and work as a team

Assumption of Risk
  None
  Shared profit and loss
  Capitation

Organizational Integration
  Informal
  Formalized
  Single corporation

Complexity
  One type of provider and/or service
  Several types
  All types

and physical integration (see Figure 13.2). Most communities have not moved very far along any dimension to achieve a higher level of organization.

Fortunately, a few examples can be found of communities where primary care networks have been established that integrated the various components of the local health system. The basic structure of the integrated system is consistent with the theory of community-oriented primary care (COPC), described below.

?a. COPC

Community assessment is a key dimension of COPC, which defines and characterizes the community so that the mix of services offered reflects both the common health problems found in it and social circumstances that influence health. These assessments of community needs are used to modify the primary care program. Program effectiveness is measured not just in terms of impact on patients but also in regard to impact on community health.

To be responsive to community needs, a health system requires the following: epidemiological analysis, community governance, and coordination of medical care and other health services with public health programs. Health professionals prefer to be both autonomous and independent, but some degree of cooperation is necessary to optimize community health. Furthermore, health providers need community support, and one way to achieve that is by means of a governing board composed of community leaders, including the local business community. The business community has a vested interest in cost-effective care, because such care can control the cost of health benefits for employees. Local government officials also wish to control the cost of health care, since taxes are never popular. Consumers want to be healthy. If providers can satisfy all of these partners, then community support is assured. Since COPC will lead to cost-effective health care, it is in everyone's best interest.

The degree to which COPC has been achieved in a local system is reflected in four functions: (1) definition and description of the community, (2) identification of community health problems, (3) modification of the health care program, and (4) measurement of program effectiveness (Starfield, 1992, p. 188). Staging criteria have been developed for each function. A community that fully performs the community definition function has a database enumerating all residents—including the addresses, telephone numbers, and demographic and socioeconomic data for each individual. Identification of health problems has been fully achieved when a community group identifies priority problems, investigates the causes of those problems, and documents current treatment patterns relating to those problems. Program modification is not being fully performed unless community and public health services as well as medical care change appropriately. Both outreach and the targeting of high-risk or priority groups within the community are necessary. Finally, effectiveness monitoring should be determined in light of program objectives, be risk-adjusted, and reveal the program's weaknesses as well as its strengths.

The COPC functions as described above will remind managers of a generic model of strategic planning: Goals and objectives are set based on data and values of the governing body, programs are redirected, and outcomes are judged against predetermined objectives. For strategic planning of a primary care network to succeed, no single partner can dominate the process. A common problem is for hospital-based planners to seek to control board membership and priority setting so that the hospital remains predominant in the local health care system. Even worse, hospital planners may initiate community health planning efforts in an attempt to shore up the role of the hospital in acute inpatient care at the expense of primary care and prevention. The consequence of such an effort is likely to be loss of legitimacy for the network and absence of community support for network initiatives. Hospital planners will have to set aside their natural tendency to want to control events and support acute care in favor of a form of leadership that supports shared goals and promotes primary care.

The fact remains, however, that in many communities the greatest reservoir of managerial experience lies in the local hospital. Leadership from this source may well make the difference in whether the network is successful. Therefore, one is forced to the conclusion that hospital executives will often be needed to play leadership roles in network development. Given a clear mission statement from the governing board of the network, and performance standards addressing community health, there is every reason to be confident that the hospital executive will bend his or her talents in the necessary direction.

❧ Performance of Primary Care Organizations

During the period 1979–82, subsidized rural primary care clinics were buffeted by a severe recession, high inflation, and significant budget cuts. Despite these difficulties, only 9 out of 193 programs studied actually closed (Ricketts et al., 1984). Programs exhibited adaptiveness and strength in a hostile environment. Interestingly, such programs benefited from being affiliated with a hospital. Clinic costs and revenue were both reduced when clinic providers used the local hospital as a free second office. However, since costs were reduced more than revenues, the financial self-sufficiency of the clinic was enhanced by the relationship (McLaughlin et al., 1985).

Clearly, primary care organizations can be durable, especially when affiliated with a hospital and receiving some public money. Looking specifically at hospital-sponsored primary care organizations, additional characteristics are also important (Shortell, Wickizer, and Wheeler, 1984). A strong hospital initial commitment to primary care and involvement of the medical director of the group in hospital decision making were important predictors of continued existence, while use of a professional rather than a bureaucratic structure, more visits per full-time equivalent (FTE) physician, use of residents, and availability of a rural or suburban site were associated with improvements in accessibility of services. Bigger clinics with low physician turnover and rural or suburban sites were more likely to contribute financially to the hospital. The financial performance of the clinic was enhanced by having more commercially insured patients, higher prices, more visits per physician FTE, multiple specialties, use of nurse practitioners and/or physician's assistants, and use of an incentive compensation plan.

A separate study of a subset of the same sample of community hospital–sponsored group practices provides another perspective on their performance. Community surveys revealed that the hospital-sponsored practices attracted people who had not previously had a regular source of care. Access and satisfaction were good. The use of inpatient services, emergency rooms, or hospital outpatient departments was not increased by the primary care programs. In short, access to primary care was improved without raising costs in other ways. The authors of this study recommended hospital-sponsored primary care programs for underserved areas.

❧ Community Governance

Primary care systems can become more organized as a result of initiatives taken by any of the participants in the system, but the local hospital may be best equipped with managerial expertise (see example 1). However, since hospital administrators are often oriented toward controlling events, they may find it difficult to play an entrepreneurial role in the development of systems that empower the community even when the hospital may be dramatically modified by the process (see example 2). Hospital administrators are more likely to approach community governance sincerely when the survival of their institutions is problematic and cooperation is one of the last remaining strategies for salvaging the situation.

Example 1: Community Leadership

Ocean County, New Jersey, has a population of 400,000 coastal residents. Many citizens are seniors, which adds a special dimension to the needs profile of the community.

Mark Pella, president and CEO of Community Medical Center in Toms River, brought together more than 80 community leaders to work on improving the quality of life in Ocean County. An external consultant was hired to facilitate the process. After an initial conference involving all participants, seven work groups were established to study transportation, teen and family issues, domestic violence, and a countywide electronic infrastructure.

Mycek, Shari. "Following the Leaders: Helping Communities Take Ownership of Their Health," *Trustee*, March 1995, pp. 6–9, Vol. 48, No. 3.

Example 2: Retaining Control

Smithville is a small town within the service area of Jonesville Medical Center. Jonesville Medical Center has been subsidizing the small hospital in Smithville for several years. Seeing the potential of using community health planning to redirect the Smithville hospital toward other purposes, the Medical Center carefully selected a steering committee in Smithville composed of likely hospital supporters and a few consumers. Only three people attended the first meeting. When asked for an explanation of the low turnout, the attendees observed that the hospitals had strategic planning processes, so another one seemed redundant. Furthermore, the planning effort appeared to be a transparent attempt to manipulate the community in a way that would solve the problems facing the hospitals rather than letting the community determine its priorities. Feeling powerless and tricked, most people did not bother to participate.

Other participants may also want to move cautiously, and for the same reasons (see example 3). As a result, one is forced to the conclusion that an informal, loosely coupled structure for the system may be the most feasible in many situations. Certainly, examples can be found of local planning boards that work to coordinate their primary care systems even without legal incorporation. In theory, these "value added partnerships" involving local business, public health programs, privately owned entities such as community health centers, and private providers such as physician practices and the hospital can be stable as long as they continue to function in the best interests of their members (Foreman and Roberts, 1992).

Example 3: Letting the Community Set the Pace

A steering committee was established in Monroe County, Iowa, to discuss formation of a local primary care network that could meet the mounting wave of managed care with clear goals. The committee was composed of representatives from local government, local physicians, the hospital board, hospital administration, economic development, a major employer, and public health.

At the outset, the group was not willing to commit itself to developing plans relating to managed care. The topic was both emotionally disturbing and technically overwhelming. The committee chose to look at planning data to gain an understanding of health problems in Monroe County. After reviewing a variety of secondary data sources, the steering committee decided that three topics required further investigation: access to primary care for children in poverty, wellness, and mental health managed care. It planned a community survey to determine consumer perceptions of problems and service needs in these areas. Coordinated implementation of some new initiatives seemed likely. The steering group was evolving into a governing board for a local primary care system.

If the local hospital is evolving into the center of a primary care system, then the hospital's board of trustees may be able to grow into a new role of community-oriented system management. However, the ability of many hospital boards to be progressive has been questioned (Griffith, 1992; Umbdenstock, Hageman, and Amundson, 1992). Creation of a new body, called a steering committee, community health planning task force, citizens' committee, or health commission may be necessary.

Community governance begins with a development process. A temporary planning body, composed of representatives of all of the stakeholders, is established in the hope that it will be sufficiently successful to continue indefinitely (see Figure 13.1). The board should be constituted in a way that will establish its legitimacy in the eyes of the larger community. After all, changes in the health care delivery system are likely to be proposed, which could lead to public outcry. Forcing changes on the community will just lead consumers to go outside the community for the services they need.

Legitimacy is a delicate issue, and one that requires an insider's knowledge of local politics. Nevertheless, some guidelines can be suggested. These include the following:

- Be sure all of the health providers are represented.
- Do not cast any health provider in a visible leadership role if cynics are likely to interpret the board as a self-serving sham. A local business leader would be an ideal chair, provided that the individual has a record of civic leadership.
- Be sure that local government is offered an opportunity to participate.
- Involve consumers. This last is a difficult issue, since on the one hand, everyone is a consumer; and on the other hand, people who are consumers without any other connection to the health system are difficult to find. Also, keep the local press and state government apprised of planning activities.
- Use an objective outsider to serve as facilitator and consultant to the development process.

After constituting the board, the first task will be to set priorities for the local health system. Several methodologies are available to lead the board to a position where it can engage in priority setting. One example is APEX-PH (Assessment Protocol for Excellence in Public Health), which was developed by the public health community. Any methodology might be appropriate if the board leadership understands that it is engaged in a strategic planning process that will examine data about the health system and interpret the data in light of community values in order to set priorities for the system.

Assembling the data for population-based strategic planning is usually called community assessment. The kinds of information required are discussed in the following section.

Once the board has been educated about the health problems facing the community, it can set priorities for what the local health system should be attempting to address. These priorities typically emphasize primary care, prevention programs, and emergency services. Task forces can be established to develop programs for addressing priority problems. Performance indicators are also needed to measure the programs' success.

The Institute of Medicine (IOM) recommended the use of 15 types of indicators for measuring the accessibility of services. These indicators have the force of expert opinion behind them. Also supporting their use is the value of some of them as measures of efficiency and quality as well as access. For example, high hospitalization rates for conditions sensitive to ambulatory care may indicate inefficient use of resources and, possibly, suboptimal care in addition to poor access to primary care. These are discussed in a later section.

ॐ POPULATION-BASED PLANNING

In accordance with the COPC concept, the primary care network should base its service mix on community needs. The data required to accomplish this should revolve around morbidity patterns (from what illnesses do people suffer?). Once these are known, services can be directed at treating the sick and preventing disease among those at risk.

Unfortunately, morbidity is difficult to measure. The menu of approaches is as follows:

1. *Demographic and socioeconomic characteristics.* Age, gender, and race are associated with morbidity rates, so collection of demographic data about the community can provide insight into service requirements. Similarly, poverty and occupational mix are also useful. Demographic and socioeconomic data are available from secondary sources, including the US Bureau of the Census. Unfortunately, complete current information is difficult to assemble for small geographic areas.

2. *Vital statistics.* Population size, birthrates, and death rates by cause (see Table 13.1, for example) are important for obvious reasons: Numbers of deaths by cause indicate which illnesses people have. However, many people suffer from acute and chronic diseases that are never listed as causes of death.

3. *Reportable disease.* Sexually transmitted diseases (STDs) and infectious childhood diseases are examples of diseases that must be reported by physicians to the health department. Most diseases, however, are not reportable. Some states will also have registries of important diseases such as cancer, birth defects, Alzheimer's disease, or trauma. Registries are valuable sources of information about disease prevalence, but their availability and completeness vary by state.

4. *Hospital discharges.* Morbidity patterns can be inferred from the discharge diagnoses of local residents. The most common diagnoses tend to mirror the most common causes of death and may reflect the most common illnesses. In addition, some conditions have been identified as "ambulatory care sensitive,"

Table 13.1   Monroe County Profile: Selected Causes of Mortality

	Total Cases in County	County Rate per 100,000	State Rate per 100,000
Malignant neoplasms	18	219.90	231.10
Benign neoplasms	N/A	N/A	16.10
Diabetes	N/A	N/A	2.50
Anemias	1	12.20	1.90
Alzheimer's disease	3	36.60	11.00
Major cardiovascular disease	47	574.10	453.20
Heart disease	34	415.30	453.20
Hypertensive heart and renal disease	3	36.60	10.80
Ischemic heart disease	25	305.40	234.60
Acute myocardial infarction	12	146.60	107.40
Old myocardial infarction and other forms of chronic ischemic heart disease	13	158.80	126.60
All other forms of heart disease	5	61.10	90.10
Cerebrovascular disease	11	134.40	74.50
Pneumonia	6	73.30	43.60
Influenza	0	0.00	1.00
Coronary obstructive pulmonary disease	6	73.30	47.30
Ulcer of stomach and duodenum	N/A	N/A	3.20
Chronic liver disease	N/A	N/A	5.60
Nephritis, nephrotic syndrome and nephrosis	N/A	N/A	7.20
Accidents and adverse effects	4	48.90	36.50
Suicides	1	12.20	11.30

Source: (U.S. Vital Statistics Tables 4 and 5, 1993)

meaning that access to good primary care can keep hospital admissions for these conditions to a minimum. Pediatric asthma is an example of a condition sensitive to ambulatory care. High discharge rates for these conditions imply that attention needs to be directed to the primary care system. Rates of common surgical procedures are also valuable, since higher-than-expected rates for procedures such as hysterectomy and mastectomy may reflect a weakness in the diagnostic process in the primary care system, a tendency to refer too readily to specialists, or a failure to detect problems early. However, only the most serious cases are hospitalized, so most illnesses are not captured by this data set.

Tables 13.2 and 13.3 are examples of how hospital discharges may be examined. Table 13.2 focuses on which case types are most common in the community, since services must be directed at common problems. Table 13.3

Table 13.2   Monroe County Profile: Most Common Case Types

Case Type	Admissions
Total number of ambulatory care sensitive	236
MDC 5–Circulatory system	242
MDC 14–Pregnancy	157
MDC 15–Newborn/neonate	130
MDC 6–Digestive system	153
MDC 4–Respiratory system	157
MDC 8–Musculoskeletal	137
Ambulatory care sensitive–chronic	132
Ambulatory care sensitive–rapid onset	102
MDC 1–Nervous system	85
MDC 19–Mental	54
Referral sensitive	65
Marker conditions	63

Total Admissions: 1,489. All ages, 1992.
Source: (Codman Research Group, Inc., 1994)

directs attention toward how the community rates compared with state averages, which may serve as benchmarks.

5. *Community perceptions.* Surveys of consumer perceptions about health status; healthy behavior; accessibility, efficiency and quality of health services; and priorities for the local health system can be conducted. Self-reported morbidity may not be completely accurate, but since perceptions drive behavior, an argument can be made for gathering this information. Unfortunately, no standard community survey form exists. Instead, many different attempts have been made to gather relevant information without making the form excessively burdensome to complete. The best approach, probably, is to seek guidance from the governing board about what kinds of information to collect, if a survey is to be conducted. For the purposes of the initial community assessment, the board needs to learn about consumer satisfaction with the accessibility of health care services. The board may also want to know where people are going for care and, if they are leaving the local market, why? Health status information may also be collected. However, it should be obtained from other sources, if possible. The board may also want to learn about the health behaviors of residents. For example, if dietary habits are poor, perhaps the primary care system should mount programs directed at changing dietary behavior. Focus groups are needed to supplement or substitute for communitywide surveys.

Table 13.3   Monroe County Profile Case Types Significantly Different from State Averages

Case Type	Significance Level	Admissions
Total Admissions	***	1,489
Total medical and surgical	***	1,113
Total medical admissions	***	792
Ambulatory care sensitive–total conditions	*	236
MDC 14–Pregnancy	***	157
MDC 15–Newborn/neonate	***	130
MDC 6–Digestive system	*	153
MDC 4–Respiratory system	*	157
MDC 8–Musculoskeletal	*	137
Ambulatory care sensitive–chronic	*	132
MDC 1–Nervous system	*	85
Adult gastro-enteritis	***	60
MDC 3–Ear, nose and, throat	***	48
MDC 9–Skin breast	**	45
Adult bronchitis/asthma	***	37
Acute myocardial infarction	**	40
Ambulatory care sensitive–chronic obstructive	**	37
Medical back problems	***	29
Ambulatory care sensitive–asthma	***	25
Other nervous system diseases	***	26
Nutr. misc. metabolic diseases	*	27
Cardiothoracic procedure	*	26
Urinary tract stones	***	21
Psychoses	•	19
Referral sensitive–coronary angioplasty	*	22
I9–Angioplasty	*	22
Pedi bronchitis/asthma	*	16
Back and neck procedures	*	19
Adult Pneumonias	•	23
Other ear nose and throat diagnoses	***	18
ACS–dehydration–volume depletion	*	18
Cellulitis	**	18
Referral Sensitive–Hip/Joint Replacement	•	20
410 chemotherapy	**	18
Chemotherapy/radiotherapy	*	18
Depressive neurosis	**	14
Lower extreme and humer pr	*	15
Appendectomy w/ appendicitis	*	13
Other musculosketal system diseases	*	16

Table continued on next page.

Table 13.3 *Continued*

Case Type	Significance Level	Admissions
Other ENT operations	*	12
19–mal. trachea/lung	*	14
Sub depend rehabilitation and detoxification		5

Significance level and relation to state average

Above state average	Below state average
*<.05	.<.05
**<.01	..<.01
***<.001	...<.0001

Source: (Codman Research Group, Inc., 1994)

Surveys cannot reach the illiterate, and response rates for many other groups may be poor. Focus groups are not regarded as being completely representative of the community from which they are drawn, but they have the advantage of producing a richer source of qualitative impressions and values than surveys can provide.

6. *Physician office billing systems.* Most people who reside in a community will visit a local physician at least once in a two- or three-year period. A bill will be generated showing the health problems addressed. Therefore, morbidity patterns can be computed from office billing systems, if their owners will share them.

All six of the data sources described above can be used to estimate morbidity patterns for a community. The costs and accuracy of each are different, and in an ideal world, all six would be used to describe the health of the community.

Once the magnitude of the community's health problems is estimated, the governing board will have to set priorities, since not all health problems are equally important. For example, the local value system may attach more importance to services for children than to mental health services. Whether or not the managers of the health system agree, in these circumstances children's health care must come first. Otherwise, the community could well withdraw its support from an "unresponsive" health care delivery system.

Priority health problems readily suggest priority health services. Once priorities are established, it will be necessary to compare priorities with the actual array of services.

For this purpose an inventory of available services is needed. For example, the distances to each of a variety of health services can be displayed as shown in Figure 13.3, with an *x* in each column showing where the service in question can be found. This approach does not allow planners to compare the volume of each type of service with the volume needed. However, no standard volume measures are available for common community-based services such as STD counseling, substance abuse treatment visits per capita, and hospice visits per terminally ill patient (IOM, 1993). Hopefully, these can be developed at some time in the near future.

In addition to examining proximity to various services, planners generally evaluate production capacity for key services. Physician services serve to illustrate the

Figure 13.3 Service Availability

Service	Local	Town A	Town B	Within 100 Miles
Primary medical care				
Hospital care				
Tertiary care				
Specialty care				
Long term care				
Emergency care				
Pharmacy				
Dentistry				
Home health care				
Other home care				
Mental health care				
Hospice				
Substance abuse treatment				
Community health nursing				
Health education				
Wellness center				
Other				

point. Figure 13.4 shows what the American Medical Association (AMA) regards as the minimum number of full-time equivalent physicians per 1,000 clients.

The key primary care provider in most locations is the family practitioner (or general practitioner) (.432 needed per 1,000). Other specialties sometimes included in primary care are general internal medicine, general pediatrics, and obstetrics/gynecology. The total number of MDs/1,000 comes out to about two per 1,000 population.

In some communities the governing board may value access to specialists more highly than these rates allow. The board may therefore choose to increase the FTE

Figure 13.4   MDs Needed in Aggressively Managed System

55% Commercial and 45% Seniors	
Specialty	**Targeted FTEs/1,000**
General practitioners/family practice	0.432
General internal medicine	0.86
Other internal medicine	0.399
Pediatrics	0.143
Obstetrics/gynecology	0.104
Psychiatry	0.048
Cardiovascular	0.060
ENT	0.075
Ophthalmology	0.020
General surgery	0.101
Orthopedic surgery	0.119
Uro surgery	0.037
Other surgery	0.048
Emergency medicine	0.020
Radiology	0.047
Pathology	0.087
Anesthesiology	0.085
Other miscellaneous	0.055
Total	1.966

Source: 1995. American Medical Association, Medicine in Transition.

devoted to specialists and reduce family practice, or it may choose to supplement primary care physicians with mid-level providers. Regardless of the final plan, the mix of providers and their availability should be consciously planned, taking into account local values as well as benchmarks provided by national organizations such as the AMA.

A similar approach can be used to plan for acute hospital beds. Often, planners assume that a total of two community hospital beds are needed per 1,000 population. Posthospital convalescent care and long-term nursing home care can take place in the same facility if more than two beds per 1,000 are available locally. Bed-to-population ratios for inpatient mental health, substance abuse treatment, and other specialized services can be based on local priorities. Numbers of FTEs devoted to services not requiring inpatient beds are also a matter for local priorities to determine. For example, community health nursing is an essential component of a primary care system. However, the extent to which community health nurses spearhead outreach programs and health education, and the degree to which they will be able to seek out vulnerable populations such as migrant labor, undocumented aliens, or the elderly will depend on local needs and priorities. No absolute "correct number" of nurses per 1,000 can be offered, just as there is no "correct" number of family practitioners per 1,000.

All of the above discussion assumes that the health system is serving a defined community. In most situations the community will be a market area consisting of a known population residing in geographic proximity. While many methods have been used to estimate "service areas," the most reasonable is to allocate zip codes or townships to a community if the plurality of residents use primary care providers in that community. This allows the compilation of micro-areas to form a denominator for population-based planning.

🙋 INFORMATION SYSTEMS AND MONITORING PERFORMANCE

The information system required by the primary care network will encompass the kinds of data used in population-based planning described above. It will also permit the network to monitor its performance, with performance being defined as provision of services directed at meeting community health needs. It is important to note that monitoring service use to assure that community needs are met also allows the organization to achieve financial control. In a capitated system, controlling the use of services is as critical as controlling the cost per unit of service, if not more so.

At first glance, it might appear that the same information used to identify community needs (i.e., morbidity, mortality, consumer perceptions) can serve to document performance. However, this is not uniformly the case, because most indicators of community health status are not sensitive to changes in the service delivery system. For example, high morbidity levels in a migrant farm labor population cannot be eliminated by increased access to primary care. However, increased access can be measured in terms of visits per capita, documenting that the network has directed its resources where they are needed. Exceptions to these rules can be found, of course. Infant mortality rates and low birthweight rates, for example, can be influenced by prenatal care.

The overall performance of the primary care system can be monitored using a standard approach derived from the health services research literature, though specific indicators can be expected to evolve over time. A commonly used approach (see Figure 13.5) is reflected in the HEDIS (Health Employer Data and Information Set). These are similar to a set of indicators recommended by the National Institute of Medicine that reflect progress toward national objectives (see Figure 13.6). The objectives are as follows:

1. To promote successful birth outcomes.
2. To reduce the incidence of vaccine-preventable childhood diseases.
3. To detect and diagnose treatable diseases early.
4. To reduce the effects of chronic disease and prolong life.
5. To reduce morbidity and pain through timely and appropriate treatment.

The IOM data set draws heavily on claims data to compute rates.

Medical care utilization rates have been used as quality indicators for several decades. For example, Paul Lembcke (1952) pioneered the use of regional utilization

---

Figure 13.5 Health Plan Employer Data and Information Set (HEDIS)

Major Quality Indicators

Preventive care and health promotion
Prenatal care
Admission and readmission rates
Outcomes for high-profile health problems
Access to providers (including urgent/emergency care)
Patient satisfaction
Detailed data on gender, age, and utilization rates
Utilization rates and costs for specific services
Analysis of high-occurrence or high-cost DRGs
Information on quality assessment and improvement

Source: 1995. American Medical Association, Medicine in Transition.

Figure 13.6 Indicators Proposed by the Institute of Medicine

1. Adequacy of Prenatal Care* (A, Q)
2. Infant Mortality Rate (A, Q)
3. Percent Low Birthweight (A, Q)
4. Congenital Syphilis Rate (A, Q)
5. Preschool Immunization Percent (A, Q)
6. Incidence of Vaccine-Preventable Childhood Diseases (A, Q)
7. Breast and Cervical Cancer Screening Rates (A, Q)
8. Incidence of Late-Stage Breast and Cervical Cancer (A, Q)
9. Continuing Care for Chronic Diseases (average number of MD contacts per year for those in fair or poor health*; proportion with no MD contacts) (A)
10. High-Cost Discretionary Care (admission rates for referral-sensitive procedures) (Q, C, A)
11. Avoidable Hospitalization for Chronic Diseases (admissions for ambulatory-care-sensitive chronic conditions) (A, Q, C)
12. Access-Related Excess Mortality* (A, Q)
13. Acute Medical Care (percent of individuals with no MD contact) (A)
14. Dental Services (average number of dental visits per year) (A)
15. Avoidable Hospitalizations for Acute Conditions (admission rates for ambulatory-care-sensitive conditions) (A, Q, C)

A = access, Q = quality, C = cost
* Not readily measured from secondary data.

Source: Modified from Institute of Medicine (1993).

---

rates as indicators of hospital quality by showing that teaching hospitals were less likely than outlying community hospitals to perform appendectomies. Furthermore, their service areas also experienced lower appendicitis death rates. The utilization rate approach to measuring quality was popularized by Wennberg and others (1973) in the United States and by Roos and others (1982, 1985, 1989) in Canada.

The IOM indicators do not address the availability and accessibility of all types of medical care. Examples of other useful indicators include travel time to hospitals and primary care, primary care providers per capita, and emergency medical services response time (see Figure 13.7). Nursing home beds per 1,000 resident population 85 years of age and over, and inpatient and residential treatment beds in mental health organizations per 100,000 population, were suggested by Aday et al. (1993) as supplemental indicators of "potential access."

Also missing from the IOM indicators are surveys of client satisfaction with the quality and accessibility of services. The IOM report recommended that additional indicators need to be developed in the following areas: HIV/AIDS, substance abuse, migrants, homeless people, people with disabilities, family violence, emergency services, postacute care services for the elderly, and prescription drugs (IOM, 1993, p. 131).

Figure 13.7   Supplemental Performance Indicators

- Hospital beds per capita (A, C)
- Travel time to hospitals (A)
- Primary care personnel per capita (A)
- Primary care physicians per capita (A)
- Specialty physicians per capita (A, C)
- Nurses per capita (A)
- Pharmacists per capita (A)
- Travel time to primary care (A)
- Dentists per capita (A)
- Nursing home beds per 1,000 people 85 years and over (A, C)
- Inpatient residential treatment beds in mental health organizations per 100,000 population (A, C)
- Home health visits per 1,000 elderly (A, C)
- Licensed mental health providers per capita (A)

- EMS response time (A)
- Hospital utilization rates for high-cost procedures (A, C)
- Hospital expenditures per capita (C)
- Physician expenditures per capita (C)
- Primary care expenditures per capita (C)
- Specialty physician expenditures per capita (C)
- Total health care expenditures per capita (C)
- Dental expenditures per capita (C)
- Mental health expenditures per capita (C)
- Dental expenditures per capita (C)
- EMS expenditures per capita (C)
- Volume in volume-sensitive conditions (Q)
- Client satisfaction (A, Q)
- Substance abuse expenditures per capita (C)

A = access, Q = quality, C = cost

Indicators of the types listed in Figures 13.6 and 13.7 are only that: indicators. They are not intended to offer positive proof of the poor performance of primary care systems. Instead, they serve as a screening mechanism. When indicator values are different from standards, closer investigation should be undertaken to verify the findings.

Careful consideration of the indicators shown in Figures 13.6 and 13.7 reveals that they are surprisingly easy to assemble. Investment in expensive software packages is not required. If the local hospital can generate discharges by diagnosis, these can be matched with population and referral-sensitive conditions. Other indicators are even more easily computed.

Not mentioned to this point are indicators of financial performance such as cost per case, net revenue, and hospital length of stay. While these measures are relevant to the financial management of an institution such as a hospital, they are less relevant to the performance of a primary care system in which the hospital is a contributory member. What drives system costs are utilization rates; and controlling the cost per unit is a problem for the hospitals, group practices, and other member agencies. Most system costs are generated by the use of specialty services outside the primary care system. If specialty use can be controlled, then cost control by local providers will be less urgent. In short, performance indicators relevant to financial control might include the following: total MD visits/1,000, specialty visits/1,000, hospitalizations/1,000, emergency department visits/1,000, total expenditures/1,000, and the cost of health insurance premiums.

This minimalist approach to management information systems is at odds with most expert opinion. The growth of managed care has given rise to calls for replacing claims data (not needed in capitated systems) with encounter data. Encounter information can become even more detailed than claims data used to be—possibly erasing the "administrative costs dividend" that proponents of managed care hoped to achieve by eliminating fee for service. Such detailed information may be useful at regional headquarters, but it is less so at the local level, since the number of cases of any given type is small. This writer remains unconvinced that detailed clinical information will save more than it costs to collect.

❧ PRINCIPLES FOR SUCCESSFUL SYSTEM DEVELOPMENT

Developing a primary care system out of the fragmented components present in most communities is a difficult task. Those who have done it successfully suggest that abiding by the following principles will increase the chances of success.

1. State at the outset that the purpose of planning is to create a shared vision of how the local system can function (Van Hook and Rosenberg, undated).
2. Expand participation beyond health care providers to include the larger community. All relevant constituencies should be represented so that the planning group will be perceived as having legitimacy. An effective chairperson is needed who is neutral, respected, and possesses group process skills (Amundson, 1991). Without local leadership, community system development efforts cannot succeed.
3. Take advantage of internal problems and external threats in a constructive way. For example, financial insolvency of the local hospital or encroachments on the local market from external provider groups can motivate communities to take planning more seriously (Coddington, Moore, and Fischer, 1994, p. 17).
4. Use a roadmap for the process. Participants will be reassured and more productive when they understand the sequence of activities (Amundson, 1993). However, the group may not be prepared to think about a major system change when it begins planning under these circumstances. It may be better just to focus on needs assessment and developing a shared vision. The group must be ready for more advanced topics before these are raised, since it can easily balk or even disband.
5. Rethink the appropriate scope of local health services. The planning group may assume that the historical service mix is reasonable for the future, unless challenged to reconsider (Amundson, 1993).

6. Analyze the health system. All major strengths and weaknesses should be identified to the greatest possible extent. These may include quality of care, local service needs, leadership, financial performance, teamwork, consumer satisfaction, and utilization patterns. Amundson (1993) recommends using an outside consultant, particularly for the needs assessment.

7. Provide briefings to the steering committee on key topics.

8. Use effective group process methods. Experience with conducting meetings, communication, team building and conflict management can all be helpful (Amundson, 1993).

9. Commit resources. Communities that are unwilling to invest in a planning process are unlikely to change. Amundson (1993) recommends that they be required to put up cash. However, if start-up funds are available from elsewhere, investment of time and energy may be a sufficient commitment from board members.

10. Continue the planning process. It is necessary to evaluate the impact of implemented plans; the planning group will need to make changes each year.

11. Take advantage of assistance from larger provider organizations. Sometimes a large hospital system will see primary care system development as being to its advantage. Empowering a community group to serve as a governing board could lead to constructive changes that could never have been forced on the community. For example, when a regional hospital has a management contract with a small hospital that is failing, it may seek to disengage to avoid losses, although fearing a backlash from the local physicians on whom it depends for referrals. Consequently, the regional hospital may choose to subsidize a planning effort without controlling the outcome, in the belief that goodwill and, possibly, rational restructuring to emphasize primary care will result.

❧ INTEGRATION WITH REGIONAL SYSTEMS

The community health system cannot exist independently of the larger health care system in which it is embedded. Local systems need big partners from whom they can acquire technical expertise and other resources, and with whom they can share financial risk.

In 1920, Lord Dawson of Penn presented a White Paper on the organization of health services in Great Britain. The report called for three levels of health services: primary health centers, secondary health centers, and teaching hospitals. Formal linkages were needed among these levels of care. This theoretical arrangement has since become the basis for regionalized health systems in many countries (Starfield, 1992, p. 4).

A more recent formulation also proposes three levels of care for regional systems (Beaulieu and Berry, 1994, pp. 270–71). At the first level, community clinics, serving about 5,000 people and spaced a 15-minute drive apart, would provide office, health education, pharmacy, laboratory, and x-ray facilities. Level II regional primary care centers, serving about 25,000 people, would add emergency care, mental health services, ambulances, public health services, periodic specialty clinics, and limited inpatient care.

Another model calls for office care, health promotion, public health, home health, pharmacy, laboratory, specialty clinics, nursing home, and dental services to be coordinated with a primary care hospital providing a few beds for observation and convalescence serving a population of about 12,000 (Merchant et al., 1994). Regardless of which model of regionalization is employed, it is clear that local primary care practices are the basic building blocks of the regional system. Secondary and tertiary care hospitals have no reason to exist beyond supporting the primary care systems in their regions. This should be kept in mind, in light of the natural tendency of referral hospitals to regard themselves as the "hubs" or centers of the system, ultimately dominating regional systems and distorting investments so that referral services are overemphasized.

The key to preventing dominance by the referral hospital, if there is one, is to design the system so that the governing boards of the primary care systems are linked into a regional system board that is distinct from the board of the referral center. One possible way to accomplish this is for the regional system board to be composed primarily of representatives of the primary care systems that make up the regional system. The immediate benefit of this design comes into play when revenue declines due to cuts in government health insurance programs or conversion to closed budgets, as has happened in many communities when aggressive managed care has taken over the market. In the absence of board representation on the part of local systems, managed care could damage local primary care systems by diverting patients to referral centers out of the community for services that could be provided locally.

Therefore, representatives of local systems may be well advised to negotiate for some or all of the following as they develop their affiliations with regional systems:

1. Maximize use of local primary care providers.
2. Include the services of essential providers such as community mental health centers and substance abuse treatment agencies in the local budget.
3. Offer residents an insurance product that is "community rated" (all enrollees pay the same premium regardless of age or preexisting conditions).

4. Allow open enrollment to the insurance plan, so that those who are ill or have low incomes can benefit from the community rating scheme.

5. Include case management in the budget of the primary care system, so that a case worker can work proactively with high-risk families.

6. Provide assistance to assure availability of primary care providers. Assistance could be in the form of recruitment, income support, or relief workers.

7. Arrange for specialty clinics to be provided locally.

8. Offer annual community health outreach programs targeted at priority problems, such as cardiovascular health, STD prevention, or drug abuse.

9. Pay malpractice insurance for health care professionals practicing locally.

❧ CONCLUSION

Turning fragmented local delivery systems into coordinated primary care systems will be difficult. Meeting this challenge involves developing nothing less than the health care delivery system of the future. Despite its difficulty, however, doing so is a necessary strategic move for local providers.

It is also an excellent way for providers to discharge their civic responsibility to function as community leaders. In the 1980s leadership seemed to have an individualistic definition. Effective leaders leaped into the competitive fray and changed their organizations by force of will, charisma, and good management. In the 1990s, leaders are empowering their workers; they lead from behind. In the year 2000 leaders will need to step back yet farther. Empowering communities means giving up control over future directions. Influence remains, but accountability moderates its force. This move takes courage, but the traditional value system of the field of health administration supports it.

Unfortunately, good intentions and skill together may not be sufficient to empower communities to govern their health care systems. Lawrence Brown and Catherine McLaughlin (1990) evaluated Community Programs for Affordable Health Care, a group of projects funded by the Robert Wood Johnson Foundation, to demonstrate the potential of effective cooperation at the local level. Brown and McLaughlin concluded that community leaders would not be likely to organize themselves into stable negotiating structures able to exercise economic discipline. Health care is big business at the local level, health care professionals have great influence, and no simple solution to the problems of access, cost and quality presents itself. Most important, the causes of inflation are found not at the community level but rather in state and federal programs, insurance company boardrooms, and regional health system headquarters.

Not everyone agrees. Robert Sigmond (1995) has articulated a powerful argument in favor of community control over and coordination of their own health care systems. Walter McNerney (1995) and Phillip Newbold (1995) have also written about the importance of community-based initiatives. Perhaps the fundamental point to be made about feasibility is that community-based health systems management is possible, given dynamic local leadership and a shared commitment to quality of life. Success is by no means guaranteed, however. That, in a nutshell, is the current challenge of health administration.

Acknowledgment

An expanded version of this chapter has been published as "Planning for Community-Oriented Health Systems." APHA, 1996.

&. REFERENCES

Aday, L. A., Begley, C. E., Lairson, D. R. and Slater, C. H. 1993: *Evaluating the Medical Care System: Effectiveness, Efficiency, and Equity*. Ann Arbor, MI: Health Administration Press.

American Medical Association 1994: Medicine in Transition: Strategies for Change.

Amundson, Bruce 1991: *Implementing a Community-Based Approach to Strengthening Rural Health Services: The Community Health Services Development Model*. WAMI Rural Health Research Center Working Paper Series #11.

Amundson, Bruce 1993: Myth and reality in the rural health service crisis: Facing up to community responsibilities. *The Journal of Rural Health*, 9, no. 3, 176–187.

Beaulieu, Joyce E. and Berry, David E. (eds.) 1994: *Rural Health Services: A Management Perspective*. Ann Arbor, MI: Health Administration Press, 270–71.

Borders, Ty 1995: *Monroe County, Iowa Health Care Needs Assessment*. Graduate Program in Hospital and Health Administration, The University of Iowa, April 16, 1995.

Brown, Lawrence D. and McLaughlin, Catherine 1990: Constraining costs at the community level: A critique. *Health Affairs*, Winter, 5–46.

Coddington, Dean C., Moore, Keith D. and Fischer, Elizabeth A. 1994: *Integrated Health Care: Reorganizing the Physician, Hospital and Health Plan Relationship*. Englewood, CO: Center for Research in Ambulatory Health Care Administration.

Foreman, Stephen E. and Roberts, Robert D. 1992: The power of health care value-adding partnerships: Meeting competition through cooperation. In Levey, Samuel (ed.), *Hospital Leadership and Accountability.* Ann Arbor, MI: Health Administration Press, 47–58.

Griffith, John R. 1992: Voluntary hospitals: Principles of the well-managed community hospital. In Levey, Samuel (ed.), *Hospital Leadership and Accountability.* Ann Arbor, MI: Health Administration Press, 47–58.

Institute of Medicine 1993: *Access to Health Care in America.* Washington, DC: National Academy Press.

Kaluzny, Arnold D. and Konrad, Thomas R. 1982: Organizational design and the management of primary care services. In Gerald E. Bisbee, Jr. (ed.), *Management of Rural Primary Care—Concepts and Cases.* Chicago: The Hospital Research and Educational Trust, 31–67.

Lembcke, Paul 1952: Measuring the quality of medical care through vital statistics based on hospital service areas: 1. Comparative study of appendectomy rates. *American Journal of Public Health,* 42, March, 276–86.

McLaughlin, Curtis P., Ricketts, Thomas C., Freund, Deborah A. and Sheps, Cecil G. 1985: An evaluation of subsidized rural primary care programs: IV. Impact of the rural hospital on clinic self-sufficiency. *American Journal of Public Health,* 75, 749–753.

McNerney, Walter J. 1995: Community health initiatives are widespread, challenging our sense of civic obligation. *Frontiers of Health Services Management,* 11, no. 4, 39–44.

Merchant, James A., Rohrer, James E., Walkner, Laurie M. and Urdaneta, Marta E. 1994: *Provision of Comprehensive Health Care to Rural Iowans in the 21st Century.* PEW/RWJ Health of the Public Report.

Miles, R. E. and Snow, C. C. 1978: *Organizational Strategy, Structure, and Process.* New York: McGraw-Hill.

Mintzberg, H. 1983: *Structure in Fives: Designing Effective Organizations.* Englewood Cliffs, NJ: Prentice Hall.

Moscovice, Ira, Christianson, Jon B. and Wellever, Anthony 1995: Measuring and evaluating the performance of vertically-integrated rural health networks. *Journal of Rural Health,* Winter, 9–21.

Mycek, Shari 1995: Following the leaders: Helping communities take ownership of their health. *Trustee,* 48, no. 3, 6–9.

Newbold, Philip A. 1995: Building Healthy Communities. *Frontiers of Health Services Management*, 11, no. 4, 45–48.

Ricketts, Thomas C., Guild, Priscilla A., Sheps, Cecil G. and Wagner, Edward H. 1984: An evaluation of subsidized rural primary care programs: III. Stress and survival, 1981–82. *American Journal of Public Health*, 74, 816–819.

Roos, N. P. and Lyttle, D. 1985: The centralization of operations and access to treatment: Total hip replacement in Manitoba. *American Journal of Public Health*, 75, 130–133.

Roos, N. P. and Roos, L. L. 1981: High and low surgical rates: Risk factors for area residents. *American Journal of Public Health*, 71, 591–600.

Roos, N. P. and Sharp, S. M. 1989: Innovation, centralization, and growth: coronary artery bypass graft surgery in Manitoba, *Medical Care*, 27, 441–452.

Sheps, Cecil G., Wagner, Edward H., Schonfeld, Warren H., et al. 1983: An evaluation of subsidized rural primary care programs: I. A typology of practice organizations. *American Journal of Public Health*, 73, 38–49.

Shortell, Stephen M., Morrison, Ellen M. and Friedman, Bernard 1990: *Strategic Choices for America's Hospitals: Managing Change in Turbulent Times.* San Francisco: Jossey-Bass.

Shortell, Stephen M., Wickizer, Thomas M. and Wheeler, John R. C. 1984: Hospital-sponsored primary care: I. Organizational and financial effects. *American Journal of Public Health*, 74, 784–798.

Sigmond, Robert M., McNerney, Walter J., Newbold, Philip A. and Altman, Drew 1995: Collaboration in a competitive environment: The pursuit of community health. *Frontiers of Health Services Management*, Summer, 11, no. 4, 5–36.

Starfield, Barbara 1992: *Primary Care: Concept, Evaluation, and Policy.* New York: Oxford University Press.

Umbdenstock, Richard J., Hageman, Winifred M. and Amundson, Bruce 1992: The five critical areas for effective governance of not-for-profit hospitals. In Levey, Samuel (ed.), *Hospital Leadership and Accountability.* Ann Arbor, MI: Health Administration Press, 47–58.

Van Hook, Robert T. and Rosenberg, Steven undated *Independent Networks: Future Directions.* Vol. 6 in a monograph series: Alternative Models for Organizing and Delivering Health Care Services in Rural Areas.

Wennberg, J. and Gittelsohn A. 1973: Small area variations in health care delivery. *Science*, 182, 1102–1107.

Motivating Effective Performance

14

Stephen J. O'Connor, University of Wisconsin—Milwaukee

Achieving organizational goals in health care depends very much on the work force's ability to perform in an effective and prompt fashion. Among the components contributing to a worker's ability to perform effectively, motivation stands out as a principal element. Consequently, one of the most significant responsibilities encountered by health care managers is the need to motivate workers sufficiently. A fundamental prerequisite to making this happen is a basic grounding in the theories, principles, and applications of human motivation. With regard to this last statement, there is both good news and bad news. The good news is that the area of motivation has garnered more attention than any other topic in the study of individual behavior. Thus, there is an extraordinarily large body of work on which to draw. The bad news is that even with this abundance of theorizing, empirical studies, and practical experience, we are still somewhat unclear and tentative as to how best to go about motivating our health care work force.

This chapter seeks to examine the concept of motivation, especially as it applies to health care organizations and to those professional and nonprofessional workers who populate them. In the process we will explore such topics as motivation and society, evolving attitudes and views about worker motivation; human needs deficiencies; the major content and process theories of motivation, and some approaches to implementing these theories; and the nature of what it means to be a professional, as well as the specific motivational challenges that poses for health care managers.

❧ MOTIVATION AND HEALTH CARE MANAGEMENT

Our current health system has been characterized as becoming increasingly *hyperturbulent* (Goes and Meyer, 1994; Shortell, 1994). As the word implies, *hyperturbulence* means that the extent and pace of change occurring in the American health system are far more than many managers are able to handle. A principal element of this rapid change appears to be an inexorable movement toward capitation, managed care, and the development of vertically integrated health networks. Purchasers of health care such as employers, insurers, governments, unions, and health coalitions are all pursuing those health care providers who offer easy access to care, a broad array of services, and exceptional value—appropriately delivered high quality at a reasonable cost. In particular, purchasers are taking an increasingly hard line toward costs. As a result, health care managers face a conundrum. On the one hand, the hyperturbulent environment is putting pressure on them to steadily improve productivity, cost efficiencies, and quality processes and outcomes (both clinical and patient-perceived). On the other hand, all of these improvements are expected to happen in an increasingly resource-scarce environment. Compounding this situation is the fact that most health care organizations are labor-intensive service businesses that rely heavily on relatively large numbers of people to meet organizational objectives. A manager's success in this type of environment requires a solid understanding of human behavior, especially motivation. Health care managers want to elicit high performance from their workers, and health care workers might be better motivated to provide a wide variety of other behaviors. Essentially, a high-performing worker or team is one that helps achieve organizational goals by delivering high-quality services in a productive and efficient manner. In addition to improving their productivity, health care managers often wish to motivate worker creativity in problem solving, promote innovativeness in creating new service products or processes, and reduce absenteeism and tardiness (Mercer, 1988). Additionally, they may be interested in trying to motivate high-quality people to seek employment with their organization, as well as to remain after they have been hired (Greenberger, Strasser, Lewicki, and Bateman, 1988).

As the work in health care organizations becomes more interdependent and team-oriented, and as concern for patient satisfaction and perceptions of service quality continues to grow (O'Connor and Shewchuk, 1995), health care organizations are seeking to develop prosocial and pro-organizational behaviors among their employees.

Interdependent work processes require team-oriented behavior, and they also require employees to work cooperatively to achieve organizational objectives. Also, as health care organizations seek to create and sustain service-oriented climates and cultures, motivating behaviors that can positively affect the quality of the interactions among workers and patients is becoming increasingly important.

❧ WORK, MOTIVATION, AND SOCIETY

Collectively, Americans tend to be a fairly hardworking lot. They generally put in more hours per week, and work more weeks per year, than most of their counterparts in developed nations around the globe. Hard work and ingenuity have always been hallmarks of the American people.

The origins of this phenomenon lie in the European Renaissance and the Protestant Reformation. These events transformed the prevailing medieval view that it was generally inappropriate for one to obtain too much gratification from human accomplishments that were not spiritually oriented. The Renaissance brought about a deep interest in the secular, nonreligious world and a new belief that human effort and earthly happiness were as essential to human existence as the need for salvation. The Reformation served to intensify this new belief system. The doctrines of Reformationists such as John Calvin and Huldrych Zwingli declared that people *"... must participate in the affairs of the world*, thereby putting forward the concept of work as a vocation in which men served God" (Herzberg, 1966, p. 23). Old notions such as choosing to live a life of poverty with few possessions (as confirmation of self-sacrifice) were radically changed. The worldview of the Reformationists held that proof of sacrifice, personal restraint, and hard work could be observed in the financial and material success of an individual. From this worldview was born the Protestant work ethic, stressing the virtues of thrift, self-discipline, and above all hard work.

This work ethic made its way to the New World with colonial immigrants and has been an integral part of the American character and outlook ever since. Even though the work values of American workers today tend to be more pragmatic and less religiously driven, many people still place a premium on success, achievement, ambition, and hard work (Myers and Myers, 1974). However, although the work ethic has served as a general cultural motivator of American society and has contributed to a productive economy and a high standard of living, its effects on individuals have not been uniformly positive. For example, workaholism is well known, and the unhealthy maladies it can bring to individuals and families are very common. Workaholics, although they tend to work very hard and long hours, are usually not proportionally more productive. Thus, while we would like to elicit greater efforts from our workers, the workaholic should not be viewed as an ultimate symbol of what greater motivation can achieve in the workplace.

From Taylor to Hawthorne: Changing Attitudes toward Motivation

By the 1700s, as the Protestant work ethic began to coincide with the British industrial revolution, notions of "economic man" began to emerge. As the spiritual and meditative *homo spiritus* was gradually replaced by a rather worldly and rational *homo economicus*, interest in all things scientific began to appear. This interest in science extended across the Atlantic with the rise of the American industrial revolution during the 1800s. Its application as a management tool in American factories came to be known as *scientific management*. While a number of individuals can be credited with introducing significant contributions to scientific management thought in the early 20th century, none is more strongly associated with that era than Frederick W. Taylor. He is probably best known for his search for efficient work methods among pig iron workers at the Bethlehem Steel Works in Pennsylvania.

Taylor espoused two major "laws" of human motivation. The first was the importance of pointing out clear individual production goals, coupled with close supervision while the work was being carried out. His second "law" of motivation stemmed from popular contemporary ideas of economic man. By harnessing a worker's natural desire for financial gain to the work activities of an organization, productivity and efficiency could be increased.

While workers were expected to do as they were told, they were not expected to have to think very hard or to be responsible for decision making. This was strictly the purview of management. Workers were clearly seen by the "scientific managers" as labor automatons—machinelike humans motivated primarily by financial reward and the creature comforts it could ultimately bring. This idea comes across in Taylor's own description of his selection and motivation of a pig iron handler named "Schmidt":

> Finally we selected one . . . as the most likely man to start with. He was a *little* Pennsylvania Dutchman who had been observed to trot back home for a mile or so after his work in the evening, about as fresh as he was when he came trotting down to work in the morning. We found that upon wages of $1.15 a day he had succeeded in buying a small plot of ground, and that he was engaged in putting up the walls of a little house for himself in the morning before starting for work and at night after leaving. He also had the reputation of being exceedingly "close," that is, of placing a very high value on a dollar.

As one man whom we talked to about him said, "A penny looks about the size of a cart-wheel to him." This man we will call Schmidt.

The task before us, then, narrowed itself down to getting Schmidt to handle 47 tons of pig iron per day and making him glad to do it. This was done as follows. Schmidt was called out from among the gang of pig iron handlers and talked to somewhat in this way:

"Schmidt, are you a high-priced man?"

"Vell, I don't know what you mean."

"Oh yes, you do. What I want to know is whether you are a high-priced man or not."

"Vell, I don't know what you mean."

"Oh, come now, you answer my questions. What I want to find out is whether you are a high-priced man or one of these chaps here. What I want to find out is whether you want to earn a $1.85 a day or whether you are satisfied with $1.15, just the same as all those cheap fellows are getting."

"Did I vant $1.85 a day? Vas dot a high-priced man? Vell, yes, I vas a high-priced man."

"Oh, you're aggravating me. Of course you want $1.85 a day—every one wants it! You know perfectly well that that has very little to do with your being a high-priced man. For goodness' sake answer my questions, and don't waste any more of my time. Now come over here. You see that pile of pig iron?"

"Yes."

"You see that car?"

"Yes."

"Well, if you are a high-priced man, you will load that pig iron on that car to-morrow for $1.85. Now do wake up and answer my question. Tell me whether you are a high-price man or not."

"Vell—did I got $1.85 for loading dot pig iron on dot car to-morrow?"

"Yes, of course you do, and you get a $1.85 for loading a pile like that every day right through the year. That is what a high-priced man does, and you know it just as well as I do."

"Vell, dot's all right. I could load dot pig iron on the car to-morrow for $1.85, and get it every day, don't I?"

"Certainly you do—certainly you do."

"Vell, den, I vas a high-priced man."

"Now, hold on, hold on. You know just as well as I do that a high-priced man has to do exactly as he's told from morning till night. You have seen this man before, haven't you?"

"No, I never saw him."

"Well, if you are a high-priced man, you will do exactly as this man tells you to-morrow, from morning till night. When he tells you to pick up a pig and walk, you pick it up and you walk, and when he tells you to sit down and rest, you sit down. You do that right straight through the day. And what's more, no back talk. Now a high-priced man does just what he's told to do, and no back talk. Do you understand that? When this man tells you to walk, you walk; when he tells you sit down, you sit down, and you don't talk back at him. Now you come on to work here to-morrow morning and I'll know whether you are really a high-priced man or not" (Taylor, 1923, pp. 43–46).

In retrospect, the work of Taylor and of the scientific management movement is often viewed disparagingly by workers and managers alike, due to its seemingly manipulative and exploitative nature. However, it is less commonly known that Taylor actually empathized more with labor than with management and that he exhibited interests in what have come to be regarded today as important human resource management issues such as performance appraisal, job analysis, job evaluation, job design, ergonomics, and selection and training (Warr and Wall, 1975). Unfortunately, his work is seldom referred to for these contributions. In addition, Taylor felt that it was *management's* responsibility to create a motivated work force. In fact, when a manager "... lamented the fact that the worker was not doing an exceptional job and that he was complaining and that he was nonproductive, Taylor countered with, 'You don't know how to manage.' He believed also that management had no right to expect the blossoming of a devotion to duty on the part of the workers; it was up to management to utilize the work force properly" (Herzberg, 1966, p. 36).

Hawthorne and a New Humanistic View of Motivation

The basic assumptions of the scientific management movement were severely challenged by a series of experiments conducted during the 1920s and 1930s at Western Electric's sprawling Hawthorne Works near Chicago, Illinois. The original purpose of these experiments was to take scientific management to an extreme, by carefully studying how changes in work processes, work environment, and compensation would affect the productivity of hourly workers who performed a variety of manufacturing tasks. The ultimate aim was to use the results of these experiments to create a physical work setting that could maximize output and productivity.

An early set of experiments focused on the relationship between levels of illumination intensity and productivity. Using careful control groups, the researchers observed that as illumination intensity increased, so did productivity. They also found that when illumination was continually *decreased*, productivity continued to rise just the same! If greater illumination intensity was not responsible for productivity increases, then what was?

Another important set of experiments took place in what was called the Relay Assembly Test Room. The researchers varied such conditions as the number, duration, and timing of rest breaks; the number of hours worked per week; and a payment scheme that was tied to the productivity of the group. Like the previous illumination experiments, productivity was observed to improve practically every time a work condition was experimentally manipulated. This was true even when the group worked a five-and-a-half day work week without any breaks (Roethlisberger and Dickson, 1939).

A later set of experiments, which used a group productivity payment scheme, was conducted in the Bank Wiring Observation Room. The very surprising findings of these experiments were that the workers did not necessarily try to maximize their payment by correspondingly intensifying their efforts (Homans, 1950; Mayo, 1960).

The results of these key experiments conducted at Hawthorne clearly revealed that the motivational principles associated with scientific management needed to be seriously reexamined. Four broad lessons related to motivation were gleaned from the Hawthorne studies. First, social factors are extremely important considerations, and work represents more than just a paycheck to most workers. Second, workers need to be treated as people with individual needs, and an individual's home or personal situation can strongly influence job performance (Mayo, 1960). The third lesson was that when people believe that someone is interested in them and the work they are doing, they will tend to respond in a positive or socially desirable manner. During the experiments at Hawthorne, work groups were under intense scrutiny by the observers who were recording their productivity. This fact alone in some measure increased productivity levels among the workers, who wanted to place themselves in a positive light. This phenomenon has since come to be known among experimental researchers as the *Hawthorne effect*. The fourth, and perhaps most profound lesson was that groups can act as potent social forces governing individual behavior (Roethlisberger, 1941). Group forces have the potential to generate enthusiasm and active participation on the job.

The highly productive work groups observed at Hawthorne were extensively involved in managerial decision-making processes, an approach very much at odds with the Taylorist view that line workers should be divorced from management decisions. At Hawthorne, the work groups themselves decided in large part how the work would be conducted, ". . . much as Schmidt did before Taylor reached him" (Leavitt, 1978, p. 298). The big differences between the findings from the studies at Bethlehem Steel and those at Hawthorne was that in the latter, workers made decisions in participative group settings. The groups appeared to act like surrogate managers, and the results in terms of human motivation were impressive.

The net effect of the studies carried out at Hawthorne was to create a major shift in the then commonly held assumptions regarding worker motivation. As a result, scientific management began to recede in popularity as it appeared that a more humanistic approach to worker motivation yielded better results, and in its place came an important new set of theories based on human needs.

❧ Motivational Processes

All of us at one time or another have probably commented on how motivated or unmotivated a particular person appeared to be. In addition, we have probably observed individuals who appeared very active and exerted a great deal of effort but in the end never seemed to accomplish much of anything, and vice versa. These observations illustrate that there are clear differences between motivation and performance. While higher motivation does often lead to greater performance, there is no universal, direct correlation between the two. High motivation is not necessarily equal to high performance (Greenberger et al., 1988). Similarly, caution needs to be exercised when labeling employees as motivated or lazy. It is important to keep in mind that performance is due not solely to personal traits or intrinsic characteristics but also to the interaction of individuals—their personal needs, experiences, expectations, physical and psychological preferences, and physical and intellectual ability and talents—with their personal situations, opportunities, and work environments.

This interactive relationship can be expressed as follows:

$$Performance = f\,(ability/talent * situation/opportunity/environment * motivation)$$

From the above equation, one can see that performance is the result of an interaction that goes beyond the merely additive. However, performance will equal zero if *any* one of its components is equal to zero, regardless of how high the other components may be. For example, what overachievers may lack in ability, they make up for in motivation and perhaps a supportive personal situation and work environment. Underachievers, on the other hand, often have the necessary ability and talent to perform, but they typically lack the motivation to do so. Thus, individual performance levels are related to (1) ability, (2) personal situation and work environment, and (3) motivation. But what exactly is motivation? Motivation can be defined as a *goal-directed, internal drive, which is always aimed at satisfying needs*. A need is a physical or psychological deficit that makes particular results or goals appealing to an individual. The need arouses the individual's internal drives and directs them toward those goals that have the capacity to satisfy it.

A simple physiological example of this needs deficiency–based definition follows. An empty stomach (unfulfilled need) stimulates hunger. Hunger serves as the impetus that activates a person to seek out a source of food to eat (goal-directed internal drive). When food is eventually found and eaten and the stomach becomes sufficiently full, the goal will be achieved. At that point the need has been fulfilled, and the motivated behavior will cease. The problem with using a physiological example such as this is that the goal attainment in this case is obvious and definitive. In the case of some psychological needs, however, the need may be just as powerful but may never be satiated enough to extinguish the goal-directed behavior. Thus, one can satisfy most physical needs such as hunger, but some psychological needs may be limitless, and therefore never really completely fulfillable. For example, if an individual is never able to absorb enough personal recognition to feel satisfied, the person's recognition-seeking behavior will never be inactivated! It is also necessary to keep in mind that because individuals may seek to direct their motivated effort toward any number and variety of goals, from a manager's perspective the quest to satisfy personal needs must be compatible with organizational goals.

Because people's needs will vary at any given time, it becomes clear that motivation is a uniquely individual and personal concept. Although we commonly speak of getting managers to *motivate* their employees, we must remember that since motivation is an internal drive aimed at satisfying individual needs, it is impossible for one person *directly* to motivate another. Nevertheless, if managers are aware of the configuration of needs operating among their employees, and if they can create work processes and structures that begin to fulfill those needs, it is certainly possible to motivate them at least *indirectly*. Actual motivation arises within people as a way to satisfy personal needs. As a result, people are self-motivated and managers can only influence this process indirectly.

&. CONTENT AND PROCESS THEORIES OF MOTIVATION

At this point, let us turn our attention to what are termed *content* and *process* theories of motivation. These theories provide managers with a basic understanding of personal needs deficiencies, and of how these needs can be transformed into motivated behavior. Content theories are concerned with the particular attributes that motivate people; they focus on *what* characteristics (content) are central to evoking certain kinds of behavior. Process theories of motivation expand on content theories by suggesting *how* specific characteristics interact (process) to bring about motivation.

Some readers may balk at having to consider motivational "theories." After all, one might argue that because professional health care managers are engaged in practice, they should save the theorizing for "ivory tower" academics, and focus instead on concrete practical applications. However, it will soon become apparent that a single "best way" to motivate health care workers does not exist. Once this is understood, we can either throw up our hands in exasperation, or we can begin to recognize the value of the various motivational theories in helping to Figure out how best to motivate workers. While the theories themselves do not offer specific practical applications, they serve as the foundation for beginning to think logically about how motivational strategies might be implemented.

The fact that adult humans have lived their lives as social beings for many years already equips them with a rich set of experiences from which to draw inferences regarding human motivation. Although we might feel that life experience has already furnished them with all they need to motivate employees, consider this: In the absence of any theoretical understanding of motivation, we tend to approach the subject based on our own firsthand experiences and those of others. From these various experiences, we develop "common sense," "rules of thumb," or "conventional wisdom" about motivation. Many times these beliefs can be invaluable and point to the truths regarding human motivation. More often than not, however, these beliefs serve us no better than old wives' tales. For every general assumption we may hold, there is often an equally compelling contradiction to that assumption. For example, reflect on the following commonsense beliefs and their contradictions (Lynd, 1939, p. 61):

1. Belief: "Education is a fine thing."
   Contradiction: "It is the practical men who gets things done."
2. Belief: "Birds of a feather flock together."
   Contradiction: "Opposites attract."
3. Belief: "Absence makes the heart grow fonder."
   Contradiction: "Out of sight, out of mind."
4. Belief: "Self-praise stinks!"
   Contradiction: "If you don't toot your own horn, nobody will!"

All of this points to the value of theory in helping us to sort out the contradictions as we seek to better understand and influence motivation. As we examine the major theories of motivation, bear in mind that all of them have been criticized to some degree; taken together, however, they do much to advance our thinking about the subject.

A good theory contains five major ingredients. First, the theory should form adequate resolving power. In other words, can it resolve the contradictions that typically arise from our commonsense beliefs? It should tell us *how* two (or more) concepts are related to one another (i.e., how rewards might be related to motivation or how motivation might be related to performance). Second, a good theory should be able to adequately explain. Adequate explanatory power should help us to answer the question, *why*? For example, why should a salary increase or monetary bonus lead, or not lead, to motivation? Third, a good theory should serve as a basis for useful *prediction*. For example, if a specific motivational intervention is applied, a good theory should allow us to predict with some degree of certainty what the outcomes might be. Fourth, a good theory should generate research. Fifth, and perhaps most important, a good theory has to be *useful!*

Content Theories of Motivation

The Hawthorne studies played a pivotal role in getting organizations to recognize the importance of social and human factors in the workplace. The *human relations movement*, which was spawned in large part by Hawthorne, served as a countervailing backlash to the perceived inadequacies of scientific management. In addition to the managerial goal of economic efficiency, good human relations also began to be viewed as an important organizational end in itself. It was from this movement that the best-known content theory of human motivation emerged: Maslow's hierarchy of needs.

Maslow's Hierarchy of Needs. Abraham Maslow developed a theory of human motivation that has come to be widely known as the hierarchy of needs. His theory, which derived principally from his experiences as a clinical professional (Maslow, 1943), fits well with our definition of motivation as a goal-directed, internal drive aimed at satisfying needs. Maslow's theory comprises three main premises. The first is that all humans at any given time have specific needs that are not fully satisfied. These unsatisfied needs result in a state of tension or discontent within a person that he or she will seek to eliminate. If the person is successful in overcoming one need, another still unsatisfied one will immediately take its place. Hence the basis for the second premise: An essentially satisfied need no longer serves as a motivator; only unfulfilled needs have the ability to provoke human action. The third premise of Maslow's theory is that human needs are ordered sequentially in a hierarchy, from lower-level to higher-level needs. Higher-level needs become operable only when those immediately preceding them have been satisfied. This process is called *satisfaction-progression*; as one set of needs is satisfied, an individual will progress to the next, higher-level set of needs, which then becomes dominant.

Maslow developed five sequential categories of needs (Maslow, 1943, 1970), arranged from lowest to highest in a hierarchy as follows:

1. *Physiological needs.* This category focuses on basic human survival and its attendant requirements for air, food, water, warmth, shelter, and clothing. These needs are so basic that the extent to which they are filled determines whether an individual will live or die.

2. *Safety needs.* As basic survival needs are satisfied, safety and security needs become activated. Immediate survival may no longer pose serious problems, but threats such as physical harm, economic hardship, deprivation, or catastrophic illness become of greater concern. From these concerns emerges a desire to protect oneself from the uncertain hazards of life.

   These safety needs are often activated in health care organizations, such as hospitals, because they have the capacity to be dangerous places. Employee fears of experiencing violence or contracting diseases such as AIDS, hepatitis, or tuberculosis can be very real. In addition to concerns for physical security, the *hyperturbulent* health care environment has created a great deal of psychological insecurity for many workers, who may fear for their jobs as their employers react to the hyperturbulence by consolidating, right sizing, and even closing. In addition, hyperturbulent change seems to make managers more likely to engage in frequent changes in policy and procedures and sometimes initiate what appear to workers as management "fads" of the month. Thus, security needs of health workers are also clearly threatened as change intensifies.

3. *Social/belongingness needs.* As the basic physiological and security needs are essentially gratified—when one has enough to eat and a fairly good sense of physical well-being—the social needs begin to predominate. Maslow (1943) termed these the love needs. This third level of the hierarchy reveals individual needs for friendship, camaraderie, affection, and social acceptance (i.e., group belongingness), as well as the reciprocation of these needs with others.

   These first three categories of needs (physiological, safety, and social) have been termed "lower-order" or "deficiency" needs because they tend to be mollified by conditions largely external to an individual person—such as shelter, income, and friends. As one basically fulfills these "lower-order" needs, new need categories (esteem and self-actualization) emerge, termed "higher-order" or "growth" needs.

4. *Esteem needs.* Satisfaction of esteem needs is achieved through a personal sense of accomplishment, independence, self-efficacy, assurance, and self-respect as well as approval, recognition, attention, and appreciation from others. Individuals

fulfill their esteem needs as they achieve a level of respect, prestige, and status among their peers.

5. *Need for self-actualization.* The need for self-actualization emerges after all the previous need categories have been fulfilled. Self-actualization means developing one's fullest possibilities through optimal use of personal abilities, talents, and skills. The meaning of self-actualization is clearly embodied in the US Army slogan, "Be all that you can be." Maslow (1943, p. 382) speaks of self-actualization as referring "to the desire for self-fulfillment, namely, to the tendency for him to become actualized in what he is potentially. This tendency might be phrased as the desire to become more and more what one is, to become everything he is capable of becoming." Needs for self-actualization are typically satisfied as individuals progress along a life journey accomplishing those things that they are best suited to do. Thus, self-actualization is an open-ended need category that is never really brought to finality or closure.

While Maslow's theory is one of the most influential motivation theories to emerge (Bowen, 1987) from the post-Hawthorne human relations movement, it has not been without its detractors. In fact, although biological, psychological, and social researchers seem to agree that people do have various needs deficiencies that they seek to eliminate, there has not been much firm empirical evidence supporting the theory as precisely espoused by Maslow (Hall and Naugaim, 1968; Wahba and Bridwell, 1987). One of the major problems with Maslow's theory has been the difficulty of clearly delineating the various levels described in the hierarchy. Thus, although the theory is as popular as ever, from a managerial perspective, this limitation makes it somewhat unsuitable for developing highly personalized motivational interventions or programs for individuals and groups. This criticism notwithstanding, Maslow's theory has been instrumental in providing expanded insight into the essence of motivation as a needs deficiency–based concept and has served as a springboard for positing and testing more complex theories of motivation.

Alderfer's ERG Theory. The criticism of Maslow's theory served as the starting point from which Clayton Alderfer sought to develop a refined and enhanced theory of motivation (Alderfer, 1972). Instead of five categories, Alderfer posited three categories of needs—*e*xistence, *r*elatedness, and *g*rowth—which gave rise to the acronym ERG, by which the theory is known. Basically, Alderfer collapsed Maslow's five sets of needs into three broader categories: (1) existence needs comprise Maslow's physiological and safety needs; (2) relatedness needs parallel Maslow's social and belongingness needs; and (3) growth needs are related to Maslow's needs for esteem and self-actualization.

To this extent Alderfer's and Maslow's theories of motivation are very similar; both see motivation as arising from the fulfillment of personal needs at both lower- and higher-order levels. But here the similarities between the theories end. While Maslow's hierarchy operates on the principle of *satisfaction-progression*, by which satisfied needs give way (progress) to a new set of needs, Alderfer postulated the dynamic of *frustration-regression*. The process of frustration-regression implies that when higher-level needs are frustrated, individuals will return to lower-level needs for satisfaction. Therefore, according to Alderfer's theory, an essentially satisfied need may actually serve as a motivator, and it is conceivable that more than one need category can be in operation at the same time. In addition, ERG theory states that growth needs actually strengthen even as they are satisfied (Mitchell, 1984). While ERG theory seems to offer a somewhat more applicable portrayal of human motivation, like Maslow's theory it has received mixed reviews when examined empirically (Schneider and Alderfer, 1973).

The theories of Maslow and Alderfer indicate that people function on different levels of the needs hierarchy and for this reason need to be viewed as being motivated differently. These disparities pose a serious challenge to management, since by definition, a motivational program directed at satisfying the needs of one group of employees may have no motivational effect on others. The hierarchical need theories of Maslow and Alderfer suggest that performance can be improved if employees have the liberty to decide how to fulfill their own personal needs. Instead of offering a single, uniform package of benefits to all employees, it may be more useful to extend the variety of benefits available and let employees choose those that best satisfy their particular needs. Also, offering some choice of work schedules, such as shortened or compacted work weeks or flexible working hours, can go a long way toward meeting individual needs.

McClelland's Three-Needs Theory.   David McClelland contributed another important content theory known as the "three needs" theory (McClelland, 1961). It is not based on a hierarchy but consists of three basic needs.

1. *Need for achievement.* The urge to excel, to strive to accomplish, to overcome obstacles, to carry out relatively difficult assignments, and to achieve with respect to a set of criteria.

2. *Need for power.* A wish to exert authority over others; the need to direct or control the actions of others.

3. *Need for affiliation.* The need for friendly and congenial interpersonal relationships with others. A desire for friendship or belonging, and avoidance of conflict. This need closely corresponds to the social and relatedness needs of Maslow and Alderfer.

According to McClelland, all three sets of needs operate simultaneously in individuals, but the intensity of these needs will differ from person to person. Furthermore, these needs are developed as people progress throughout their lives.

Need for Achievement.   Individuals with strong achievement needs see success in personal feats. For them, this need is satisfied by constantly striving to do things better. They prefer to take *personal* responsibility for determining solutions to problems and carrying out the work that needs to be done. They seek challenges that are moderately difficult, and they avoid those that appear inordinately easy (very high probability of success) or hard (very low probability of success). In addition, high achievers actively seek out feedback as to how they are performing with respect to themselves and others, in order to gauge how well they are performing. The extent to which these attributes exist within a work setting will serve to motivate employees with high achievement needs.

McClelland studied the achievement need extensively, not only with respect to individual and organizational performance but in regard to entire national economies as well. He asserted that the impulse in individuals to achieve was largely not inherited but rather parentally and culturally determined. In fact, McClelland developed training programs aimed at teaching people to think like individuals with high achievement needs. He also studied the correlation between the need for achievement, as exemplified through the content of popular children's stories and songs in a variety of countries (developed, undeveloped, contemporary, ancient), with ensuing rates of national economic growth. His findings showed that when people and cultures consistently thought about doing better, they actually did better, at least economically (McClelland, 1987).

Need for Power.   The need for power relates to the desire to be in control and to have some degree of influence over others. Power in this sense is related not to tyrannical behavior but to a wish "to have impact, to be strong and influential" (McClelland and Burnham, 1995, p. 128). Individuals with high power needs tend to favor more aggressive, position-oriented circumstances where they have the opportunity to "take charge" and influence others to carry out organizational objectives.

The three needs of power, achievement, and affiliation have been broadly examined in terms of job role success, especially the relationship between managerial and nonmanagerial roles. Interestingly, although a strong need for achievement appears to correlate with individual, organizational, and even national performance, it does not necessarily lead to managerial effectiveness. This is because individuals with high achievement needs tend to be more concerned with their own individual excellence, not necessarily with trying to induce others to achieve similarly high levels of success.

Chusmir (1986) scored over 70 different health-related occupations in terms of the degree to which they satisfied needs for achievement, power, and affiliation (see Table 14.1). His study revealed that the health care occupations that appeared to fulfill the achievement need best were those of technician (i.e., dialysis, electrocardiographic, surgical, hematology/serology) and technologist (i.e., medical, radiologic, nuclear medicine).

Power needs tend to be more closely related to success in the managerial role. In fact, the most successful managers tend to have fairly strong power needs and relatively weak affiliation needs (McClelland, 1975; McClelland and Burnham, 1995). Interestingly, the health care jobs that seem best able to satisfy power needs and least able to satisfy affiliation needs (see Table 14.1) are primarily the management roles (i.e., hospital administrator, nursing school dean). Higher needs for power may actually serve as a determinant of management effectiveness.

Holland, Black, and Miner (1987) examined 668 hospital administrators in terms of career success. The criteria for success included hospital size, compensation, years as chief executive officer (CEO), years in other positions, and the number of years it took to become CEO. Their most notable finding was that those individuals who scored highest in terms of managerial success had "a stronger willingness to impose wishes on others (power motivation) and [were] more competitive (in work-related situations as well as in games). They also show[ed] a stronger willingness to stand out from the work group (to be unique) and [to] have a more favorable attitude toward authority Figures" (Holland, Black, and Miner, 1987, p. 62).

Need for Affiliation.   The need for affiliation has received far less attention than the achievement and power needs. This may be due to the fact that strong achievement needs result in high performance and that strong needs for power are necessary for managerial effectiveness. Those harboring high needs for affiliation tend to be less content with, or successful in, management jobs because they place an especially high premium on social harmony. The types of activities and decisions (i.e., terminating, disciplining, critically evaluating, allocating resources, etc.) that a manager must carry out do not always allow for consistently smooth interpersonal relations.

As McClelland and Burnham (1995) state, "[t]he top manager's need for power ought to be greater than his or her need for being liked" (p. 126). However, this traditional mark of the successful manager may slowly be changing. In the future, strong needs for affiliation may become a much more important requirement for managers. This is especially true in health care, where teamwork is increasingly required to carry out administrative functions adequately. Individuals with stronger affiliation motives bring benefits to this area by being more cooperative and accommodating. As such, they may seek to alleviate dysfunctional conflict and bring together groups with diverging outlooks and interests (O'Connor, Shewchuk, and Raab, 1992).

Table·14.1 Health care motivation profiles of over 70 health-related occupations in terms of the degree to which they satisfy needs for achievement, power, and affiliation

Job title	DOT code	Need profile	Ach	Aff	Pwr
Hospital administration and operations					
Hospital administrator, superintendent, coordinator rehabilitation services, emergency medical services coordinator, sanitarian	117	Pwr	2	1	4
Coordinator auxiliary personnel	127	Pwr	2	1	5
Supervisor, volunteer services, food service, ward service, tray line, floor housekeeper, manager	137	Ach and Pwr	3	2	3
Executive chef	161	Ach	4	1	2
Central supply supervisor	164	Balanced	2	2	2
Medical services administrator, hospital record administrator, communications coordinator, assistant hospital administrator, executive housekeeper, librarian, director food services, director volunteer services, building superintendent, laundry superintendent	167	Pwr	3	2	4
Hospital insurance representative	267	Pwr	3	2	4
Hospital collection clerk	357	Ach	4	2	2
Cook	361	Ach	4	2	2
Hospital admitting clerk, cashier, insurance clerk, receiving clerk, ward clerk	362	Ach	4	2	2
Medical record technician, x-ray file clerk, medical service technician	367	Balanced	3	3	3
Ambulance attendant, emergency medical technician	374	Aff	1	4	1
Ward supervisor, ward attendant, psychiatric aide	377	Aff	2	4	2
Linen room attendant, clerk, checker, exchange attendant	387	Aff	2	3	2
Television rental clerk	467	Aff	2	3	2
Food tray assembler	484	Aff	0	3	0
Formula maker, formula room worker	487	Aff	1	3	1
Diet clerk aide	587	Aff	1	2	0
Hospital attendant	674	Aff	0	3	0
Hospital entrance attendant, messenger, admitting office guide, food service worker, tray line worker	677	Aff	1	3	0
Ambulance driver	683	Pwr	1	1	2
Central supply worker, cleaner, clothes room workers	687	Aff	4	0	2
Medical and dental technology					
Medical technologist, teaching supervisor	121	Ach	4	0	2
Medical technologist, chief	161	Ach	5	1	2
Radiologic technologist, chief	162	Ach	5	1	2
Chemistry, microbiology, technologists, orthotist, prosthetist	261	Ach	5	1	2
Cytotechnologist	281	Ach	3	1	1
Medical, nuclear medicine, hematology serology, tissue technologists, orthotist, prosthetist assistant	361	Ach	4	2	2
Dialysis, electrocardiographic technicians, electroencephalographic, radiology, x-ray technologists	362	Ach	4	2	2
Ultrasound technologist	364	Ach	4	2	2
Surgical technician	374	Aff	1	4	1

Table continued on next page.

Table 14.1   Continued

Job title	DOT code	Need profile	Ach	Aff	Pwr
Medical and dental technology					
Medical lab assistant or technician, hematology or serology technician	381	Aff	3	2	1
Cephalometric analyst	384	Aff	1	3	1
X-ray developing machine operator	685	Aff	0	1	0
Laboratory assistant	687	Aff	1	2	0
Nursing					
Dean, school of nursing, educational consultant, state board nursing; directors: community health nursing, educational community health, nursing service, occupational health nursing, school of nursing, executive director nurses association	117	Pwr	2	1	4
Nurse instructor	121	Pwr	4	0	2
School nurse, community health staff nurse	124	Pwr	1	1	3
Head nurse, nurse supervisor, nurse consultant	127	Pwr	2	1	4
Nurse practitioner, nurse midwife	264	Balanced	2	2	2
Nurse anesthetist	371	Ach and Aff	3	3	1
General duty nurse, office nurse, private duty nurse, staff nurse, licensed practical nurse	374	Aff	1	4	1
Therapists					
Coordinator, rehabilitation services	117	Pwr	2	1	4
Occupational, physical, manual arts, recreational therapists	124	Pwr	1	1	3
Art, music therapists	127	Pwr	2	1	4
Hypnotherapist	157	Ach	4	1	1
Industrial therapist	167	Pwr	3	2	4
Physical therapist assistant	224	Pwr	1	1	3
Corrective or respiratory therapist	361	Ach	4	2	2
Assistant therapy aide	377	Aff	2	4	2

Source: Chusmir, L. H. (1986). How fulfilling are health care jobs? *Health Care Management Review,* 11(1), p. 30.

Nevertheless, many patient-oriented jobs contain strong motivational content, which can satisfy affiliation needs. Table 14.1 indicates that the motivational profile comprising the most common types of nursing jobs is highest in affiliation and lowest in achievement and power.

Herzberg's Motivation-Hygiene Theory.   Frederick Herzberg proposed a slightly different theory of motivation, which he labeled the *motivation-hygiene* theory (Herzberg, Mausner, and Snyderman, 1959; Herzberg, 1968). It contends that employees' attitudes toward work are formulated as a direct result of their experiences with it. When individuals maintain good attitudes toward work, they should be satisfied and motivated. Alternatively, if their attitudes are not good, they will be dissatisfied and unmotivated.

While this may seem intuitively obvious, the interesting twist proposed by Herzberg was that the work factors contributing to job satisfaction were demonstrably *different* from those contributing to job dissatisfaction.

Herzberg tested his theory by asking people, initially several hundred accountants and engineers in the Pittsburgh area, to recall carefully those times when they felt especially satisfied at work and those times when they felt especially dissatisfied at work. The results of this and several other studies tended to confirm Herzberg's initial theoretical proposition. Five factors emerged as relating to job satisfaction: achievement, recognition, the nature of the work itself, responsibility, and advancement/growth. These factors, which Herzberg termed *motivators*, are intrinsically tied to the basic content of the work itself. In contrast, the factors relating to job dissatisfaction—such as company policy and administration, supervision, working conditions, salary, and interpersonal relations—tended to be external to the job. Herzberg termed these factors *hygienes*. Hygienes are more preventive and environmental in nature; however, despite the degree to which these factors may be fulfilled on the job, they will not serve to improve satisfaction, only to prevent dissatisfaction. According to this theory, for job satisfaction to improve, the intrinsic motivators need to be present. When the motivators are absent, *satisfaction* may not exist, but *dissatisfaction* should not occur as a result.

Herzberg's theory asserts that the factors producing dissatisfaction are independent and distinct from those that lead to satisfaction. The motivators are responsible for building job satisfaction; and the hygienes, or lack of them, are instrumental in creating job dissatisfaction.

Like the other content theories of motivation, Herzberg's theory has received its fair share of criticism. These criticisms tend to center on four primary concerns. First, his initial findings were derived from a study carried out on two groups—accountants and engineers—whose work content is more professional in nature and consequently not representative of, nor generalizable to, all work settings. Second, Herzberg's findings may have been strongly influenced by the fact that people tend to attribute poor outcomes (dissatisfaction) to others and good outcomes (satisfaction) to themselves. Third, serious controversy exists as to whether job satisfaction and dissatisfaction are indeed two distinct and separate notions, and the results of research into this debate have been thoroughly confusing. While some studies appear to confirm the theory (Herzberg, Mausner, and Snyderman, 1959), others refute it (Pinder, 1984). For example, some motivators and hygienes have been observed to contribute to satisfaction and dissatisfaction simultaneously (House and Wigdor, 1967)! Fourth, because Herzberg's theory focuses on job satisfaction, one major assumption is that satisfaction leads to motivation and productivity.

In spite of these criticisms, Herzberg's motivation-hygiene theory is very well known and popular. Its widespread appeal is due to the relative ease by which managers can understand the theory and translate it into everyday operational use. The theory suggests two key ways to motivate employees. First, do not ignore the hygienes. Make sure they are operating at a level that will neutralize employee dissatisfaction. If not, workers may attempt to constrict output, undermine various work processes, and generally feel discouraged on the job. Nonetheless, because the presence of hygiene factors can never lead to job satisfaction and motivation, nothing will be gained by overemphasizing them. Second, change job content so that workers have the opportunity to experience the motivating factors. Efforts to redesign, enrich, and enlarge health care jobs are direct attempts to make them more satisfying and motivating. It can become extremely difficult to motivate some health care workers because their jobs often become boring and routine. For example, the work of some clinical laboratory personnel can be extremely tedious and predictable because it is often narrow and specialized, whether by disease, causative agent, type of clinical specimen, or type of test performed. For a laboratory worker, much of the work performed and skills involved are standardized. Some of the work must conform to exacting prescribed standards, creating strict routines. Other tasks become standardized through the repetition of a test.

Because this type of work condition may not have high potential to motivate, one way to overcome this problem is to enlarge the job horizontally so that the worker accomplishes a wider variety of tasks. If the scope of the job is further extended vertically (job enrichment) the worker not only has a greater variety of tasks but also exerts more control over them.

One study of 522 health administrators examined the relative perceived importance of a variety of variables in terms of influencing them to remain (retention) in current administrative positions, or to be recruited (recruitment) into new ones (Fottler, Shewchuk, and O'Connor, 1993). Of the 13 variables considered, four were consistently viewed as being the most important in terms of both retention and recruitment (see Figures 14.1 and 14.2). These variables were (1) freedom in decision making, (2) opportunities for personal growth, (3) caliber of the management team, and (4) opportunities for advancement. Interestingly, the variable perceived as being *least* important relative to both retention and recruitment was appearance of the physical work environment. As mentioned previously, health care managers want to motivate excellent people to seek positions with, as well as remain with, their organization after they are hired. These results and others (Alpander, 1985, 1990; Longest, 1974) corroborate to some limited extent the greater importance of *motivators* and the lesser importance of *hygiene* factors in terms of what motivates individuals in health care organizations.

Summary of the Content Theories. The four content theories described above give emphasis to the significance of satisfying human needs in order to bring about motivation.

Figure 14.1 Relative ratings of 13 job attributes considered "very influential" in persuading health administrators (N = 522) to maintain employment with their current organization

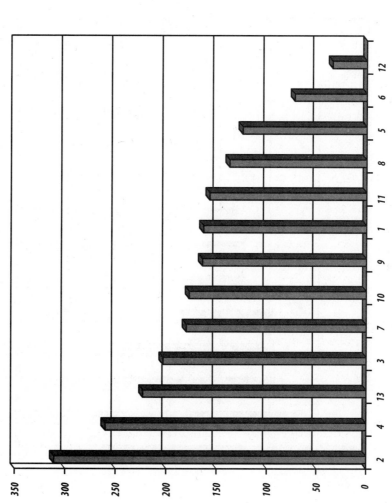

1 - Salary

2 - Freedom in decision making

3 - Opportunities for advancement

4 - Opportunities for personal growth

5 - Chance to serve humankind

6 - High job profile

7 - Organization's reputation

8 - Organization's financial condition

9 - Geographic location

10 - Institutional mission/values

11 - Corporate culture

12 - Appearance of the physical work environment

13 - Caliber of the management team

Source: Fottler, Shewchuk, and O'Connor (1993).

Figure 14.2 Relative ratings of 13 job attributes considered "very influential" in persuading health administrators (N = 522) to seek employment with another organization

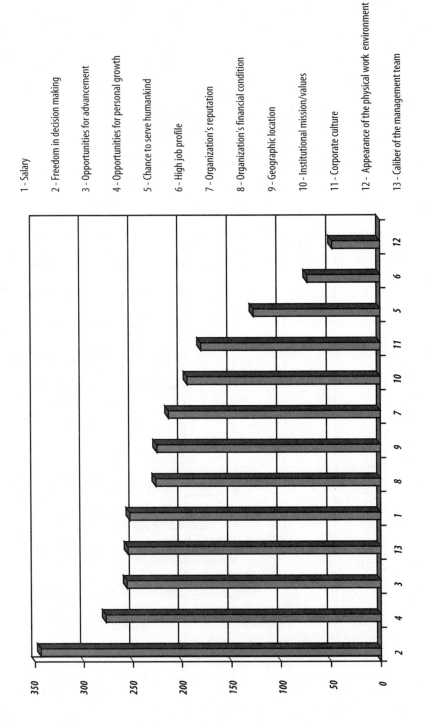

1 - Salary

2 - Freedom in decision making

3 - Opportunities for advancement

4 - Opportunities for personal growth

5 - Chance to serve humankind

6 - High job profile

7 - Organization's reputation

8 - Organization's financial condition

9 - Geographic location

10 - Institutional mission/values

11 - Corporate culture

12 - Appearance of the physical work environment

13 - Caliber of the management team

Source: Fottler, Shewchuk, and O'Connor (1993).

There are similarities and variations among them. Alderfer's ERG theory is a direct extension of Maslow's hierarchy of needs. ERG theory condensed Maslow's five needs down to three and operationalized the motivating capability of the needs a little differently. Whereas the needs present in Maslow's hierarchy are viewed as being static and operating sequentially, from bottom to top (*fulfillment-progression*), ERG theory offers a slightly more adaptable model based on the prescript of *frustration-regression*.

Herzberg's two-factor theory of motivators and hygienes further extends the theories of Maslow and Alderfer. The motivating factors tend to indulge the higher-order needs, whereas the hygienes tend to satisfy most lower-order ones.

Finally, McClelland's three-needs theory focuses on the needs for achievement, power, and affiliation. Health care jobs vary extensively in terms of how well each of these needs is fulfilled.

The content theories of motivation can provide health care managers with an excellent sense of *what* specific work factors and conditions may serve to kindle worker motivation. Unfortunately, the content theories do not serve to explain *how* these elements interact and move people to select particular goals or behaviors. It is the process theories of motivation that attempt to answer these questions and to which we now turn.

Process Theories of Motivation

The process theories of motivation go beyond the content theories by suggesting *how* specific characteristics within a person interact (process) to bring about motivation. The process theories discussed in this section are expectancy, equity, goal setting, and reinforcement.

Expectancy Theory.   Expectancy theory is one of the most influential process theories of motivation. Developed by Victor Vroom in the 1960s, this theory goes beyond viewing employees as fundamentally driven by needs (Vroom, 1964). Expectancy theory sees workers as having the capacity to select behaviors based on their beliefs that (1) effort will lead to performance and (2) their performance will lead to desired personal outcomes. The major elements that make up the process of expectancy theory are expectancy, instrumentality, and valence.

Expectancy is the linkage between effort and task performance. It is the individual's subjective probability that a given level of effort will lead to successful task performance (a first-level outcome). This probability can range from zero (no hope of successfully performing, regardless of how much effort is expended) to one (perception that a particular effort will always lead to performance). Expectancy is an individual's answer to the question, will my efforts result in performance?

Instrumentality serves to link job performance to various second-level outcomes. It is the individual's perceived probability that a particular job outcome will occur as a direct result of performance. Job outcomes involve both positive occurrences (pay raises, promotions, etc.) as well as negative ones (reprimands, firings, etc.). Instrumentality is a person's answer to the question, will my successful performance on the job result in my preferred outcomes?

Valence is a person's preference for a particular job outcome. It is a probability that can range from –1 to +1. Valence is the answer to the question, how much do I value this outcome?

According to expectancy theory, motivation derives from the interaction of expectancy (*E*), instrumentality (*I*), and valence (*V*). This relationship can be expressed as follows:

$$\text{Motivation} = E \,{*}\, I \,{*}\, V$$

It is important to recognize that if *any* one of these components is perceived as being low or absent, then motivation for that particular task will also be low or absent. The example that follows applies expectancy theory to physician motivation.

A physician is involved in a new, long-term disease management program for her patients with diabetes. The health maintenance organization (HMO) for which she works wants the disease to be managed in such a way that it is kept under control so that patients can maintain a higher quality of life and longer-term costs do not rise as a result of the need for more extensive medical interventions. Using the basic process of expectancy theory in Figure 14.3 as a model, we can examine the extent to which

Figure 14.3 General process of expectancy theory

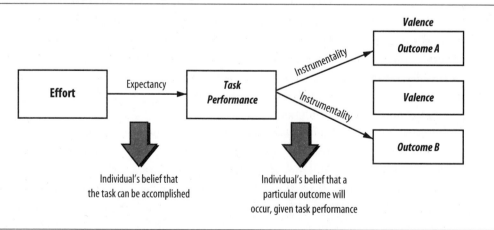

this physician might be motivated to actively follow the disease management guidelines. Will her efforts lead to performance? Her expectancy probability is very high that this will occur. The physician is very confident that between her own knowledge and the detailed guidelines for managing the disease given to her by the HMO, she will be able to do a good job of keeping her diabetic patients' disease under control.

The HMO, though, while exhorting the physician to follow the new diabetes management guidelines, uses primarily financial incentives to motivate physician behavior. The HMO uses a holdback, bonus pool of dollars in which the physician can share at the end of the year. The more dollars the physician saves the HMO over the course of the year, the bigger the pool—and the bigger the bonus check at the end of the year.

The physician has high expectancy for performing effective diabetes disease management. But the disease management guidelines require her to get patients to test their blood sugar levels four times per day using testing strips that cost over $100 per month, and frequently to order relatively expensive laboratory tests, glaucoma screenings, and podiatric referrals throughout the course of a year. The physician thus recognizes that despite effectively managing diabetes among her patients (high performance), she will very likely not be able to share in any financial bonuses disbursed at the end of the year. This is an outcome that she does not prefer (negative valence). In this case the linkage between performance and outcome, or instrumentality, is very high but the outcome has a strong negative valence. Because the outcome (specific, short-term economic incentive) is not related to performance in this instance, the physician's motivation to accomplish effective, long-term diabetes management has been severely diminished. In the future, HMO administrators may wish to assign greater weight to quality indicators as a condition of sharing in the financial pool.

While expectancy theory serves as an excellent model for getting managers to think about how rewards, performance, and effort are linked, it also has several drawbacks. First, expectancy theory rests on an individual's *personal* desire to perform, and the amount of effort they are willing to expend attempting to reach performance goals. Unfortunately, a clear consensus does not always appear as to what establishes *volition* to perform or performance *effort* among people carrying out particular tasks. For this reason, effort can be troublesome to gauge precisely. Second, the theory is predicated on rational, conscious decision making, assuming that individuals consciously evaluate the outcomes (good and bad) that will result from their choice to perform. While this process may work most of the time, it does not hold up for all individuals and situations; rational calculations are not always correctly made, and some choices to perform may be unconsciously motivated (D'Aunno and Fottler, 1993). For example, the HMO physician may continue to work very hard at controlling her diabetic patients' disease even in the face of performance outcomes that do not reward such behavior—probably because she is able to obtain other preferred outcomes, such as a strong sense of achievement and satisfaction with being able to effectively help people.

Health care managers can learn several lessons from expectancy theory. First, management needs to define expected levels of performance This is important because workers need to know what is expected of them in order to perform. Second, what management expects in terms of job performance must actually be realistic and achievable; otherwise, workers will soon realize that regardless of how hard they try, rewards will never be forthcoming. Third, it is important to ascertain which second-level outcomes individual workers value most highly. This information can be learned by asking them personally or through a survey, or by watching how they respond to different types of rewards over time. Fourth, it is important to assess carefully whether the reward structure is at odds with desired behavior. This very common problem has been referred to as the folly of rewarding A while hoping for B (Kerr, 1975). The HMO, in our example, created positive expectancies for physician performance but imposed a reward system that directly subverted these expectancies. Also, as mentioned earlier, many of the work processes in health care organizations are becoming more interdependent, requiring employees to become more team-oriented and to work cooperatively. While *individuals* may have high expectancies to perform, their positive efforts may be seriously jeopardized by other members of the team who are unable or unwilling to contribute effectively to group performance. Thus, it is important not to penalize workers who are unable to perform due to factors beyond their control.

Adams's Equity Theory. Equity theory originated during the 1960s (Adams, 1963). Adams's theory states that people are concerned with the rewards they receive not only in an absolute sense but in a comparative sense as well. Equity theory views the association between workers and employers as a relationship based on trade-offs, whereby workers are induced to make contributions or inputs based on an expectation that they will receive something of value in return. The theory further contends that workers will assess their circumstances relative to others and make a personal judgment based on this comparison as to whether or not they are being treated equitably given their level of contributions.

Essentially, equity theory asserts that a person compares his or her ratio of contributions (inputs) to rewards (outputs) with relevant others. This comparison will result in perceived inequity if the individual feels that he or she is receiving fewer or greater rewards from the situation than another individual who is making an equivalent contribution. On the other hand, a feeling of equity will develop if the individual feels that his or her ratio of contributions to rewards is equivalent to that of another person. Further, the disequilibrium brought about by inequity results in a tension or conflict that an individual will seek to eliminate. Individuals are thus motivated by their desire to reduce tension and restore equity. They can accomplish this by (1) changing their own inputs or outputs, (2) cognitively adjusting their perceptions of their own or others' inputs and outputs, (3) getting others to change their inputs or outcomes, (4) finding a new job that restores equity, or 5) substituting a new comparison standard.

Equity theory tells us that people will compare themselves with others in terms of inputs and outputs. If they feel that inequity exists, they will be motivated to restore equity on their own. Thus, the major message of this theory is that managers need to diminish actively any sense of *real* or *perceived* inequities that employees may harbor. In some cases equity may very well need to be restored by improving wages or other rewards. In other cases it may be a matter of rectifying misperceptions regarding equitable treatment.

Locke's Goal-Setting Theory.　One process theory of motivation that has received a great deal of recent interest is goal-setting theory. First proposed by Edwin Locke in the 1960s (Locke, 1968), goal-setting theory is considered to be among the most valid and generalizable motivation theories (Baron, 1991), and it is perhaps the most useful one from both a practical and research perspective (Pinder, 1984). Goals serve explicitly to inform employees what needs to be accomplished on the job and how much energy it will take to do it. Goals are defined as "desired outcomes in terms of level of performance to be attained on a task rather than the desire to take specific action" (Locke and Latham, 1990a, p. 24). It is thus an individual's *intention* to attain developed goals that can serve as a principal determinant of motivation.

According to this theory, motivation to reach a goal will increase as the goal itself becomes more precise and harder to achieve. In fact, this general relationship has been observed in essentially hundreds of field and experimental studies (Locke and Latham, 1990a). Thus, individuals should be expected to exhibit higher levels of task performance when goals are relatively *specific* and *difficult* than when they are vague or simple, as in the commonly recommended aphorism, "Do your best, that is all anyone can ask for."

Although goals appear to have the ability to elicit motivated performance, they will not function properly unless people are both conscious and accepting of them. When individuals know their organization's goals, they have a better idea of what is expected of them because they have a clearer sense of what needs to be done. However, unless these goals are personally accepted as legitimate and doable, their effect on motivating performance will be minimal at best. A goal viewed as impossible to achieve will rarely instill the motivation necessary to attain it (Locke, 1982). This is also true for goals that are very easy to achieve. Consequently, goals need to be specific, relatively difficult (not impossible), and endorsed by the people expected to act on them. Since goals need to be accepted, do individuals who actively participate in the setting of goals exhibit higher performance than those who receive them from management? The research findings on this question are not very clear (Latham, Steele, and Saari, 1982; Locke and Latham, 1990b). In some cases participation in goal setting has been shown to lead to better performance, and in other cases externally furnished goals have also resulted in better performance. However, *acceptance* of goals will generally increase to the extent that an individual is actually involved in the process of setting them. This participative type of goal setting is often observed, for example, in the hospital strategic planning process, whereby senior managers typically develop specific operating objectives jointly with frontline managers.

Feedback on goal attainment is considered as critical to bringing about motivation as the selection of suitable goals. Because feedback allows a person to evaluate progress toward a goal, it can act as an excellent tool for directing behavior. It has been observed that self-created feedback has a much stronger effect on motivation than feedback from external sources (Ivancevich and McMahon, 1982). Finally, even when clear goals are lacking, the presence of feedback can still positively influence employee motivation (Becker, 1978).

Skinner's Reinforcement Theory.   Reinforcement theory is based heavily on the work of B. F. Skinner (1953). This theory is much more behaviorally directed in its approach than the more cognitively directed expectancy or goal-setting theories. For example, where reinforcement theory contends that behavior is conditioned by reinforcement, goal-setting theory argues that the behavior of an individual is more intentionally directed and is strongly influenced by various psychological elements such as personal temperaments, expectations, and affect. Reinforcement theory is also termed operant conditioning and behavior modification.

In reinforcement theory there is always a stimulus, a response to the stimulus, and a consequence. It is the consequences that serve to reinforce behavior. These consequences are of three major types: (1) positive reinforcement, (2) negative reinforcement, and (3) punishment. People consistently tend to engage in those behaviors that result in valued or pleasurable consequences (positive reinforcement). Positive reinforcers include such things as peer recognition, performance-based pay, etc. When a specific behavior is no longer positively reinforced with valued consequences, people tend to avoid it. This situation is known as negative reinforcement or as nonreinforcement. Punishment differs from negative reinforcement in that it is an active consequence aimed at reducing or extinguishing a specific behavior. Negative reinforcement (nonreinforcement), on the other hand, is simply the removal of positive reinforcers to an earlier learned response.

Consequences can be applied to reinforce or change behavioral responses in a variety of ways, known as reinforcement schedules, of which there are four main types.

1. *Fixed interval.* In this schedule the reinforcement occurs after a precise period of time. For example, an employee receives a pay check on a weekly or biweekly basis.
2. *Variable interval.* Here the consequences to a response occur after the passage of variable time intervals. For example, government radiological safety inspections of hospitals for proper storage and handling of therapeutic radioisotopes such as radium, cesium, and iridium generally occur at such intervals; that is, unannounced and at any time.
3. *Fixed ratio.* According to this schedule, a consequence occurs after a specific number of correct behaviors take place. For example, an HMO that markets its Medicare product to individuals uses this type of schedule when it pays a bonus every time the salesperson signs up 20 new subscribers.
4. *Variable ratio.* This reinforcement schedule differs from fixed ratio schedules in that consequences result after a *variable* number of appropriate behaviors occur. It is the power of variable reinforcement schedules that makes gambling (i.e, playing slot machines, black jack, or lottery games) so addictive. The variable ratio schedule is considered one of the most potent reinforcers.

Reinforcement theory has shown itself useful in explaining such things as absenteeism, tardiness, work effort, and the amount and caliber of work performed (Landy and Becker, 1987). Despite this, two major criticisms have been leveled at this theory. The first is that extensive management use of reinforcers can be viewed as coercive. To this extent the theory is somewhat reminiscent of the scientific management approach, which sought "one best way" to increase worker productivity by finessing various factors such as reinforcers. Reinforcement through the use of positive and negative reinforcers will very likely be futile if management alone determines how these methods will be devised. Employee contribution to the design of these systems is extremely important if they are to be effective.

The second criticism of reinforcement theory centers on the fact that it tends to be very limited in its attention to human psychology and emotion. This may be a vestige of the fact that Skinner's empirical studies of reinforcement theory rely largely on pigeons, not humans. For example, the theory does not provide much understanding of worker job satisfaction (Landy and Becker, 1987). D'Aunno and Fottler (1993) sum up this criticism of reinforcement theory as follows: "People are often portrayed as somewhat mindless robots in pursuit of rewards. This critique is similar to a critique of expectancy theory: that is, it views people as very rational in pursuit of valued outcomes. The difference here is that critics of expectancy theory argue that it does not even give people credit for thinking" (p. 72).

Summary of the Process Theories. The process theories of motivation emphasize the processes or sequences of how individual motivation is initiated, supported, or impeded. Expectancy theory proposes that motivation arises from an individual's assignment of probabilities to two relationships: (1) that effort will result in performance (expectancy) and (2) that effort will relate to specific outcomes (instrumentality). It is, therefore, highly internally focused. Equity theory, on the other hand, is more externally focused, with motivation stemming from individual comparisons with others. Unfairly or inequitably viewed comparisons create a state of psychological tension or disequilibrium that individuals are motivated to reduce or eliminate.

Goal-setting theory differs from both expectancy and equity theory in that it regards the principal determinant of motivation as an individual's conscious desire to reach developed goals. Reinforcement theory suggests that motivation is not so much purposely intended as dependent on the conditioning of behaviors through the application and timing of various positive and negative consequences.

Like the content theories, none of the process theories is a complete and perfect model of human motivation. Each has its attendant strengths and weaknesses. However, knowledge of these process theories, in conjunction with the content theories, can serve as an excellent basis for health care managers to better understand and influence motivation in their organizations. In fact, because motivational problems are often multidimensional, using a combination of motivational techniques is often preferable to using a single method (Locke and Latham, 1990b).

Motivating Effective Professional Performance

The next section briefly explores what it means to be a professional and the essential role that autonomy plays in this definition. The ensuing discussion examines how several of the motivational theories might be applied to professional workers, and in the process provides a better insight into how best to motivate them. In particular it considers intrinsic rewards (especially recognition) and feedback.

A profession can be thought of in terms of (1) who its members are (selection, licensure, and cohesion), (2) what they know (their knowledge base and standards), (3) why they act as they do (service orientation and code of ethics), and (4) how they direct their activities (occupational autonomy and impact on social policy) (O'Connor and Lanning, 1992). Of the various components that make up a profession, the amount of autonomy or self-direction appears to be the defining characteristic (Haug, 1988).

Health care organizations are heavily populated with such autonomous professionals, ranging from accountants to information systems specialists, from senior executives to clinical psychologists, social workers, optometrists, podiatrists, medical doctors, nurses, and others. Because so many of the patient care activities that take place in health care organizations are conducted by clinical professionals, we will focus our attention on them.

Economic and Intrinsic Rewards.   Herzberg's *motivation-hygiene* theory proposes that intrinsic factors associated with work are more motivating to workers than extrinsic factors such as money. Because health care is viewed by society as an especially cherished and important social good that restores health and relieves human suffering, it has the potential to offer workers strong intrinsic rewards deriving from the nature of the work itself, recognition, and opportunities for professional advancement. As such, "if health workers . . . are committed to alleviating suffering, it behooves management to give these workers a sense of efficacy, a sense that their devotion is not in vain" (Benveniste, 1987, p. 43). Research tends to confirm the significance of Herzberg's motivating factors in providing those things that health care professionals value most highly in their work (Alpander, 1985, 1990; Guy, 1985; Fottler, Shewchuk, and O'Connor, 1993).

During the 1800s and early 1900s, one of the chief activities of hospital administrators was that of pinching pennies (Schulz and Johnson, 1983). Nurses' salaries tended to be extremely low, and administrators rationalized that because the caring and humanistic rewards inherent in nursing were so high, greater extrinsic rewards such as salary were surely unnecessary. Unfortunately, many nurses (predominantly women) worked long and hard for unconscionably low wages, not because the intrinsic rewards were so powerful but because so few alternative employment opportunities were available to them. More recently, as women have experienced a greater variety of employment options, hospitals have recognized that money (an extrinsic factor) can play an important role in motivating professional nurses.

According to Herzberg's theory, money is not a motivator but a hygiene. If it is not adequately present, it should serve to dissatisfy and demotivate; if it is amply present, it should not result in satisfaction or motivation, only in the neutralization of dissatisfaction. It is certainly true that financial rewards will indeed create dissatisfaction among professionals if they believe them to be inadequate relative to their contributions. However, a very important caveat is in order: *Money can also act as a form of recognition*, that is, it has the capability to act as a motivator.

It has been said that "money is as money does." Amply educated professional workers who are already earning sufficiently good incomes typically do not seek greater financial reward exclusively for what it will buy them. Rather, because many health professionals have fairly high needs for achievement, money acts as as a symbolic but tangible recognition of their success, competence, and achievement.

> The logic is certainly simple enough: one who learns more, grows more, accomplishes more, and takes on more responsibility is therefore worth more. In at least token fashion, a pay raise acknowledges this belief. The individual pay raise may not be particularly large, but the mere fact of its granting is often the periodic reinforcement that one may need to continue believing that one's worth is being recognized. . . . Additional money remains far more important for what it symbolizes—recognition, reward, and reaffirmation of worth—than for what it buys (McConnell, 1984, p. 93).

Even though money has been characterized as a hygiene or dissatisfier, among health professionals it takes on greater importance because it is an indicator of recognition, and recognition may be one of the most important motivators operating among this group of workers. In fact, research suggests that recognition is the most critical motivating factor for employees of American hospitals (Alpander, 1985). Table 14.2 shows how the major motivational elements at work in American hospitals correlate with one another. Recognition correlates positively and significantly with job importance, opportunities for advancement, individual growth, a belief that effort will result in performance, and the expectation that performance will be rewarded (Alpander, 1985).

Recognition, therefore, one of Herzberg's satisfiers, appears to be one of the most powerful tools for motivating health care workers. A variety of methods are available by which individuals can be recognized, including the use of money. An old saying warns, "Never ridicule a recognition." For example, Baptist Medical Center in Oklahoma City recognizes employees through ceremonial programs called Top Gun awards. Employees spend hours preparing for these ceremonies by constructing sets and creating costumes around a *Star Trek* theme. The hospital president once opened the ceremonies with these words: "These are the voyages of the Starship Boobyprize, en route to the northwest sector of Galaxy OKC (Oklahoma City) in search of excellence in healthcare" (Lutz, 1990, p. 30). To outsiders not familiar with this hospital, this activity may seem silly or childish; however, although the ceremony is undoubtedly unusual, it is an intensely serious matter because it constitutes a very public recognition of hospital employees.

The hyperturbulent health care environment has been putting pressure on health care organizations to become more productive, efficient, and concerned with quality. Physicians play a central role in this regard because most of the clinical work that is carried out is done so at their behest. For this reason, managers must have the ability to influence those unfavorable physician behaviors that result in such things as

Table 14.2 Pearson correlations between various motivational elements in American hospitals.

	Age 1	Service 2	Education 3	Importance of job 4	Security 5	Fairness 6	Advancement 7	Recognition 8	Belongingness 9	Personal Growth 10	Physical Condition 11	Co-workers 12	Superiors 13	Iv$_a$ 14	Iv$_b$ 15	E$_1$ 16	E$_2$ 17	V$_R$ 18
1		.3018*																
2					−.4208*	−.4180*												−.4220*
3					.5980**		−.4168*											
4					.6018*			.5581*										
5						.6161**												
6																		
7								.4780*										
8													.5827*					
9																		
10								.5982**										
11																		
12																		
13																		
14																.6700**		
15																		
16								.6083***										
17								.5902*										.7510**
18																		

* p < 0.5   ** p < .01

Iv$_a$ = Intrinsic satisfaction the employee is getting while performing
Iv$_b$ = The task satisfaction the employee receives after task performance
E$_1$ = Expectancy level that the effort will lead to successful task performance
E$_2$ = Expectancy level that successful task performance will be rewarded
V$_R$ = Perceived value of the reward

Source: Alpander, G. G. (1985). Factors influencing hospital employee motivation: A diagnostic instrument. *Hospital & Health Services Administration*, 30(2), p.75.

unnecessary diagnostic testing, excessive resource consumption, and low ratios of quality outcomes to resources consumed.

Attempting to motivate physicians can be a difficult task because medicine represents the quintessential profession, and physicians are trained and socialized as professionals to think independently and to act with lots of individual discretion and autonomy in the work that they do. As such, physicians typically do not take kindly to managerial intrusions into their work. However, these interventions are usually necessary to control costs and quality from an organizationalwide or communitywide perspective.

The professional elements of autonomy and discretion do not mix well with frequent organizational performance evaluations. Furthermore, these types of evaluations, if and when they exist, tend to discourage professionals such as physicians from learning and risk-taking behaviors. For this reason, informal types of rewards seem better suited to them, but these still may not be enough to motivate behavioral changes, especially if the physicians in question are nonsalaried, independent entrepreneurs or contractors.

Nearly all physicians, as a result of their high achievement needs and professional socialization, are very much concerned with the quality of care delivered to their patients and truly want to perform excellent medicine. However, they cannot evaluate how well they are doing in a vacuum. They must be able to compare their performance with their own past performance and with that of their counterparts, and to benchmark norms. This is where goal-setting and reinforcement theory, especially feedback, can play a major role in changing and sustaining behavior (Dyck, Murphy, Murphy, et al., 1977; Berwick and Coltin, 1986).

Often, special groups of physicians and managers will specify the actions or behaviors that need to be adopted, for example, by issuing practice guidelines or disease management criteria to serve as baseline behavioral goals. On their own, guidelines may have some impact on behavior, but as many health administrators can attest, they are often greeted with resistance or hostility and do very little to bring about quick and comprehensive changes in practice. However, when appropriate consequences (both desirable and undesirable to the physician) are linked to these guidelines, and an information system is put in place to provide timely and useful feedback, desired practice behaviors are more likely to occur. For professionals like physicians, frequent and high-quality informational feedback provides them with a clear sense of how they are doing; it also helps to reduce the uncertainty, risks, and anxiety associated with engaging in unfamiliar behavior patterns and to build their confidence that they are doing things right (Kongstvedt, 1993).

Three important cautions need to be carefully considered when using feedback. The first is that the feedback data need to be truly helpful and useful in order to motivate physician behavior. This means that the feedback must be correct, given at frequent and specific time intervals, and contain an array of financial, utilization, and quality-related information. It should help a physician to track his or her own progress over time and also compare it with his or her peer group (Braham and Ruchlin, 1987). "If the only data [managed care] physicians get are letters at the end of the year informing them that all of their withhold is used up, they can credibly argue that they have been blindsided" (Kongstvedt, 1993, p. 92), and most likely they will be less motivated to follow performance guidelines in the future.

The second concern is that feedback data need to be clearly related to what is important, because this is where people will direct their energy (Charns and Smith Tewksbury, 1993). If the feedback comprises primarily cost and economic data, that is probably where the bulk of the professional's attention and motivation will be directed. This is also true when quality measures are used as feedback information. If the measures are not exact and thorough indicators of quality, then the professional's motivation to improve on the indicators could result in no net improvements in real quality. This situation has been likened to climbing the signposts instead of following the road (Lanning and O'Connor, 1990). This particular problem will be further compounded if positive rewards are directly related to improvements observed in the faulty feedback information.

Finally, feedback given to physicians should not be classified as being good or bad. Because they are highly trained professionals, health care managers should expect "that each individual will draw the appropriate conclusions from his or her feedback report" (Braham and Ruchlin, 1987, p. 12). Professionals such as these do not need to be punished through public embarrassment or reprimand. In most cases it will be clear to them when they have missed the mark.

❧ Conclusion

The 1990s will challenge the ability of managers to motivate health care workers, especially as the hyperturbulent environment continues to demand higher levels of efficiency, productivity, and quality from its providers. These types of demands are made even more difficult by the fact that they are expected to occur with fewer resources and within extremely labor-intensive organizational settings.

For health care managers, one very important way to combat these environmental demands effectively is to gain a basic understanding of human motivation and to apply that knowledge in such a way as to encourage higher performance from workers. Because a single best way to motivate, or a grand theory of motivation, will not be forthcoming in the near future, it is probably wisest to think about the issue from a number of different perspectives. As individual motives are so very personal, and because of the wide diversity of professional and nonprofessional jobs present in health care organizations, a manager will need to draw on a variety of motivational approaches to be effective at addressing unique personal and organizational needs. This chapter has explored (1) the changing health care environment and its requirements for a highly motivated work force, (2) evolving views as to how workers should best be motivated, (3) the essential content and process theories of motivation, and (4) what it means to be a professional and some implications of this definition in terms of motivating health care workers.

🙠 REFERENCES

Adams, J. S. (1963). Toward an understanding of inequity. *Journal of Abnormal and Social Psychology, 67* (November), 422–436.

Alderfer, C. P. (1972). *Existence, relatedness, and growth: Human needs in organizational settings*. New York: The Free Press.

Alpander, G. C. (1985). Factors influencing hospital employee motivation: A diagnostic instrument. *Hospital and Health Services Administration, 30*(2), 67–83.

Alpander, G. C. (1990). Relationship between commitment to hospital goals and job satisfaction: A case study of a nursing department. *Health Care Management Review, 15*(4), 51–62.

Baron, R. A. (1991). Motivation in work settings: Reflections on the core of motivational research. *Motivation and Emotion, 15*(1), 1–8.

Becker, L. J. (1978). Joint effect of feedback and goal-setting on performance: A field study of residential energy conservation. *Journal of Applied Psychology, 63*(4), 428–433.

Benveniste, G. (1987). *Professionalizing the organization: Reducing bureaucracy to enhance effectiveness*. San Francisco: Jossey-Bass.

Berwick, D. M., Coltin, K. L. (1986). Feedback reduces test use in a health maintenance organization. *Journal of the American Medical Association, 255*, 1450–1454.

Bowen, D. D. (1987). Retrospective comment. In Boone, L. E., and Bowen, D. D. (eds.), *The great writings in management and organizational behavior*, 2nd ed. (pp. 121–122). New York: Random House.

Braham, R. L., and Ruchlin, H. S. (1987). Physician practice profiles: A case study of the use of audit and feedback in an ambulatory group practice. *Health Care Management Review, 12*(3), 11–16.

Charns, M. P., and Smith Tewksbury, L. J. (1993). *Collaborative management in health care: Implementing the integrative organization.* San Francisco: Jossey-Bass Publishers.

Chusmir, L. H. (1986). How fulfilling are health care jobs? *Health Care Management Review, 11*(1), 27–32.

D'Aunno, T. A., and Fottler, M. D. (1994). Motivating people. In Shortell, S. M., and Kaluzny, A. D. (eds.), *Health care management: organization design and behavior*, 3rd ed. (pp. 57–84). Albany: Delmar Publishers.

Dyck, F. J., Murphy, F. A., Murphy, J. K., Road, D. A., Boyd, M. S., Osborne, E., De Vlieger, D., Korchinski, B., Ripley, C., Bromley, A. T., and Innes, P. B. (1977). Effect of surveillance on the number of hysterectomies in the province of Saskatchewan. *New England Journal of Medicine, 296*(23) 1326–1328.

Fottler, M. D., Shewchuk, R. M., and O'Connor, S. J. (1993). Relative importance of work-related variables on the recruitment and retention decisions of health care executives. In Schnake, M. (ed.), *Southern management association proceedings* (pp. 483–485). Valdosta, GA: Southern Management Association.

Goes, J. B., and Meyer, A. D. (1994). *Health care reform and industry hyperturbulence: Lessons learned from California and Minnesota.* Presented at the 1994 Academy of Management Meeting. Dallas, TX.

Greenberger, D., Strasser, S., Lewicki, R. J., and Bateman, T. S. (1988). Perception, motivation, and negotiation. In Shortell, S. M., and Kaluzny, A. D. (eds.), *Health care management: A text in organization theory and behavior* (pp. 81–141). New York: John Wiley and Sons.

Guy, M. E. (1985). *Professionals in organizations: Debunking a myth.* New York: Praeger.

Hall, D. T., and Naugaim, K. E. (1968). An examination of Maslow's need hierarchy in an organizational setting. *Organizational Behavior and Human Performance, 3*(1), 12–35.

Haug, M. E. (1988). A re-examination of the hypothesis of physician deprofessionalization. *The Milbank Quarterly, 66* (Supplement 2), 48–56.

Herzberg, F. (1966). *Work and the motivation of man.* Cleveland, OH: The World Publishing Co.

Herzberg, F. (1968). One more time: How do you motivate employees? *Harvard Business Review, 46*(1), 53–62.

Herzberg, F., Mausner, B., and Snyderman, B. (1959). *The motivation to work.* New York: John Wiley and Sons.

Holland, M. G., Black, C. H., and Miner, J. B. (1987). Using managerial role motivation theory to predict career success. *Health Care Management Review, 12*(4), 57–64.

Homans, G. C. (1950). *The human group.* New York: Harcourt, Brace.

House, R. J., and Wigdor, L. A. (1967). Herzberg's two-factor theory of job satisfaction and motivation: A review of the evidence and criticism. *Personnel Psychology, 20*(3), 369–389.

Ivancevich, J. M., and McMahon, J. T. (1982). The effects of goal-setting, external feedback, and self-generated feedback on outcome variables: A field experiment. *Academy of Management Journal, 25*(2), 359–372.

Kerr, S. (1975). On the folly of rewarding A, while hoping for B. *Academy of Management Journal, 18*(4), 769–783.

Kongstvedt, P. R. (1993). Changing provider behavior in managed care plans. In Kongstvedt, P. R. (ed.), *The managed health care handbook.* 2nd ed. Gaithersburg, MD: Aspen Publishers.

Landy, F. J., and Becker, W. S. (1987). Motivation theory reconsidered. In Cummings, L. L., and Staw, B. M. (eds.), *Research in organizational behavior,* Volume 9 (pp. 24–35). Greenwich, CT: JAI Press.

Lanning, J. A., and O'Connor, S. J. (1990). The health care quality quagmire: Some signposts. *Hospital and Health Services Administration, 35*(1), 39–54.

Latham, G. P., Steele, T. P., and Saari, L. M. (1982). The effects of participation and goal difficulty on performance. *Personnel Psychology, 35*(3), 677–686.

Leavitt, H. J. (1978). *Managerial psychology,* 4th ed. Chicago: University of Chicago Press.

Locke, E. A. (1968). Toward a theory of task motivation and incentives. *Organizational Behavior and Human Performance, 3*(2), 157–189.

Locke, E. A. (1982). Relation of goal level to performance with a short work period and multiple goal levels. *Journal of Applied Psychology, 67*(4), 512–514.

Locke, E. A., and Latham, G. P. (1990a). *A theory of goal setting and task performance.* Englewood Cliffs, NJ: Prentice Hall.

Locke, E. A., and Latham, G. P. (1990b). Work motivation and satisfaction: Light at the end of the tunnel. *Psychological Science, 1*(4), 240–246.

Longest, B. (1974). Job satisfaction of registered nurses in a hospital setting. *Journal of Nursing Administration, 4*(3), 46–52.

Lutz, S. (1990). Hospitals stretch their creativity to motivate workers. *Modern Health-care, 20*(9), 20–33.

Lynd, R. S. (1939). *Knowledge for what? The place of social science in American culture.* Princeton, NJ: Princeton University Press.

Maslow, A. H. (1943). A theory of human motivation. *Psychological Review, 50*(4), 370–396.

Maslow, A. H. (1970). *Motivation and personality,* 2nd ed. New York: Harper and Row.

Mayo, E. (1960). *The human problems of an industrial civilization.* New York: Viking Press.

McClelland, D. C. (1961). *The achieving society.* New York: Van Nostrand Reinhold.

McClelland, D. C. (1975). *Power: The inner experience.* New York: Irvington Publishers.

McClelland, D. C. (1987). That urge to achieve. In Boone, L. E., and Bowen, D. D. (eds.), *The Great writings in management and organizational behavior,* 2nd ed. (pp. 384–393). New York: Random House.

McClelland, D.C., and Burnham, D. H. (1995). Power is the great motivator. *Harvard Business Review, 73*(1), 126–135.

McConnell, C. R. (1984). *Managing the health care professional.* Rockville, MD: Aspen Publishers.

Mercer, A. A. (1988). Commitment and motivation of professionals. In Fottler, M. D., Hernandez, S. R., and Joiner, C. L. (eds.), *Strategic management of human resources in health services organizations* (pp. 181–205). New York: John Wiley and Sons.

Mitchell, T. R. (1984). *Motivation and performance.* Chicago: Science Research Associates.

Myers, M. S., and Myers, S. S. (1974). Toward understanding a changing work ethic. *California Management Review, 16*(3), 7–19.

O'Connor, S. J., and Lanning, J. A. (1992). The end of autonomy? Reflections on the postprofessional physician. *Health Care Management Review, 17*(1), 63–72.

O'Connor, S. J., and Shewchuk, R. M. (1995). Doing more with less, and doing it nicer: The role of service orientation in health care organizations. In Moore, D. P. (ed.), *Academy of Management Best Paper Proceedings 1995* (pp. 120–124). Vancouver, BC: Academy of Management.

O'Connor, S. J., Shewchuk, R. M., and Raab, D. J. (1992). Patterns of psychological type among health care executives. *Hospital and Health Services Administration, 37*(4), 431–447.

Pinder, C. C. (1984). *Work motivation.* Glenview: Scott, Foresman.

Roethlisberger, F. J. (1941). *Management and morale.* Cambridge, MA: Harvard University Press.

Roethlisberger, F. J., and Dickson, W. J. (1939) *Management and the worker—An account of a research program conducted by the Western Electric Company, Hawthorne Works, Chicago.* Cambridge, MA: Harvard University Press.

Schneider, B., and Alderfer, C. P. (1973). Three studies of measures of need satisfaction in organizations. *Administrative Science Quarterly, 18*(4), 489–505.

Schulz, R., and Johnson, A. C. (1983). *Management of hospitals,* 2nd ed. New York: McGraw Hill.

Shortell, S. (1994). *Organized delivery systems as a response to industry hyperturbulence.* Presented at the 1994 Academy of Management Meeting. Dallas, TX.

Skinner, B. F. (1953). *Science and human behavior.* New York: The Free Press.

Taylor, F. W. (1923). *The principles of scientific management.* New York: Harper and Brothers Publishers.

Tubbs, M. E. (1986). Goal-setting: A meta-analytic examination of the empirical evidence. *Journal of Applied Psychology, 71*(3), 473–483.

Vroom, V. (1964). *Work and motivation.* New York: John Wiley.

Wahba, M. A., and Bridwell, L. G. (1987). Maslow reconsidered: A review of research on the need hierarchy theory. In Steers, R. M., and Porter, L. W. (eds.), *Motivation and work behavior* (pp. 51–67). New York: McGraw Hill.

Warr, P., and Wall, T. (1975). *Work and well-being.* Baltimore, MD: Penguin Books, Inc.

Index